# Public Health
# in
# America

This is a volume in the Arno Press series

# PUBLIC HEALTH
# IN
# AMERICA

Advisory Editor

Barbara Gutmann Rosenkrantz

Editorial Board

Leona Baumgartner
James H. Cassedy
Arthur Jack Viseltear

See last pages of this volume
for a complete list of titles.

# HUMAN HEALTH

ROBLEY DUNGLISON

ARNO PRESS

A New York Times Company

New York / 1977

Editorial Supervision: JOSEPH CELLINI

---

Reprint Edition 1977 by Arno Press Inc.

Reprinted from a copy in
The University of Pennsylvania Library

PUBLIC HEALTH IN AMERICA
ISBN for complete set: 0-405-09804-9
See last pages of this volume for titles.

Manufactured in the United States of America

---

**Library of Congress Cataloging in Publication Data**

Dunglison, Robley, 1798-1869.
   Human health.

   (Public health in America)
   Published in 1835 under title: On the influence
of atmosphere and locality.
   Reprint of the ed. published by Lea & Blanchard,
Philadelphia.
   1. Hygiene.  2. Climatology, Medical.
I. Title.  II. Series.
RA775.D78   1977         613      76-25660
ISBN 0-405-09815-4

# HUMAN HEALTH:

OR

THE INFLUENCE OF ATMOSPHERE AND LOCALITY; CHANGE OF AIR AND CLIMATE; SEASONS; FOOD; CLOTHING; BATHING AND MINERAL SPRINGS; EXERCISE; SLEEP; CORPOREAL AND INTELLECTUAL PURSUITS, &c. &c. ON HEALTHY MAN; CONSTITUTING

## ELEMENTS OF HYGIENE.

BY

ROBLEY DUNGLISON, M. D.,

PROFESSOR OF THE INSTITUTES OF MEDICINE, &C., IN JEFFERSON MEDICAL COLLEGE OF PHILADELPHIA, LECTURER ON CLINICAL MEDICINE, AND ATTENDING PHYSICIAN TO THE PHILADELPHIA HOSPITAL, SECRETARY OF THE AMERICAN PHILOSOPHICAL SOCIETY, &C. &C.

A NEW EDITION,

WITH MANY MODIFICATIONS AND ADDITIONS.

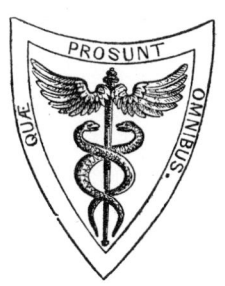

PHILADELPHIA:
LEA & BLANCHARD.

1844.

ENTERED, according to the Act of Congress, in the year one thousand eight hundred and forty-four, by ROBLEY DUNGLISON, in the Clerk's office of the District Court of the Eastern District of Pennsylvania.

GRIGGS & CO., PRINTERS.

# PREFACE.

SINCE the author published the first edition of this work, the subject of Hygiène has been more extensively and practically regarded, and, in many of its relations, has received the fostering care of governments. To this circumstance we are indebted for interesting sanitary inquiries, and valuable reports, and for various excellent contributions to vital statistics. These results of the researches of able investigators have modified materially many of the views which had been generally entertained in regard to the salubrity or insalubrity of different callings, and have led to a greater degree of attention on the part of philanthropists to the domestic condition of the poorer classes, to which rather than to their industrial relations, it would seem that many of the evils must be ascribed.

In this country, and in Great Britain, Hygiène has not usually formed a distinct branch of medical instruction; but on the European continent it constitutes a separate department; and since the time of M. Hallé more especially, public and private Hygiène have formed part of the curriculum of study at the *Ecole de Médecine* of Paris; "public hygiène" being understood to comprise the study as it concerns man collectively; whilst "private hygiène" applies to him individually. It is obvious, however, that this separation must often be forced and unnatural; although in many cases a clear line of demarcation may be drawn. A modern able writer, Dr. A. Combe, in his "Principles of Physiology," has deplored the ignorance of the profession, which is the necessary result of the little attention that has been paid in the schools to the subject. "The prominent aim of medicine," he remarks, "being to discriminate, and to cure *disease*, both the teacher and the student naturally fix upon that as their chief object; and are, consequently, apt to overlook the indirect, but substantial aid, which an acquaintance with the laws of health is calculated to afford, in restoring the sick, as well as in preserving the healthy from disease. It is true, that almost every medical man, sooner or later, works out this knowledge for himself; but in general, he attains it later than he ought to do, and seldom so completely as he would have done had it been made a part of his elementary education, to which he saw others attach importance." "In my own instance," Dr. Combe adds, "it was only when entering upon practice, that I had first occasion to feel, and to observe the evils arising from the ignorance which prevails in society in regard to it."

The Author has subjected the first edition of this work to a complete revision, and has endeavoured to notice, in this edition, the recent researches of distinguished hygienists. He has had a twofold object in view, as he had in preparing the first edition,—to produce a work which might serve the student as an accompaniment to the observations on Hygiène, that are made in Lectures on the Institutes of Medicine— and one which might equally enable the general reader to understand the nature of the action of various influences on human health, and assist him in adopting such means as may tend to its preservation. Hence the Author has avoided introducing technicalities, except where they appeared to him to be indispensable, or strongly indicated.

109 South 10th St.         ROBLEY DUNGLISON.
*July*, 1844.

# CONTENTS.

## CHAPTER I.

ATMOSPHERE AND LOCALITY.

### SECTION I.

Influence of the atmosphere, and of local characteristics on the salubrity of different places.—Atmospheric air—always constituted alike—pressure of the atmosphere—range of the barometer—effects of augmented density—pressure in mines unattended with danger—effects of diminished density, especially when suddenly experienced—effects of the air at great heights above the surface of the earth—height of the barometer at different elevations—errors on the subject of animal and vegetable existence at great elevations—effects of elevated temperature on human health—effects of diminished temperature - Page 13

### SECTION II.

Hygrometric state of the atmosphere—effect of the degree of dryness of the air on the cutaneous, and pulmonary transpirations—mode in which the air acts as an irritant to wounded and burnt surfaces—moist air a better vehicle for animal, vegetable or mineral exhalations—atmospheric vicissitudes frequently the source of disease—Russian vapour bath—vicissitudes from cold to heat the source of disease—atmospheric vicissitudes necessary to full mental and corporeal development—effect of light, and of electricity on the functions - - 38

## SECTION III.

Changes in the air by respiration—black hole at Calcutta—black assize of Oxford, &c.—effects of carbonic acid gas—carburetted hydrogen—sulphuretted hydrogen—animal and vegetable exhalations—endemic, epidemic, and other influences—malaria—its nature not known—does not arise from vegetable putrefaction singly—nor from animal putrefaction singly—nor from aqueous decomposition singly—nor from all these combined—conflicting opinions upon the subject—nature of the emanations, that cause other endemic diseases, likewise unknown—our ignorance of the origin of epidemic, and contagious disease  58

## SECTION IV.

Powerful influence of locality on man—comparative salubrity of different soils—comparative mortality of different countries—mortality and longevity of the counties of England and Wales—mortality, and longevity not always in a like ratio—longevity in different counties of Virginia—insalubrity of great towns—comparative mortality of different cities—the human species, especially the young, require a pure air—great improvement in the value of life—salutary effects of change of air—effect of winds—action of the heavenly bodies on man  -  95

## SECTION V.

Effect of the seasons—comparative mortality amongst adults and children—winter residence for the consumptive—France and Italy—Madeira—Canaries—the Azores—Bahamas—Bermudas—West Indies—Havanna—Vera Cruz—Cumana—Peru—Chili, &c.—Effects of a Sea voyage—climate of Florida, &c.—Saint-Augustine, &c.—comparative merits of seaside and inland situations—due succession of seasons necessary for full mental and corporeal development—effects of unseasonable weather  -   -   -   -   -  137

# CHAPTER II.

## FOOD.

### SECTION I.

Difference between the elements of animal and vegetable bodies, not great—definition of aliments—digestive apparatus of an animal indicates its food—natural food of man—sketch of the physiology of digestion—singular case of fistulous opening into the stomach, with experiments—classification of aliments—fibrin—albumen—gelatin—osmazome—fat and oil—fecula—mucilage—sugar—terms nutritious and digestible not convertible—proper digestive texture of food      179

### SECTION II.

Animal aliments—quadrupeds—character of their meats according to age, sex, food, climate and season, fatness or leanness, incipient putrefaction, mode of slaughtering, &c.—birds; white fleshed, dark fleshed, aquatic and rapacious—effect of feeding, or killing, &c.—reptiles—fish—ichthyophagi—fancied evils of a fish diet—fondness of the ancients for fish—poisonous fish—esteemed parts of fish—effects of feeding, castration, age, season, crimping, &c.—shell fish—crustacea—insects - - - - - - -      204

### SECTION III.

Milk—various kinds—frangipane—cream—butter—cheese—buttermilk—eggs—vegetable aliments—congenerous vegetables possess similar virtues—farinaceous vegetables—bread—maccaroni—vermicelli—buckwheat—millet—cassava flour—potato—rice—Indian corn—sago—tapioca, &c.—leguminous vegetables—peas, beans, &c.—different kinds of kernels—potherbs—beet, carrot, parsnip, radish, leek, lettuce, cucumbers, cabbage, &c.—mushrooms—fruits—preserved fruits      236

vi                    CONTENTS.

## SECTION IV.

Condiments; saline, aromatic, and oily—sugar—salt—salt indispensable—vinegar—pickles—verjuice—capers, &c.—aromatic condiments; much used in torrid climes—oily condiments; butter; oil—preparation of food—object of cookery—roasting—broiling—boiling—baking—frying, &c., sauces    -    -    -    -    -    266

## SECTION V.

Of drinks—physiology of thirst—digestion of liquids—effects of drinking on the digestive function—cold drinks—hot drinks—water; its nutritive properties; different kinds—mode of rendering potable—juice and infusions of animal and vegetable substances; raspberry and strawberry vinegar—lemonade—toast-water—barley and rice water—gruel—tea—coffee; chocolate—cocoa—whey, soda water    -    -    280

## SECTION VI.

Simple fermented liquors—bad effects of their abuse—wines—their sensible, and chemical properties—proportion of alcohol in different fermented liquors—brisk wines—Burgundy wines—claret wines—Oporto wines—Spanish wines—Madeira wines—wines of the Rhine, and Moselle,—sweet wines—cider—malt liquors—distilled fermented liquors—liqueurs    -    -    -    -    -    -    305

## SECTION VII.

Alimentary regimen best adapted for man—evils of too great a quantity of food—proper number of meals—sudden changes of regimen unwholesome—regimen must vary according to different circumstances—best regimen for developing the full powers—training—how practically effected—tobacco—history of its introduction—its effects on the functions—snuffing—smoking—chewing    -    -    -    322

## CHAPTER III.

#### CLOTHING.

Substances used for clothing—wool—silk—hair—down, &c.—influence of the colour, shape, pressure, &c. of vestments—of individual vestments—particular applications, and precautions—adaptation of clothing to temperature, &c. - - - - - 340

## CHAPTER IV.

#### BATHING AND MINERAL SPRINGS.

Ancient baths—different kinds of baths—functions of the cutaneous envelope—effects of bathing on the functions of the skin—cold bath—warm bath—hot bath—tepid bath—sea bathing—manner of bathing—time of bathing—duration of the bath—vapour bath—shower bath—affusion—ablution—douche—footbath—practices accessary to bathing—flagellation—friction—shampooing—kneading—anointing—mineral springs - - - - - - 358

## CHAPTER V.

#### EXERCISE.

Effect of posture on certain of the functions—shock produced by exercises—active exercises—their effects on the functions—exercise should be accompanied with mental amusement—travelling exercise—walking—leaping—running—dancing—the chase—fencing—boxing—wrestling—singing—declaiming—reading aloud, &c.—passive exercise, or gestation—riding in a carriage, litter, palanquin, sedan chair, &c.——sailing, &c.—exercises of the infant—tossing—rocking, &c.—indolence, and its evils - - - - - 376

## CHAPTER VI.

#### SLEEP.

Objects of sleep—evils from protracted watchfulness, and from too much sleep—temperature of the room—state of the bed—position, &c.—proper time for retiring to rest—time to be consumed in sleep—early rising—siesta. - - - - - - 392

## CHAPTER VII.

#### CORPOREAL AND MENTAL OCCUPATIONS.

Influence of professions limited to a few circumstances; exposure to vicissitudes; variations of temperature; mineral and other exhalations, &c.—literary pursuits not often the cause of disease—head affections ascribed to them—imagination said to act injuriously on the body—duration of life amongst authors—bad effects of too early application—necessity of health for the full exercise of the intellect—intense mental excitement injurious—effects of emotions, when inordinate 405

## APPENDIX.

Deposition involving questions regarding the effect of draining a malarious soil—table of the mean temperature, &c., of the seasons, in different places in America, Europe, &c.—tables of the temperature of St. Augustine, &c. during certain months—mean temperature, &c. of corresponding months in certain winter retreats—temperature, &c. of Campeche, and of Santa Cruz—table of the comparative digestibility of different alimentary substances - - - 431

# HUMAN HEALTH.

The human body is composed of various organs, differing essentially from each other in their anatomical conformation, and in the functions which they have to execute. When all these functions are harmoniously performed, *health* is the result; but if any one or more experiences aberration, *disease* is induced. This aberration is indeed itself a state of disease.

The object of *Hygiène* is to inquire into the circumstances that may promote health or give rise to such aberration; or, in other words, into the influence of physical, and moral agents on healthy man; and thence to deduce the best means for preserving health, and for developing all the healthful energy of which the functions are capable.

## CHAPTER I.

ATMOSPHERE AND LOCALITY.

SECTION I.

Influence of the atmosphere, and of local characteristics on the salubrity of different places.—Atmospheric air—always constituted alike—pressure of the atmosphere—range of the barometer—effects of augmented density—pressure in mines unattended with danger—effects of diminished density, especially when suddenly experienced—effects of the air at great heights above the surface of the earth—height of the barometer at different elevations—errors on the subject of animal and vegetable existence at great elevations—effects of elevated temperature on human health—effects of diminished temperature.

In entering upon the investigation of various circumstances that affect human health, none, perhaps, demands an earlier consideration than the influence of the atmosphere, and of the local characteristics, which occasion such a diversity in the salubrity of different countries, and districts of the same country. Whilst we observe the inhabitants of the more mountainous regions enjoying robust health, those of the lower districts near the ocean, or dwelling on the banks of the larger streams, are found to be liable to diseases, which are endemic, or the products of such situations; and daily observation instructs us, that the air of the city is not possessed of all those advantages, for the preservation of health, which are afforded by the more pure air of the country.

We find, again, that particular regions of the globe are liable to diseases known only to them :—the base of lofty mountains constitutes a locality, almost every where favourable to the development of *Goître* or swelled neck: the smiling plains of Italy are saddened by the prevalence of the pellagra—a loathsome cutaneous affection; and those of the torrid zone are affected with the yellow fever. All these diseases are produced by local causes, originating in the particular state of the atmosphere—as regards its barometrical, thermometrical, hygrometrical, and electrical conditions, singly or combined—and in the existence of certain emanations from the soil; which last, indeed, in the minds of some have been looked upon as the sole cause of the difference of salubrity between different countries.

Where a particular affection is universally prevalent in a locality, it must be presumed, that the *constitutio aeris* is always favourable, and unites with certain local influences to maintain the necessary causation; but where we observe a district—previously healthy, perhaps even signalized for its salubrity—devastated by a malignant disease, as by typhus, a precise union of the requisite *constitutio aeris* and local influences must exist, for the time, to induce it; and the reason why it never recurs in such a district, or does so only after a lapse of years, is owing to the necessary catenation of causes not again supervening. In this way we account for the appearance of yellow fever occasionally in our seaports, and for its annual presence in the torrid regions of the globe.

Unfortunately, it is easier to suggest the influences that occasion endemics and epidemics, than it is to explain their precise nature or operation. On the main points of meteorology we are signally deficient in information. There are, doubtless, physical circum-

# ATMOSPHERIC PRESSURE. 15

stances, which determine the shape of to-day's clouds, and a knowledge of which might have enabled us to prognosticate their presence, but this knowledge is far beyond our limited powers in the present state of science.

Still more restricted is our acquaintance with the meteorological conditions that affect human health; nor can we indulge an expectation that future improvements in science will enable us to possess any accurate knowledge on the subject. There are many interesting points, however, connected with the matter, which we do know, and on which we possess much information of an interesting character. Let us first inquire into the properties of the air we breathe, and the influence of its various and varying conditions on the health of man.

The air, which every where surrounds the earth to the height of fifteen or sixteen leagues, and the total mass of which constitutes the atmosphere, is a ponderable, perfectly elastic fluid, invisible in small masses, insipid and inodorous. It consists, chemically, of twenty parts of oxygen to eighty of nitrogen, and these proportions have been found to exist in the air whencesoever taken,—whether from the summit of Mont Blanc, the top of Chimborazo, the sandy plains of Egypt, or from an altitude of 23,000 feet in the air. In addition to these chief constituents, carbonic acid can always be detected, the proportion being estimated by Dalton at not more than the $\frac{1}{1000}$th, or $\frac{1}{1400}$th of its bulk. It holds also water in a state of vapour, caloric, the electric fluid, and a multitude of matters continually emanating from the earth or from its animal or vegetable occupants. Hydrogen in the proportion of 1 part in 1000 has been found in the air of Paris; and sulphurous acid gas in that of London.

The pressure of the atmosphere at the level of the sea results from the whole weight of the atmosphere, and is capable of sustaining a column of water thirty-four feet high, or one of mercury of the height of thirty inches,—as in the barometer. This is equal to about fifteen pounds avoirdupoise on every square inch of surface, so that the body of a man of ordinary stature, the surface of which Haller estimates at fifteen square feet, sustains a pressure of 32,400 pounds. This enormous pressure is not felt, in consequence of the cavities of the body, and of the bones being filled with incompressible fluids capable of sustaining every kind of pressure, or with air, equally elastic with that without, and which counterbalances the outward pressure, so that no inconvenience is experienced.

But even this pressure is not so extraordinary as that to which certain of the inhabitants of the water are habitually subjected. Water is 811 times heavier than air, and sea water, from its saline impregnation, has a greater specific gravity than distilled water; so that fish, under ordinary circumstances, have to force themselves through an element between 8 and 900 times heavier than air, and consequently, more resisting to them than air is to us. But certain sea fishes live at a great depth,—3,000 feet, for example, beneath the surface. In such case, they are loaded with the weight of a column of water 3,000 feet high, and nearly 80 times heavier than that of the atmosphere. Yet they exist, and move about in the fluid with the greatest celerity, owing to their being filled internally with liquids, which resist the pressure from without, by reason of their impenetrability; so that, as Biot remarks, their membranes are no more injured by it than the thinnest pellicle would be, if forced down to the same depth; and the facility of their movements is explained in the same manner as the ease with which we travel through the air surrounding us,—that the body is equally pressed upon in all directions.

The range of the barometer varies from about 28 inches to 31; and if the changes be not extremely sudden between these extremes, the human frame is not very liable to suffer, but if we descend far below the surface of the earth, or ascend to a great height in the air, changes,—especially if the range has been to a great extent, and suddenly experienced,—will be produced in many of the functions, and more or less indisposition be occasioned.

Our acquaintance with the effect of great augmentation in the density of the air is more limited. The only means we possess of observing it is in mines penetrating far beneath the surface; and perhaps in no case have these exceeded a league, and that not in perpendicular depth; whilst the phenomena, attendant upon a sudden passage into a rarer atmosphere, have been observed at nearly 23,000 feet or upwards of four miles perpendicular height. Where the weight of the air is much increased, as in mines, it is fair to presume that the respiration must be slower, on account of the same quantity of oxygen being contained in a smaller bulk of air. It has been presumed, also, that the greater density of the air may constrain the inspiratory movements, so as to render them less frequent; but this, although specious, is conjectural. It certainly does not seem, that any augmented pressure, hitherto experienced in subterraneous excavations, has been attended with danger.

Experiments with the diving bell would shed some light on the effect produced by suddenly augmented density of the air; but here a source of fallacy exists in the air being rapidly deteriorated by respiration,—the oxygen disappearing, and carbonic acid, which is directly unfavourable to animal life, taking its place. From this change, the respiratory movements would be soon deranged, and the effect of deficient aeration of the blood be speedily apparent.

About the time the cholera first made its appearance in England, it was observed by Dr. Prout (*Bridgewater Treatise*, Amer. Edit. p. 197, Philad. 1834) that there was a positive increase in the weight of the air, similar to what might be supposed to be produced by the diffusion of a heavy gaseous principle through the lower regions of the atmosphere. Hence he inferred, that the cause of cholera was a poisonous body analogous to malaria, whose high specific gravity, and feeble diffusive powers kept it near the earth's surface, along which it insensibly crept, especially in low and damp situations. He very properly, however, does not lay much stress on this inference.

More numerous opportunities present themselves for witnessing the effect of a diminution in the density of the air. If an animal be placed under the receiver of an air-pump, and the air be exhausted, the air within the body, being no longer counterbalanced by the pressure of that without, expands; the animal appears inflated, and soon dies. In the mammalia, birds, fishes, &c. death is occasioned from this cause, as well as from the want of a due quantity of oxygen in the rarefied air surrounding them; but the amphibious animal, which is capable of subsisting for a long time without air, appears to be but little incommoded by its removal.

Many fishes are provided with an apparatus, called the *swimming-bladder*, which regulates their specific gravity according to circumstances, and if they be placed under the receiver of an air-pump, the air in the bladder dilates until the bladder bursts, after which they are unable to rise in the water, but crawl, as it were, along the bottom. Similar results would seem to occur to many kinds of fish, when taken at great depths, or even at the depth of from 70 to 100 feet. So long as they remain at the depth to which they are accustomed, the air of the swimming-bladder has the degree of compression, and elasticity necessary for supporting the column of water constantly pressing upon them; but if they be suddenly raised to the surface, the bladder swells and bursts, and the air which it contained, occupying 80, or 100 times more space, fills the cavities of the body, forces the stomach out of the mouth, and kills them: under such circumstances they float after death on the surface. It is only, however, when the pressure is suddenly removed, that these phenomena are witnessed. When the transition is more tardy, the animal possesses the power of regulating the quantity of air contained in this receptacle, so that no evil results.

Effects of a similar kind would be produced in the human body by any very sudden abstraction of the ordinary atmospheric pressure. It is the pressure of the air that prevents the escape of the fluids contained in the vessels; and if it be largely diminished, hemorrhages are apt to occur from those parts of the body, where the vessels are least protected by the textures in which they creep, as in the windpipe, and mucous membranes generally. The effect of diminished pressure on a part of the body is well exemplified by the application of a cupping glass.

The inconveniences, sustained on ascending lofty mountains, are partly owing to the rapid passage from a denser to a rarer medium. Some, however, have affirmed, that they are altogether dependent upon the fatigue induced by the ascent. Bouguier, Haller, Rudolph Meyer and others are of this opinion, and the Abbé Ferrara asserts, that none but invalids are incommoded in ascending to the summit of Etna. Londe, too, affirms that he has scaled the highest peaks of the Pyrenees, without experiencing any inconvenience, except what arose from the excessive cold, and that the acceleration of respiration, and circulation ceased after resting for some time; whence he likewise infers, that the effects are to be ascribed solely to the violent exercise of the ascent. On the other hand, we have the testimony of De Sayve, De Saussure, Hamel, Raymond, Von Humboldt, and numerous others to show, that fatigue could have had little or no agency; and what strikingly exhibits the accuracy of their deduction is, that the same inconveniences were sustained by Gay Lussac in his celebrated aerial voyage, when he ascended to the height of 21,735 French feet. (Levy, *Traité d' Hygiène Publique et Privée*, ii. 373, Paris, 1844.)

The indisposition experienced under such circumstances is extremely common in South America, and is there termed *Sorocco*. A German traveller (*Meyen*) thus describes the effects produced on his party, during an expedition to the mountains of Peru.—" We were tormented with a burning thirst, which no drink was able to assuage: a slice of water-melon which we had brought with us was the only thing we could relish, whilst our people ate garlic and drank spirits, maintaining, that this was the best way to guard against the effects of the journey. We kept on ascending till two o'clock in the afternoon. We were already near the little ridge which extends W. S. W. from the summit of the mountain, when our strength at once abandoned us, and we were overtaken by the disease *Sorocco*. The nervous feverishness under which we had suffered from the first had been gradually becoming worse and worse, and our breathing became more and more oppressed; fainting, sickness, giddiness, and bleeding at the nose came on; and in this condition we lay a considerable time, until the symptoms grew milder from repose, and we were able to descend slowly."

It is from the feelings experienced at such lofty elevations, that legitimate deductions, with regard to the effect of the air at great heights, can alone be drawn. At lesser elevations the uneasiness sustained may be so trifling as scarcely to be felt by the robust; and hence the testimony of those, who have ascended the Himālā mountains, or the Andes, is infinitely more satisfactory than that of the traveller who has merely climbed to the summit of the Pyrenees, the most elevated point of which is not more than 10,722 feet; whilst the Chipea-Pic, of the Himālās, reached by Captain Gerard, is 19,411 English feet; and Humboldt, on Chimborazo—the highest of the Andes—attained a height of 19,374 English feet.

These facts exhibit the inaccuracy of the idea of Cassini, that no animal can exist at the height of 2,446 toises,—15,640 feet English. (*Elémens d' Hygiène*, par E. Tourtelle, tom. i. p. 233; 3ème edit. 1815.) The observers, sent out to measure the earth under the equator, lived for a considerable time on the summit of Pichincha, 15,939 feet above the level of the sea, and consequently 300 feet above the point mentioned by Cassini; and the same gentlemen, whilst encamped upon the mountain, frequently observed vultures soaring at the height of

1,300 feet above them,—or in an atmosphere, where the mercury of the barometer was below fourteen inches. The remark of Cassini was founded on the presumption, that the atmosphere, at the height of 15,640 feet, is one half rarer than at the level of the ocean, and on the fact, that if the air be suddenly dilated to one half the density under the receiver of the air-pump, an animal placed under it dies. Such might be the effect upon man if the density were as suddenly diminished, but we have multitudes of instances to show, that there is within him a capability of resisting injurious influences to a surprising extent, provided the system has even a short time for accommodating itself to the new circumstances, under which it may be placed. Even the small period that elapses in the ascent of a balloon to this giddy elevation is sufficient for the purpose; and death, we have seen, did not result where the elevation, attained in this manner, was even 6,095 feet greater than that indicated by Cassini as the limit of animal existence.

The highest town, of any extent, on the earth is Potosi, in Bolivia, celebrated for the mines in its vicinity. It is 13,265 feet above the level of the Pacific ocean. Two hundred years ago, it is said to have contained 160,000 inhabitants, but the number is not now greater perhaps than 12,000. Perhaps the highest inhabited spot on this hemisphere is the farm of Antisana in Quito, the elevation of which is 13,400 feet. Yet the human family are capable of subsisting at these lofty elevations with the same facility as amidst the arctic snows when once habituated to them;—inconvenience being felt by new settlers only, and even these, by the gradual ascent, have the different organs accommodated to the new external relations.

We have no observations to guide us regarding the comparative frequency of respiration and circulation in those who inhabit such elevated districts. The effect of a sudden change from a denser to a more rarefied atmosphere quickens, as we have seen, both one and the other, but much of the effect probably soon subsides. It is reasonable to presume, that the respiration is permanently more rapid, in consequence of the rareness of the atmosphere requiring a greater number of inhalations, or in other words a greater quantity of air to produce the same effect in supplying the wants of the system. Nor are we better informed regarding the disposition to particular diseases, occasioned in the inhabitants of such regions, or whether there be any, that can be legitimately ascribed to a permanent residence in an atmosphere more dense or more rare than that at the level of the ocean.

From what has been already observed, a sudden transition from a dense to a rarer atmosphere must be unfavourable for such as are liable to hemorrhage from the mucous membranes, and especially from the lungs; and it is presumable, that it might lay the foundation for serious chest affections; but this could only happen where the change had been rapid and considerable, and perhaps could scarcely apply to those, who have been born, and bred at such elevations as the town of Potosi. The truth indeed appears to be, that changes in the density of the air, if not greatly above or below the ordinary, and not rapidly induced, are not attended with any marked effects upon human health : and that, in many instances, phenomena are ascribed to this cause, which are more properly referable, perhaps, to other meteorological conditions existing together with, or independently of, barometrical changes.

At the level of the sea, in this climate, the average height of the barometer is about thirty inches. At the height of 23,000 feet, its mean elevation is about 12.95 inches. Its height is different at different altitudes, and therefore the remark of M. Londe, that the density of the air, best adapted for human health, and longevity, ought not to cause the mercury to fall much under twenty-eight French inches, (nearly thirty inches English,) and that an elevation of 2,075 *mètres*—about 6,800 English feet—above the level of the sea, is unfavourable to health, is untenable. The cities of Quito and Cuenza are at greater elevations than this, and Potosi at double the height.

The elevated regions of Asia, however, afford us most striking examples of the impropriety of deducing general inferences of the kind alluded to. In the valleys and ridges of the lofty Himālā mountains, immense tracts, which, according to seeming analogy, ought to be entirely barren, or perpetually enveloped in snow, are richly covered with vegetation; abound in animals, and are scattered with villages. Marang, a large village, 8,500 feet above the sea, enjoys a mild climate. During eight days spent there by Captain Gerard, the temperature varied from 58° to 82° of Fahrenheit, and flies were extremely troublesome. At the village of Zon-Ching, 14,700 feet high, in latitude 31° 36′ N., and which was at one time considered to be in the region of perpetual congelation,

Mr. Colebrook found the hills clothed with Tartaric furze. The banks of the river were covered with grass turf, and prickly bushes; around, the land was verdant; and flocks of sheep were browsing, and deer leaping. On the crest of the Huketo pass, 15,786 feet high, Captain Gerard observed Yaks, (*Bos Poëphagus*, a remarkable bovine animal—the *grunting-ox* of Shaw and Pennant,) and horses, feeding on the surrounding heights, and found the climate pleasant, the temperature being 57° Fahrenheit. On Zinchen, 16,136 feet high, and on the neighbouring mountains, horses were galloping about in all directions, and feeding on the very tops of the heights. Kites and eagles were soaring in the air; large flocks of small birds, like linnets, were flying about, and locusts leaping among the bushes. At the village of Pui, at an elevation of 13,600 feet, there were cultivated fields of barley and turnips. A little lower, the ground was covered with thyme, sage, and many other aromatic plants, besides juniper, sweet-brier, and gooseberries; and vineyards and groves of apricots were numerous; and, lastly, near the village of Nako, in the midst of the Himālā range, situate 12,000 feet above the sea, in the heart of an abundant population, Gerard found the grain in August already yellow, with a broad sheet of water, surrounded by tall poplar, juniper, and willow trees of prodigious size. "Here," he remarks, "are produced most luxuriant crops of Barley, wheat, phaphur (*polygonum*,) and turnips, rising by steps to nearly 700 feet higher than the village, where is a lama's residence, inhabited throughout the year. The fields are partitioned by dykes of granite. At Taz-hi-gang they are enclosed by barberry and gooseberry bushes." (*British India*, by Murray, Wilson, &c.— Harpers' edit. vol. iii. p. 205.)

Yet, late French writers on hygiène copy implicitly from their predecessors, that no trees are found anywhere at the height of 2,000 toises, (12,790 English feet)—and that at 2,300 toises, (14,708 English feet) there is no trace of vegetation. On the northern side of the Himālās, fine birches are found at 14,000 feet, and *tama* bushes, which furnish excellent firewood, at 17,000 feet.

Even the sanitary depôts for those suffering under the diseases of the lower, and hotter parts of India, are situate, in some instances, higher than the point assigned by M. Londe as the limit of human salubrity. Dargeeling, in the Sikkim mountains, 330 miles from Calcutta, has been recommended as a sanitarium. Its height is about 7,218 feet above Calcutta, and its mean temperature is calculated to be 24° below that of Calcutta, and only two degrees above that of London. A convalescent retreat has also been provided at Simla, a station among the hills between the Suttledge and Jumna, near Sabhatto, 7,500 feet above the level of the sea.

The temperature of the atmosphere has probably a more extensive influence in modifying human health than its density. The range within which life can be maintained is great, and the vicissitudes are numerous and sudden. In our climate, the changes occasionally amount to 40 or 50° and even more in twenty-four hours.

The capability of existing amidst the snows of the frigid zone, or in the burning equatorial climes, is one of the great characteristics of the human race; and it is surprising to reflect on the quantity of heat, that must be constantly elicited, in the former case, to resist the external cold. In the temperate, and the colder regions of the globe, where the thermometer rarely attains the temperature of man, —that is 98 or 100°,—the body must be constantly parting with its coloric and where the spirit in the thermometer has stood at 72° below the zero of Fahrenheit's scale,—as it did during the journey of Captain Back in the northern regions of this continent,—the expenditure, in spite of appropiate clothing, must have been immense. It would seem, however, that in such cases the organs of calorification take upon themselves an increased action; and perhaps if the temperature of a resident in these inhospitable regions were observed, it would be found that the heat of his blood is some degrees higher than that of the inhabitants of the more temperate, and the torrid regions. Analogy and observation lead, at least, to such a conclusion. The quadrupeds of the frigid zone have a temperature higher than those of any other region of the globe. Captain Lyon found the temperature of an arctic fox, recently killed, to be $106\frac{3}{4}$ Fahrenheit, when that of the atmosphere was—14°.

On the other hand, the capability of resisting high elevations of temperature is great. In the author's treatise on *Human Physiology*, (5th edit., Philad. 1844.) numerous instances are adduced of the impunity with which air, at a temperature of 300° and upwards, has been breathed for some time; but this is a temperature to which we are not liable to be exposed, except for purposes of science, or of public exhibition. In Virginia, the thermometer scarcely ever rises to blood heat. In many parts of the state, there are a few days when it attains to 94°—and occasionally to 98°; but in South Carolina, it has been seen as high as 115°; as well as in the Llanos or plains near the Orinoco; and it appears to have been as high as 116° at Fort Gibson, on the 15th of August, 1834. In Africa, according to a letter with which the author was favoured many years ago, by the Chevalier Isoard, of Paris, the mercury is sometimes seen at 125°. The highest temperature of British India is met with in the Great Western Desert, and other sandy districts, at the level of the sea, or nearly so,—as the Circars and the Lower Carnatic. Elphinstone observed the thermometer at 112° in the Western Desert: Heyne, in the Northern Circars, saw the mercury at midnight at 108°, and at 8 A. M. at 112°; and it is affirmed to have been noted as high as 130°. (Professor Jameson, *British India*, vol. 3, p. 170.) This is probably the most elevated temperature that has ever been noticed in any region, whilst—72° may be regarded as the point of greatest observed depression;—the observed range of the thermometer, consistent with prolonged human existence, comprising, therefore, at least 200°.

The following table of the highest temperature observed in different climates is given by M. Arago. (See *Annuaire du Bureau des Longitudes*, 1825,—and *Elémens de Physique*, &c.—par Pouillet, tom. iv. p. 637—2de édit. 1832.)

| PLACES. | MAXIMUM OF HEAT. | NAMES OF OBSERVERS. |
|---|---|---|
| Equator, | 101° | Humboldt. |
| Surinam, | 90° | |
| Oasis of Mourzouk, | 130° | Ritchie and Lyon. |
| Pondicherry, | 112° | La Gentil. |
| Madras, | 104° | Roxburg. |
| Beit-el-Fakih, | 101° | Niebuhr. |
| Martinique, | 95° | Chauvalor |
| Manila, | 111° | Le Gentil. |
| Antougil, (Madagascar,) | 113° | do. |
| Gaudeloupe, | 101° | Le Gaux. |
| Vera Cruz, | 96° | Orta. |
| Isle of France, | 91° | Cossigny. |
| Philæ, (Egypt,) | 110° | Cautelle. |
| Cairo, | 104° | do. |
| Bassora, | 114° | Beauchamp. |
| Paramatta, (New Holland,) | 106° | Gen. Brisbane. |
| Cape of Good Hope, | 111° | La Caille. |
| Vienna, (Austria,) | 96° | Broquin. |
| Strasburg, | 96° | Herrenschneider. |
| Paris, | 101° | |
| Warsaw, | 93° | Deljue. |

| PLACES. | MAXIMUM. | NAMES OF OBSERVERS. |
|---|---|---|
| Franecker, (Holland,) | 94° | Van Swinden. |
| Copenhagen, | 92° | Bugge. |
| Nain, (Labrador,) | 82° | De La Trobe. |
| Stockholm, | 94° | Ronnoss. |
| Petersburg, | 87° | Euler. |
| Abo, | 94° | Lèche. |
| Iceland, (Eyafjord,) | 69° | Van-Sheels. |
| Hinsden, (Norway,) | 77° | Schytte. |
| Melville Island, | 60° | Parry. |

In those cases, in which the heat of the atmosphere is greater than that of the blood, a compensating power is exerted by the organs of calorification, so that the heat of the system is but little modified by it.

The human body is capable of being penetrated by the caloric from substances exterior to it as those substances are themselves; but, within certain limits, it possesses the faculty of resisting heat, and retaining the same temperature. It has been elsewhere shown, that even when the temperature of the atmosphere is not higher than our own, a sensation of unusual warmth is experienced, yet no caloric is communicated to us. The cause of the feeling is, that we are accustomed to live in a medium of a less elevated temperature, and consequently to give off caloric habitually to the atmosphere. (See the author's *Human Physiology*, 5th. edit. i. 104 and ii. 186. Philad. 1844.)

In this climate the body is constantly parting with caloric, and in order to diminish the expenditure, and to obviate the sensation of cold we have recourse to clothing, and during the colder seasons to artificial warmth; yet there is a range of temperature in which, clothed as we are, no sensation of cold is experienced, even although heat may be disengaged from the body to some extent. The *comfortable point* varies in different climates and seasons; and is greatly dependent upon the temperature which has previously existed. In this climate, it may be placed perhaps between 70° and 80°. If, however, the thermometer has ranged as high as 98°, or upwards, and has maintained this elevation for some time, a depression of fifteen or twenty degrees imparts an uncomfortable sensation of cold; whilst we often observe in spring, an elevation from 30° or 40° to 75° or 80° produce an oppressive feeling of heat. The arctic navigators, after having lived for some days in a temperature of

15° or 20° below 0, considered the air mild, and comfortable when the mercury rose to zero.

We may consider, then, that it is natural for man to be subjected to a constant abstraction of caloric, and that his organism is adapted accordingly; but if, from any cause, the organs of calorification should become deranged, so that external heat, greater than that of the body, could produce its ordinary effects by conduction or radiation, or both, as it does on inanimate objects, so as to raise the temperature twelve or fourteen degrees, the individual would die. On the other hand, if the abstraction of heat from the frame were excessive, so that the calorific agents could not supply the matter of heat as rapidly as it is expended, the temperature would fall; the fluids would congeal, and, when the temperature of the whole body was depressed to 79°, death would ensue. It would appear, consequently, that the temperature of the animal body may be lowered beyond the natural nearly twice as much as it can be raised, consistently with the persistence of vitality. (Edwards, *On the Influence of Physical agents on life*,—Hodgkin and Fisher's translation, p. 197.)

Independently of all other considerations, the heat of the torrid regions of the globe appears to be positively detrimental to animal health. The constant excitement induced by the elevated temperature disposes the intestines to assume a morbid condition under favouring excitant influences. In this way we account for the various derangements in the mucous membrane of the intestinal tube, which are so frequent in warm climates, and seasons;—diarrhœa, dysentery, cholera, &c. with those universal attendants upon inflammation of the upper portion of the small intestine,—liver diseases. These are so common, that it is rare to meet with a case of fever in tropical regions, not accompanied by bilious derangement. The excitement, prevailing in that portion of the intestinal canal into which the biliary ducts pour their bile from the liver extends along those ducts, and arouses the liver to inordinate secretion, or produces other functional, or organic disease in that viscus. This state of irritation of the duodenum, induced too often by undue quantity, or quality of aliment, is that of nine-tenths of the affections termed *bilious*. A person, after having dined heartily on a substance difficult of digestion, is affected with heart-burn, distention, flatulence, great uneasiness, and constant eructation; yet, although the cause is manifest, he prefers to have the symptoms ascribed to a predominance of bile, rather than to a circumstance, the belief in which would tend to curtail him in the slightest degree of his enjoyments.

Fevers, dysentery, liver disease in some shape, with every variety of bowel affection, may be regarded as the diseases of hot climates. That hepatic disease is capable of being induced by heat alone, we have proof in the animal kingdom. The celebrated *Pâtés de foies gras*, prepared at Strasburg, and Metz, which are so much esteemed as to be sent as far as Paris, Vienna, St. Petersburg, and are frequently seen on the festive tables of this country, are prepared from the livers of geese, artificially enlarged by means of heat. The animal is crammed with food, kept from drink, nailed to a plank by the webs of its feet, and placed quite close to the fire: in due time, the liver becomes greatly enlarged, and scarcely ever fails to acquire the condition so prized by the gourmand.*

In many of the unhealthy districts of India, animals, as the dog, are frequently affected with the endemic liver diseases,—so strongly do the morbific causes act on the animal economy in these insalubrious situations.

Similar remarks to those made regarding the effect of an atmosphere of diminished density on the respiratory function are applicable here. Warm air, being more dilated than cool, contains less oxygen in the same bulk; and, consequently, a greater number of inspirations is necessary to effect the requisite aeration of the blood. Such, at least, would be the result if the temperature were to change suddenly from a cold to a comparatively warm point; but it seems

* The following extract from the *Almanach des Gourmands*, is written with the *goût* of an amateur. "Ce qui mérite a l'oie toute la reconnaissance des véritables gourmands, ce qui lui assigne un rang très distingué parmi les volatiles, ce sont *des foies*, dont on fabrique à Strasbourg ces pâtés admirables, le plus grand luxe d'un entremêts. Pour obtenir ces foies d'une grosseur convenable, il faut sacrifier la personne de la bête, Abondée de nourriture, privée de boisson et fixée près d'un grand feu, au devant duquel elle est clouée par les pattes sur une planche, cette oie passe, il faut en convenir, une vie assez malheureuse. Ce seroit même un supplice tout-a-fait intolérable pour elle, si l'idée du sort qui l'attend ne lui servoit de consolation. Mais cette perspective lui fait supporter ses maux avec courage; et lorsqu'elle pense que son foie plus gros qu'elle même et lardé de truffes, revetu d'une pâte savante ira porter dans toute l'Europe la gloire de son nom, elle se résigne à la destinée et ne laisse pas même couler une larme."

probable, that under the protracted influence of an elevated temperature, the hurry of respiration subsides; the point of indispensable aeration is depressed; the lungs become less active; and less oxygen is consumed,—the consumption being always found to keep pace with the degree of muscular exertion, and being, by many distinguished physiologists, considered dependent upon it. It is well ascertained, that the consumption of oxygen is largely augmented by muscular exertion, when not pushed to the extent of inducing fatigue. Séguin found it increased four fold.

The effect of an elevated temperature in diminishing its consumption has been proved by experiments on animals. Crawford found that a Guinea pig, confined in air at the temperature of 55°, consumed double the quantity which it did in air at 104°. He also found that the venous blood, when the body was exposed to a high temperature, had not its usual dark colour; but, by its florid hue, indicated that little change had taken place in its constitution in the course of circulation. This was probably owing to diminished nervous power, which, as every circumstance appears to show, is considerably depressed when the body is exposed to great heat; and the difficulty of breathing, and sense of suffocation, which are observed to supervene under such circumstances, are probably referable, not to rarefaction of the air, but to debility of the inspiratory muscles, owing to the enervating effects of the elevated temperature on the brain. In this way we may account for the great lassitude, and yawning induced by the summer heats, as well as for the languor and listlessness, and the indisposition to mental or corporeal labour, which are so characteristic of those who have resided for a length of time in torrid climes. How many individuals have sailed from their country to the scorching presidencies of British India, in the full possession of youthful energy—intellectual as well as corporeal—and have returned to the land of their nativity, after a lapse of some ten or twenty summers, so thoroughly changed, as hardly to have one characteristic remaining, and seeming to be devoid of all power of actively exerting either mind or body!

We can thus understand, that warm climates may be unfavourable to those who are predisposed to diseases of the brain, especially to such as are characterized by debility and mobility of the nervous system—as paralysis, epilepsy, mania, &c. The author has met with some cases of hemiplegia in young men between 20 and 30, developed by a brief residence in India; and the injurious effects of the climate of the East, on those who have any tendency to mental derangement, have frequently been noticed. On these unfortunate individuals heat probably acts in two ways:—by augmenting the mobility of the nervous system, and by keeping up constant excitement.

A recent writer, M. Rostan, (*Art.* Air. *in Dict. de Médecine*) asserts, that warm climates are beneficial to the scrofulous, rickety, scorbutic and rheumatic; but, as regards the first three, we suspect he has not much ground for the assertion. Scrofula and rickets are but little dependent upon temperature, if they can be regarded as at all so. They, as well as scurvy, would seem rather to be excited by confined and deteriorated air, and by privation of light. Hence, the first two are most common in manufacturing establishments, whilst the third is chiefly seen on board ships, and in penitentiaries. It is indeed but rarely met with, since its grand cause,—that of restricting individuals, compelled to inhabit a confined space, to one sort of diet, it matters not whether animal or vegetable,—has been obviated by a more varied supply; and since a better system of ventilation and cleanliness, has been established. At one time, scurvy was the scourge of ships on long voyages; and as these were frequently to the North, it was imagined that a cold atmosphere was an exciting cause, or greatly favoured its production; whilst the main cause was wholly overlooked.

Rickets, once so common in England as to have obtained the name "*English Disease*," is now extremely rare;—and in many climates of a similar temperature is, like scrofula, uncommon. It is by no means frequent in the United States. We have the best evidence, however, of the incorrectness of M. Rostan's observation regarding the good effects of an elevated temperature on scrofula, in the remarks of Dr. Whitelaw Ainslie, a physician of great respectability, and much experience in the diseases of Southern India, to the medical staff of which he belonged. He observes, that perhaps of all disorders, that to which the climate of India proves most *ungenial* is scrofula. "No young man," he says, "with an hereditary tendency to this complaint, should, on any account, be sent to India, where *we have never known one individual* with the malady in his habit, who enjoyed tolerable health for ten months together. Soldiers, so tainted, are fit for nothing but lumbering up an hospital; and, for the most part, after lingering a few years, burdens to themselves and to their regiments, they fall a prey to the most frightful and ravaging ulcers. How this baneful effect of a hot climate, upon persons so unfortunately predisposed, is to be accounted for, it may be difficult to say, as the state of darkness, in which we have so long wandered, regarding the proximate cause of affections of this nature, leaves us little more than a conjecture. One thing is certain, that as laxity of the solids, and a general deficiency of bodily vigour, are known to be the constant concomitants of the complaint, such a condition will be greatly increased by extreme heat, which enervates in no common degree." (*British India*, vol. III. p. 269.)

Rheumatism is the only affection referred to by M. Rostan, which is benefited by a warm climate. But, although the warmth of the day may be beneficial in these cases, great caution is necessary not to sleep out in the open air, during the heavy dews that fall in the torrid regions. Moreover, although warmth is favourable in these cases, it does not seem that heat is equally so. When rheumatism is connected with an irritable condition of the digestive organs, or a relaxed state of the system, a torrid climate has been found to disagree. In many of the West India Islands, rheumatic affections are by no means uncommon, and it is affirmed, that even acute rheumatism is not rare. In Jamaica, however, rheumatic affections would seem to be much less prevalent amongst the British Troops than in the windward and leeward cammand, or in Great Britain (Sir James Clark, *Sanative Influence of Climate*, p. 311, Lond. 1841.)

Gout, a congenerous disease, attacking similar structures, is not encouraged by a hot climate. This has been particularly noticed in those, who have left the temperate regions to reside in the torrid zone, and who have been subject to this affection. They have generally long intervals between the fits; and these, when they do occur, are usually slight.

It is on those predisposed to consumption, that a warm climate acts most beneficially. Although that formidable disease, which destroys so large a proportion of the inhabitants of the temperate regions of the earth, is met with in torrid climes, it cannot be called a disease of such climes. In the West India islands the cases are comparatively few, and wherever the mean temperature approaches 80° and upwards, it can scarcely be said to be endemic. From this cause, as well as from the greater equability of the temperature of the warmer regions of the earth, the physician is in the habit of recommending those, who are strongly predisposed to consumption, to pass the season of coldness, and vicissitude, in a warm climate; and even when tubercles exist in the lungs, but have not proceeded to suppuration, we have sufficient evidence of the good effects of such a course: but where consumption is confirmed; when tubercular matter is evidenced in the expectoration; and when, along with this, an examination of the chest by the ear, or stethoscope, indicates that cavities exist there, or that a considerable portion of the lungs is incapable of respiration, no good is to be anticipated from a change of climate: on the contrary, the disorder is often hastened to a fatal termination by the enervating influence of excessive heat. A fearful responsibility consequently rests on the medical adviser, who is inexcusably culpable if, owing to insufficient examination, he hurries away an unfortunate sufferer to a distant, and foreign country, far removed from his family, his friends, and the various comforts, and associations which *home* affords, under the delusive hope of restoration, when the disease has made such serious inroads. It has been frequently affirmed, that when the physician discovers that all his endeavours have proved unavailing for arresting the mischief, he sends the victim on this forlorn hope, careless of the results,—and the opprobrium may have attached to an unfeeling and inconsiderate adviser; but the error is more commonly one of ignorance, arising from insufficient examination, and hopes are indulged, that the extent of mischief *may* not be as serious as it appears, and that a change to a warm and equable atmosphere may possibly restore all to its former integrity. Since the improvements introduced into the diagnosis of chest diseases, these errors are much less venial, and therefore less common, than they were formerly.—But we shall have to recur to this topic hereafter.

Such are the chief effects of warmth, considered singly, on human health, and on the play of several of the functions,—as proved by direct observation, and by just theory. Writers on this subject have not confined themselves, however, to this mode of investigation, but have wandered into the regions of fancy and conjecture. Thus, we are told by one writer, that "sleep is the sole desideratum with the inhabitants of the torrid regions; and that they are lazy, feeble, idle, ignorant, and cruel, and consequently tyrants or slaves: and that such is, in fact, the lot of the Turk, the Asiatic, and the African." (Rostan, *loc. citat.*) Such deductions can only be drawn from a very limited view of anthropology; and the writer would have discovered, had he extended his inquiries, that to the extreme north of Europe, and even in its more temperate regions, and still more in the cold districts of northern Asia, and at the far extremities of our own continent, both north and south, people may be found possessing most, if not all, of the characteristics which he ascribes to the influence of elevated temperature.

To the young, and the vigorous, a moderately depressed temperature is agreeable, and exciting. The first effect is to diminish the circulation in the capillary or small vessels of the surface, and to interfere somewhat with the process of cutaneous calorification, so far at least as regards those parts that are not well protected by appropriate clothing against the coldness of the atmosphere; but reaction soon succeeds, either spontaneously, or aroused by exercise, and an agreeable glow follows the state of diminished calorification. This excited action at the sentient extremities of the nerves is appreciated by the brain, which responds to the stimulus; the play of the nervous system becomes more energetic, and every function under its presidency acts in consequence, with more than usual vigour; perception is more acute; reflection more ready; and the nutritive functions are more vigorously accomplished, with the exception of the cutaneous transpiration, which is necessarily less. The secretion from the kidneys is, however, so largely augmented as to compensate for the defective depuration by the skin. A table, formed by Lining from experiments made in South Carolina, shows, that during the warm months the perspiration largely exceeds the renal secretion, whilst in the colder months the reverse holds good.

|            | Renal Secretion. | Perspiration. |
|------------|------------------|---------------|
| December,  | 70.81            | 42.55         |
| January,   | 72.43            | 39.97         |
| February,  | 77.86            | 37.45         |
| March,     | 70.59            | 43.23         |
| April,     | 59.17            | 47.72         |
| May,       | 56.15            | 58.11         |
| June,      | 52.90            | 71.39         |
| July,      | 43.77            | 86.41         |
| August,    | 55.41            | 70.91         |
| September, | 40.60            | 77.09         |
| October,   | 47.67            | 40.78         |
| November,  | 63.16            | 40.97         |

The effects, described above, are such as are produced by a moderate cold,—for example between 30 and 45° of Fahrenheit's scale,—provided the exposure has not been too long continued, and due exercise and clothing have been employed. When, however, the body is subjected even to this temperature, and *à fortiori* to a lower, without the necessary endeavours to counteract its influence, the subcutaneous circulation is impeded; secretion, and calorification are retarded, or arrested; the skin becomes rough; and the blood circulates in greater quantity in the interior of the frame, so that inflammatory or subinflammatory affections are apt to supervene, especially in the air tubes, the lining membrane of which, in consequence of the diminished cutaneous exhalation, and circulation, has its vessels probably more engorged; hence the different forms of bronchitis,—cough, winter cough, &c.—which prevail during the colder seasons, and prove so fatal to the aged especially.

It was asserted by Dr. Beddoes—and experience has corroborated his assertion,—that during the coldest months there is regularly the greatest number of deaths amongst those above sixty years of age; and Dr. William Heberden, Jr., a learned and accurate observer,—who published some interesting observations on the *Climate and Diseases of London*,—has observed, that one of the first things, that must strike every mind engaged in the investigation of this subject, is the effect of a severe frost on old people. "It is curious," he remarks, "to observe, among those who are said in the bills to die above sixty years of age, how regularly the tide of mortality follows the influence of this prevailing cause; so that a person used to such inquiries may form no contemptible judgment of the severity of any of our winters, merely by attending to this circumstance."

These views are somewhat applicable to our own climate. We should not, however, be justified in according with Beddoes, that "during the coldest months there is regularly the greatest number of deaths among those aged above sixty, and the fewest in the middle of summer." On the contrary, next in fatality to the pulmonary affections, induced by the severity of winter's cold, we would class the disorders of the lining membrane of the intestinal canal occasioned by excessive heat, which are highly dangerous in advanced life, owing to the exhaustion they occasion in a frame, whose elasticity has been diminished by prolonged exertion.

These facts should induce the elderly individual to adopt every precaution, during winter, to keep the cutaneous exhalation and calorification—not now effected as in youth—active by appropriate clothing (especially when subjected to exposure,) and by a well regulated temperature in his apartment. Nor is less attention required in the state of first childishness,—in infancy. Direct observation shows that the function of calorification is less perfectly accomplished the nearer to birth; and that the compensating power, which we notice to be possessed by the older child, and by the adult, exists to a limited extent only for some time after birth;—the temperature of the infant rising and falling according to the greater or less elevation of that of the medium which it respires, or in which it is placed,—and in this respect resembling somewhat the cold, rather than the warm-blooded animal. In this tender state, exposure to a cold atmosphere is apt to produce local irregularities in the action of the vessels, and various congestive or inflammatory disorders, which the tender organism is not calculated to withstand; and accordingly it is found, that exposure to a cold atmosphere proves very fatal to infants not properly protected against its deranging influence.

Except in such cases, however, a pure, dry, cold air invigorates the frame; and if we find that, during the season at which depressed temperature prevails, more indisposition exists, the circumstance may be explained more satisfactory by other mutations in the atmosphere, in combination with diminished temperature, or alone.

When the temperature is still more depressed than in the case we have considered, and the frame is not sufficiently protected against its influence, very different phenomena occur. Instead of an invigorating action, the nervous system becomes torpid: the brain ceases to be affected by impressions from without, and an irresistible desire for sleep comes on, which if indulged, becomes the sleep of death, and is perhaps one of the easiest modes in which life becomes extinct.

A striking instance of this occurred during one of Cook's voyages, when the ship Endeavour was on the coast of Terra del Fuego. Sir Joseph Banks, Dr. Solander, and others, in making a botanical excursion, were overtaken by night on the hills, and although Dr. Solander had warned them of the dangers of lying down to sleep when they felt benumbed, emphatically remarking, " whoever sits down will sleep, and whoever sleeps will wake no more," he himself became so overpowered as to find the desire for sleep irresistible, and insisted on being permitted to lie down. He was allowed to do so for five minutes, and when aroused after this brief repose he had almost lost the use of his limbs, and the muscles were so shrunk that his shoes fell from his feet. Several of the party began to lose their sensibility, after an exposure to the cold of near an hour and a half, but the fire recovered them. Two blacks, however, who remained in the cold asleep perished.

The effect of severe cold has been often witnessed in expeditions to the North Pole; and captain Parry (*Expedition to the North Pole,* i. 108,) thus describes the condition of some of his crew on their return to the ship, after long exposure to cold. "When I sent for them into my cabin, they looked wild, spoke thick and indistinctly, and it was impossible to draw from them a rational answer to any of our questions. After being on board for a short time, the mental faculties appeared gradually to return with the returning circulation, and it was not till then, that a looker-on could easily persuade himself that they had not been drinking too freely." "I have more than once," he adds, "seen our people in a state so exactly resembling that of the most stupid intoxication, that I should certainly have charged them with that offence, had I not been quite sure, that no possible means were offered them in Melville Island to produce any thing stronger than snow water."

But the most memorable instance of mortality, from excessive cold, combined also with privation of food, occurred in the disastrous campaign of Napoleon, in 1812, against Russia. During the bivouacs of the army at Miedneski, in the nights of the 8th and 9th of December, the thermometer was as low as—27° and—32° of Fahrenheit. The horses died in great numbers, and the soldiers, who were without furs or cloaks, were struck with stupor if they took the least rest. Death, in these cases, according to the veteran surgeon, Larrey, was preceded by pallor of the countenance; by a kind of idiocy; difficulty of articulation; defective vision, and sometimes a total loss of the sense; and in this way they continued to march supported by their comrades or friends. The action of their muscles was greatly enfeebled; they staggered like drunken men; and the debility went on augmenting until they fell—a certain evidence of the total extinction of life. The uninterrupted, and rapid march of the soldiers in a body compelled such as could not keep up to quit the centre of the column, and proceed along the sides of the road; but when separated from the close column, and left to themselves, they soon lost their equilibrium, and fell into the ditches filled with snow, in which they could scarcely raise themselves. They were immediately attacked with a painful torpor, which rapidly became converted into a state of lethargic stupor, and in a few moments they had terminated their miserable existence.

There is one remark made by this distinguished surgeon, (*Mémoires de Chirurgie Militaire*, tom. iv. p. 125,) which is worthy of remembrance;—namely, that the French and the inhabitants of southern Europe, contrary to what has been imagined, suffered less from the severe cold of Russia, than their German, and Dutch allies, who dwell in a cold and moist climate, but one nearer in character to that of Russia than the climate of southern Europe. The Hollanders of the third regiment of grenadiers of the guard, consisting of 1787 officers and soldiers, were almost entirely destroyed,—not more than forty-one having returned to France two years afterwards; whilst two other regiments of grenadiers, composed of men almost all born in the southern provinces of France, saved a large portion of their soldiers;—a circumstance perhaps to be in some measure explained by the greater moral energy of the southern Europeans elicited by their fine sky, and peculiar national habits than of the Hollanders, who are proverbially more apathetic. For this reason, we can understand, why they should likewise be more affected with nostalgia, the *maladie du Pays* of the French; or, as it is more appropriately called by the Germans, H e i m w e h, ' *Homeache*,'—a species of melancholy, produced by an inveterate, and corroding desire to return to the " dear green valley of their native stream," and which has often induced permanent mental derangement and suicide.

These facts have led a recent writer (Guerard, Art. *Froid.*, in *Dict. de Med.* xiii. 520, Paris, 1836) to the general inference, that circumstances connected with the individual are even more powerful than physical circumstances themselves; and that although the effect of depressed temperature varies according to the intensity and duration of the cold, its state of tranquillity or agitation, and the proportion of vapour which it contains, it is at least equally modified by the age and sex of the individual, his temperament, moral disposition, the exercise which he takes, and the regimen to which he is subjected. Thus, whilst Franklin, Parry, Ross, Scoresby, and others were exposed for whole months to a temperature from 50 to 70° below the zero of Fahrenheit's scale, without the health of the men suffering materially, the fatal campaign of 1812, alluded to above, destroyed the *élite* of European nations in the army,—although the temperature was not depressed below —37°,—owing to dejection of spirits, privation of food, constant marching, the debilitating effects of all these influences being added to that of a rigorous winter.

## SECTION II.

Hygrometric state of the atmosphere—effect of the degree of dryness of the air on the cutaneous, and pulmonary transpirations—mode in which the air acts as an irritant to wounded and burnt surfaces—moist air a better vehicle for animal, vegetable, or mineral exhalations—atmospheric vicissitudes frequently the source of disease—Russian vapour bath—vicissitudes from cold to heat the source of disease—atmospheric vicissitudes necessary to full mental and corporeal development—effect of light, and of electricity on the functions.

THERE is another condition of the atmosphere, which, singly, or combined with those that have been mentioned, must exert considerable influence over the functions. It has, indeed, been regarded as the most injurious to human life of all the physical qualities of the air. We allude to the *hygrometric*. Air possesses the property of dissolving water; and consequently all liquid bodies, when exposed to it, experience evaporation,—the amount varying according to the degree in which water is already contained in the air. Even during the driest weather, water is always present in the atmosphere, although its proportion is constantly fluctuating; and if we reduce the temperature of the air sufficiently, we can always cause it to be precipitated in the form of dew. This is the cause why our vessels, containing iced water, are covered with moisture on the exterior, in the very driest days of summer;—a circumstance which has given occasion to an ingenious hygrometer, invented by Mr. Daniell for indicating the precise point, at which dew is deposited in various conditions of the atmosphere.

The quantity of water, contained in a cubic foot of air charged with moisture, at 65° of Fahrenheit, is, according to De Saussure, eleven grains; but the air is perhaps never wholly saturated. From a comparison of numerous observations, Gay Lussac affirms, that the mean hygrometric state of the atmosphere is such, that it holds just one half the moisture necessary for its saturation.

The amount of aqueous vapour in the atmosphere is very variable owing to the continual change of temperature to which the air is subject. The quantity of water, that may be extracted by hygrometric bodies from 100 cubic inches of air, at 57°, is 0.35 of a grain; but, according to Clement and Desormes, at 54° Fahrenheit, only 0.236 of a grain can be detached by exposure to chloride of calcium, which, when placed in the air, attracts moisture from it, and is hence said to be *deliquescent*.

When we ascend to great heights in the atmosphere, the hygrometer gradually falls, except in passing through clouds, which consist of water in the state of vesicular vapour. In the celebrated aerial voyage of Gay Lussac, he found the air to contain but one eighth of the moisture necessary for saturation. This is perhaps the greatest degree of dryness ever noticed.

It has been a question with physiologists, whether the air abstracts moisture from the animal body as it does from inorganic substances. They who think, that the cutaneous and pulmonary transpirations are mere transudations, or dependent upon a physical permeation of fluid from within the appropriate vessels to without, and independently of all vital agency, believe in the affirmative, whilst they who regard those transpirations as altogether vital, consider that no such physical effect can result. Others again, with more propriety, believe that they are partly dependent upon physical evaporation, and partly upon vital secretion (*Human Physiology*, 5th edit. ii. 253, Philadelphia, 1844.)

Were we indeed, to grant the position, that the cutaneous, and pulmonary transpirations are produced by vital agency alone, and in no respect to be assimilated to physical transudation, a great agency, in modifying the quantity of these transpirations, must be ascribed to the varying condition of the atmosphere as regards moisture. If the air be dry its power of absorption is greater: the perspirable matter evaporates as soon as it is secreted; but when the air contains such moisture, the perspirable matter does not readily evaporate, but accumulates on the surface in a sensible state. In the former case, we should expect the activity of the exhalants to be increased by the ready removal of the secretion, and in the latter to be diminished for opposite reasons.

From what has been said, it can be easily understood, why, in a warm, moist air, we seem to perspire more than in a hotter and drier, although we are really exhaling less. It is asserted by Schmidtmeyer, that in the climate of Chili, notwithstanding the very high temperature in summer, the perspiration passes off so entirely in the insensible form, that, during the most violent exercise, it might be doubted whether any perspiration whatever exist.

If the air be greatly charged with moisture, especially during the heat of summer, owing to a diminution of the cutaneous, and pulmonary transpiration—the evaporation of which constitutes a cooling process—we feel languid, and listless, with an indisposition to every mental or corporeal exertion. This is the cause why we suffer little more during the hot summers of this country, than in those of Great Britain, where the air is always more loaded with humidity, although the thermometer may be fifteen or twenty degrees higher here than there.

Again, when we are exposed to a moist temperature, much greater than that of the body, we may seem to perspire profusely, whilst the cutaneous moisture may be chiefly owing to another cause. In certain experiments, instituted by Dr. George Fordyce, and Sir Charles Blagden with heated air, they found, in a temperature of 260° of Fahrenheit, that small quantities of water in metallic vessels speedily boiled, and that streams of moisture ran down the whole surface of the body; but, that this was merely the vapour of the room, condensed by the cooler skin, the temperature of which was probably only raised a few degrees above the ordinary standard, was proved by the fact, that when a Florence flask, filled with water of the same temperature as the body, was placed in the room, the vapour condensed in like manner upon its surface, and ran down in streams. On the other hand, when the air is cold, and moist,—owing to aqueous vapour being a better conductor of caloric than air, the heat is abstracted in greater quantity from the frame, and we feel more chilly than the temperature, it would seem, is calculated to explain; and therefore, more liable to have those disordered, and irregular actions induced, which give occasion to different febrile and inflammatory disorders.

It has been already said, that at great elevations the air is extremely dry; whilst the pressure is much diminished. On these accounts human bodies dry with extreme rapidity. This dry air M. Gay Lussac found, at the height of upwards of 21,000 French feet, to be extremely disagreeable in respiration; owing, as he conceived, to the desiccation produced in the lungs. M. Edwards also ascribes the uneasy sensations, experienced on the tops of lofty mountains, to the augmented evaporation from the lungs, produced by diminished atmospheric pressure and the great dryness of the air. This great dryness at high elevations was appreciated by Garcilasso de la Vega. " It is a well known fact," he observes, " that the Adelanta do Don Diego de Almagro, on his march towards Chili, when, as is probable, he was led by his guides over the highest plain of Tacora, lost more than 10,000 Indians, 150 Spaniards, and a number of horses, all of whom fell a sacrifice to hunger, thirst, and this disease. The soldiers on that memorable expedition built themselves walls of the dead bodies of their comrades merely to protect themselves against the drying effect of the wind."

But facts,—as M. Edwards has judiciously remarked,—connected with an excessive evaporation from the lungs may be observed in other than elevated regions. In winter, when, during a very sharp cold, an apartment is warmed by means of a stove, a painful sensation is experienced, by many persons, in the chest. The air, in a frost, contains scarcely any watery vapour, and the heat of the stove, by augmenting the temperature of the air, increases its capacity for vapour, so that a much greater evaporation is produced than in summer. It is an old and general custom to place upon the stove a vessel of water to remedy the inconvenience, and it is advantageous. (Edwards, *op. citat.* p. 263.)

It is probably in this way, that air acts as an irritant to a wounded, and ulcerated surface; and the great improvement, that has taken place in the management of such cases, has consisted in carefully excluding air, the admission of which occasions a rapid evaporation of the moisture covering them, and excites irritation in the vessels, whose office it is to effect the reparatory process. The same principle of management prevails whenever the skin is extensively inflamed, as in ordinary cases of erysipelas or Saint Anthony's fire, or in cases of burns and scalds. In the latter especially, if the contact of air be carefully excluded, the mischiefs, that might otherwise have resulted, are completely obviated. In this way, we account for the advantage derived from enveloping a burnt, or scalded limb in cotton wool; or from covering it with cloths, moistened in a thick liniment—as that composed of lime-water and oil—capable of filling up the areolæ of the rag, and thus of completely preventing the admission of air, and the desiccation which would inevitably result from it.

The barometric, and thermometric influences of the air are exerted with more or less energy upon the animal system, according as its hygrometric condition is more or less considerable,—that is, according as it is dry, or damp. Dry air, for example, is heavier than moist, inasmuch as watery vapour is lighter than air in the proportion 625 to 1,000. When the air, consequently, is highly charged with moisture, the mercury in the barometer falls; and, on the other hand, when it is dry, the mercury rises. We have seen, again, that our sensations of heat and cold, are greater when the air is damp, owing to the presence of water between its particles adding to its conducting power; and lastly, that as the dissolving power of the air augments in proportion to its dryness, and temperature, its action upon the fluids of the body must be less in a moist, than in a dry atmosphere.

It may be remarked, by the way, that a moist atmosphere is better adapted than a dry one to dissolve various animal, vegetable, or mineral substances, which are susceptible of volatilization. We have many instances to prove, that volatilizable substances are sooner converted into the gaseous state under such circumstances. Lime-burners are well aware, that limestone can be burnt, and reduced to the state of quicklime, much sooner in moist than in dry weather; and, in the latter case, they not unfrequently place a pan of water in the ash pit, the light vapour of which,—lighter, as we have seen, than atmospheric air,—assists in carrying off the carbonic acid gas, which is heavier. Camphor is found to volatilize with much greater celerity in damp situations, and every one has noticed the fragrance of a garden after a summer's shower. There are certain bodies, too, which require the presence of moisture for their escape:—thus, the odorous particles of argillaceous substances are quiescent until they are breathed upon, or, in other words, until they become moistened by the fluid exhaled from the lungs, or by moisture of some kind, after which the mineralogist readily recognises their characteristic odour. Every one must have noticed how powerfully the stench of putrid ditches is conveyed to the olfactory organs in summer, previous to rain, when the air becomes charged with moisture, and how readily offensive substances are detected in a fog by the same sense.

The agency of moisture is doubtless also concerned in the conveyance of various emanations from the soil, which produce endemic disease. It has long been noticed, that whilst the inhabitants of a plain, on the level of a marshy land, have escaped diseases that are known to be produced by the emanations from such land, or by *malaria*,—as it has been termed by the Italians,—those dwelling on neighbouring elevations have suffered extensively. Observation would seem to have shown, that this malaria is somewhat heavier than atmospheric air; but as watery vapour is incessantly exhaled from the surface of the earth under the influence of solar heat, and as this vapour possesses so little specific gravity, it takes up the heavier miasms along with it, and, under favourable circumstances, they are deposited on the elevations.

Similar remarks apply to the communication of the matter of contagion, which would appear to be modified in its activity by the degree of moisture in the atmosphere influencing its solubility and volatility; but on this topic our evidence is not quite as satisfactory. The same may be said of epidemic influences, of which our ignorance is unhappily so profound. It may be remarked, as some corroboration of this view, that the Harmattan, a wind which blows periodically from the interior of Africa towards the Atlantic ocean, and which is characterized by its extreme dryness, is asserted to put an end to all epidemic, and contagious affections,—even to small pox; and it is said that, at such times, the disease is not easily communicable by art. It is proper to observe, however, that the moist Sirocco has been said to interfere with the operation of vaccination and of inoculation for the smallpox and to render it inert; but, as Dr. John Davy (*Notes on the Ionian Islands and Malta*, vol. i. p. 270. Lond. 1842,) has suggested, many mistakes respecting the Sirocco of the Mediterranean, have probably arisen from confounding it with the dry Harmattan. His observations did not lead him to ascribe any such properties to the Sirocco; and that the remark was not correct in regard to its interfering with vaccination he was assured by a very experienced vaccinator.

We shall find, hereafter, that humidity modifies the action of atmospheric electricity on the animal body, as well as the electrical condition of the body itself.

It has been already seen, that in the varying atmospheric conditions, which have been considered, the system has the power of accommodating itself to the changes, provided they are not too extensive or sudden. But if the mercury were to vary from twenty-eight inches to thirty-one at once, it is difficult to say what might be the effects of the sudden vicissitude. Or again, if the temperature should suddenly rise from $-72°$ to $130°$ of Fahrenheit, as a natural consequence of this rise the barometer would fall; and from these combined causes,—even from the vicissitude of temperature taken singly,—man would perhaps cease to exist. Vicissitudes in the hygrometrical state of the atmosphere could probably be borne with the greatest impunity.

It can rarely happen, that these vicissitudes in the barometric, thermometric, and hygrometric states of the air are experienced singly. It has already been seen, that as we ascend in the air, the atmosphere necessarily becomes lighter, the mercury of the barometer consequently descends, and at the same time greater and greater coldness is experienced according to the elevation; so that if we are ascending high mountains we ultimately attain the regions of perpetual congelation. We have seen, also, that at very great elevations, the air is much drier, and that inconvenience is sustained from this cause. High up in the atmosphere we have, consequently, a combination of of a low state of barometric, thermometric, and hygrometric conditions.

When the air is warm, it is more expanded, the barometer therefore sinks in it, whilst a larger quantity of aqueous vapour can be held in the invisible state than when the temperature is lower.

These facts will show, that the different atmospheric modifications, which have been considered, may be variously circumstanced, so as to give rise, as will be seen hereafter, to much of that peculiarity observed in different climates, and to the various mutations experienced in the air of the same district. Vicissitudes in temperature are most appreciable by our senses, and to them, consequently, our attention is most frequently directed. A rapid alternation from heat to cold is felt most disagreeably, and we are disposed to refer numerous morbid conditions to it, especially if the cold be attended with dampness, which it is sure to be, if the vicissitude has been very sudden. During the state of warmth, a large quantity of vapour may be retained in the air in an insensible form, which becomes apparent if the temperature suddenly subsides to an unusually depressed point. Robust individuals may experience these alternations without detriment, but the delicate,—they who are liable to internal affections, on slight irregularities,—often suffer greatly. It has been supposed that much of this effect is owing to a sudden check to perspiration; but the system generally accommodates itself so that the depuration, previously accomplished by the skin, takes place to a considerable extent from other outlets. Thus, the air may continue, as it often does in winter in this climate, for days together, greatly below the freezing point, and yet no evil, under ordinary precautions may result from protracted exposure to it. It does not, indeed, appear probable, that many of the maladies, so often ascribed to depressed temperature, or to taking cold, are owing to mere diminution in the general cutaneous exhalation, but rather that they are ascribable to local irregularities of the capillary system of vessels, between all the parts of which there is such an extensive and intimate sympathy, that if one part be irregularly affected, another portion of the system—more disposed than the rest, owing to inappreciable circumstances, to morbid derangement—becomes itself morbidly implicated. The probability of some evil resulting from getting the feet wet is proverbial; yet the effect, immediately produced by exposure, implicates but a slight extent of surface: still, if twenty people be exposed to this cause of disease, upwards of two-thirds will probably be attacked with inflammation, or irritation somewhere. One may have one form of catarrh, another may have a second, another inflammatory sore throat, another inflammation of the lungs, another inflammation of the bowels, and so on, according as the capillary system of one part in any individual is more liable, at the time, to take on increased action than the rest.

It has been generally asserted by writers, that a sudden vicissitude from heat to cold is likely to affect the bowels by driving in the perspiration, and occasioning it to settle on the lining membrane of the intestinal tube. This does not appear to be philosophical, although the fact of diarrhœa supervening under such circumstances may be indisputable. The mucous membranes essentially resemble the skin in function, but they differ greatly in one respect. The cuticular covering of the skin impedes the absorption of substances from without, whilst the mucous membrane of the intestinal canal has the important office of absorbing all substances possessed of the necessary degree of tenuity. It is an absorbing, as well as an exhaling, membrane. It is probable, that where a bowel affection results from exposure to cold, in the mode just mentioned, the excited action of the exhalants is caused by the lining membrane of the intestines sympathizing with the irregular action of the cutaneous capillaries, so that the membrane is not in a simple state of healthy exhalation, occasioned by the *driving in* of the cutaneous transpiration, but actually labours under inflammatory excitement or irritation,—for such is always present, to a greater or less extent, in these cases, produced in the same manner as where a distant organ becomes irritated, in consequence of an irregular action of the capillaries of the feet, as in the case assumed above.

It need scarcely be remarked, that these effects, as well as all those that are produced by atmospheric vicissitudes, affect the feeble, the convalescent, and those debilitated, and irritated by previous evacuations, or disorders, more than the healthy.

During the winter season we frequently pass from a heated atmosphere, at 80° or upwards, to one of 32°, on leaving a crowded apartment, and often without adopting the necessary protections against cold; and many a lovely victim has recorded the danger of such a transition to the delicate; yet it is surprising that the mischief is not even more extensive. There seems to be much less danger, in these cases, from passing into the open air, whilst the system is strongly heated, than after we have waited, as is the common practice, until we have become cool. Whilst the skin is hot, and dry, the whole capillary system is in a state of activity, and if we pass into the cold, whilst this activity exists, we are better able to resist its depressing effects, and, accordingly, every one must have noticed, that he has suffered less from cold under such circumstances, than when he has waited until the organs of calorification have begun to act with less energy. The experiments of M. Edwards (*Op. citat.* p. 125,) show how those, who are liable to frequent exposure to severe cold, are rendered more capable of bearing it, by subjecting themselves, in the intervals, to a high temperature,— the effects of which are continued beyond the time of its application. Let it be borne in mind, however, that the above observations do not apply to that state in which the activity of the vessels has begun to subside in consequence of perspiration, which is a cooling process, having been established. In such case, the heat is undergoing resolution, and if we then expose ourselves to cold,—owing to that cause, as well as to the irregular capillary action, apt to be excited by cold and dampness,—we have disease induced, much in the same way as when the feet are exposed to cold and moisture. The morbid condition is not, however, excited by the check given to the sensible perspiration, but is owing to irregular local action of capillaries, which, as has been already said, is one of the most common causes of morbid conditions of the various structures.

That the sudden application of cold, when the body is highly excited, is not of itself likely to produce disease, provided the application be general, is proved by the effects of the Russian vapour bath. Of this Dr. Traill, of Edinburgh, has given a description from personal observation, and experience. On one occasion, Dr. Traill observed the temperature of the room, and noticed the effect of the heated vapour on the pulses of himself, and of two other bathers. The heat is generally from 133° to 144° of Fahrenheit. On the occasion alluded to by Dr. Traill, it ranged in the bath during his stay from 126° to 135°; but this temperature is far short of that, mentioned by Acerbi, to which the Finnish baths are elevated, (158° and 167°) of Fahrenheit. The effect of the bath is to accelerate the pulse, but the degree of this acceleration differs in different individuals, according to their excitability. The pulse soon regains its natural standard after leaving the bath, and, when Dr. Traill took it in a highly feverish state, he was, within an hour after, entirely free from fever. "On bathing a second time," says Dr. Traill, "I was accompanied by the same two friends: our pulses were about seventy-four in a minute. On just coming out of the bath, Dr. Traill's pulse was 116, Mr. Johnson's 88, Mr. Palk's 88. A quarter of an hour afterwards, while on the couch, they were as follows: Dr. Traill's 114, Mr. Johnson's 88, Mr. Palk's 88. After being dressed, and sitting in an adjoining coffee-room, perhaps one hour after the bath, Dr. Traill's beat 88, Mr. Johnson's 88, Mr. Palk's 80."

Whilst exposed to the great heat above mentioned, a powerful affusion of cold water is made upon the naked bodies of the bathers from a shower bath in the ceiling, and this is said to be remarkably grateful. "It is, indeed," says Dr. Traill, "scarcely possible to describe the effect, which is highly exhilarating and refreshing." Acerbi mentions, that some of the harness of his carriage having given way in the neighbourhood of one of the Finnish baths, the bathers ran out, although the ground was covered with snow, and, after having afforded them the necessary assistance, returned to their luxurious enjoyment.

But, although vicissitudes from heat to cold are generally regarded as most frequent sources of disease, they cannot take place from cold to heat with perfect impunity. In certain cases, indeed, we observe the most disastrous effects produced;—on exposing a frozen limb, for example, to the fire. In such case, the limb is in a state of suspended animation; the vessels are no longer pervious to blood; the nervous energy in the part is in a state of torpidity; and, if the limb be exposed to external heat, the vessels, continuous with the obstructed capillaries, have their action excited; inflammation results at their living extremities, and the congelation becomes converted into irrecoverable mortification.

" Wo to the man," says Larrey, (*Op. cit.*) in his description of the unfortunate campaign to which allusion has been made, " benumbed by cold; whose animal functions were nearly annihilated, and whose external sensibility especially was extinct, if he suddenly entered too warm a chamber, or approached too close to the large fires of the bivouac. The more prominent parts, benumbed, or frozen, and at a distance from the centre of the circulation, were struck with gangrene, which supervened on the instant, and developed itself with such rapidity, that its progress was sensible to the eye;—or, the individual was instantaneously suffocated by a kind of turgescence, which appeared to attack the pulmonary and cerebral systems. He perished as by asphyxia. In this way died the *Pharmacien-en-chef* of the guard, M. Sureau. He had arrived at Kowno without accident, except that his strength was diminished through cold and hunger. An asylum was offered him in a very warm room in the *pharmacie* of the hospital. He had not been many hours, however, in this new atmosphere, before his limbs, which had lost all sensation, became tumefied and puffy, and soon afterwards he expired in the arms of his son, and of one of his colleagues, without the power of utterance. Individuals were often noticed to fall stiff dead into the fires of the bivouac; and every one, who approached near enough to heat his frozen hands and feet, was struck with gangrene, wherever the cold had annihilated the vital properties."

The prevention of such effects is obvious. It is to avoid all external warmth, until sensibility and circulation have been somewhat restored in the frozen parts, by friction with substances, the temperature of which is little, if at all, elevated beyond that of the parts themselves; and, where the individual has been long exposed to a depressed temperature, not to take him too hastily into a warmer. When the effect of depressed temperature upon the extremities is to a less extent, diminishing merely the calibre of the vessels, and they are exposed, under such circumstances, to the heat of the fire, increased action takes place in the unaffected extremities of the blood vessels that are continuous with the affected capillaries; blood is forced into them in undue quantity so as to over-distend them, and inflammation results, constituting the affection known by the name of *chilblains.*

It need scarcely be added, that a sudden and rapid change from cold to heat may develope irritations, and inflammations in various structures, according to their predisposition, at the time, to be morbidly affected; and that hemorrhages and other affections, occasioned by heat, and by diminished atmospheric pressure, might be the result in such cases.

When the air from being dry becomes moist, affections are apt to be developed, which are the product of moist air; and these, it will be recollected, differ according as the moisture is accompanied with elevation, or depression of temperature. No inconveniences result from a sudden vicissitude from a moist to a dry air, so far as mere moisture is concerned. It has been already shown, that at high elevations much inconvenience is experienced from this cause; but in such case the dryness is extreme, and there are deranging influences of a barometric and thermometric kind operating at the same time. The remark is applicable only to the ordinary vicissitudes from moisture to dryness, which are experienced in any given locality.

It must not be presumed, that these vicissitudes in the physical characters of the air, when within the bounds of moderation, are detrimental to man. Without the changes effected by the seasons, animals would be deprived of the support they derive from the vegetable kingdom; and it is probable, that if we lived in the state of perpetual spring, which has been imagined by poets as best adapted for animal existence and comfort, our enjoyments would be much less than they are at present. How unvaried would seem the succession of day after day! How devoid should we be of that buoyancy, and elasticity, which we experience when the moisture of a foggy morning is dispelled by the rays of the sun, and all is life and gaiety!

It may be said, indeed, that we should experience none of the langour and lassitude, which a heavy, louring, atmosphere induces. This is true;—but all our pleasures are relative, and the same intensity of comfort could not exist, if all were sameness. We should become lazy and listless; worn out with *ennui,* or depressed with melancholy; and as the stimulus would be wanting, which the constant mutation of the physical agents around us is perpetually applying to the frame, so as to maintain its various functions in energetic activity, we might probably be liable to more derangements than affect us at present, under all our atmospheric vicissitudes. These very mutations have indeed been regarded by one of the most distinguished of British philosophers, Sir Humphry Davy, as a cause of the mental activity, which he considers to characterize his countrymen. "Of all the climates of Europe," he remarks in his "*Consolations of Travel,*" "England seems to me most fitted for the activity of the mind, and the least suited to repose. The alterations of a climate so various and rapid continually awake new sensations; and the changes in the sky, from dryness to moisture, from the blue ethereal to cloudiness and fogs, seem to keep the nervous system in a constant state of excitement. In the changeful and tumultuous atmosphere of England to be tranquil is a labour, and employment is necessary to ward off the attacks of ennui. The English nation is pre-eminently active, and the natives of no other country follow their objects with so much force, fire, and constancy."

The vicissitudes of the temperate regions of the globe are so numerous, and often so unexpected, that it is impossible for us to guard well against their injurious effects. Some persons endeavour, as they say, to fortify their children from early infancy, so that they may resist them, or be less affected by them than others with whom the same plan has not been pursued. It need scarcely be said, that all undue clothing, and residence in heated apartments without change, must be liable to the objections we have urged against an unvaried condition of the physical influences around us; but at the same time it is not every infant that will bear the plans, which are employed by some parents to harden them;—such as bathing every morning in cold water; exposure to the air at all temperatures; light clothing—even when the air is cold, &c. Many an infant has fallen a victim to this dogged persistence in error. Two fifths, at least, of mankind die of acute diseases, and a large majority of these are induced by exposure to cold. If, however, the infant be habituated to daily tepid bathing, and ablution, for a time, and the temperature of the fluid be gradually depressed, until cold water alone is used; and if it be comfortably clothed with flannel next the skin, and be sent into the fresh air, whenever the weather is serene, even if the temperature should be somewhat depressed, it may be accustomed to exposure as far as is prudent, and better adapted for bearing with impunity the vicissitudes of the weather, than where it is immured under the circumstances just mentioned.

Similar remarks apply to the adult, who can expose himself to cold air with impunity under ordinary precautions, provided he does not accustom himself to dwell in too heated apartments. But we shall have occasion to recur to this subject under another head.

Independently of the qualities of the air, which have engaged attention, a marked influence on the animal economy is exerted by different fluids of which it is the vehicle. Light is one of these, which is a healthful stimulant to the skin, as it is a special stimulant to the organ of vision. This stimulation is not felt under ordinary circumstances, but when we leave an obscure place to enter into the bright glare of day, when the brain is affected with any febrile, or insane delirium, or the eye with inflammatory excitement, it is strikingly manifested. Plants, deprived of light, become white, blanched, or *etiolated*—as it has been termed—and they acquire, at the same time, an excess of aqueous, and saccharine particles. This is shown in the common practice of blanching celery. Captain Parry found, that the cress he raised during the polar winter was devoid of its usual colour; and common plants, which have vegetated in mines, or in excavations deprived of the solar light, have been so changed as to be scarcely recognizable.

This kind of *etiolation* is observed also in man, especially in such as pass their lives in dark places, as in mines. The inhabitants of a crowded city may, in this way, be distinguished from those of the country. "When a gardener," says a recent writer on this subject, (Dr. James Johnson, " *Change of Air*", p. 8, American edition,) " wishes to etiolate, that is to blanch, soften, and render juicy a vegetable, as lettuce, celery, &c. he binds the leaves together, so that the light may have as little access as possible to their surfaces. In like manner, if we wish to etiolate men and women, we have only to congregate them in cities, where they are pretty securely kept out of the sun, and where they become as white, tender, and watery as the finest celery. For the more exquisite specimens of this human etiolation, we must survey the inhabitants of mines, dungeons, and other subterraneous abodes—and for complete contrasts to these, we have only to examine the complexions of stage-coachmen, shepherds, and the sailor 'on the high and giddy mast.'"

It is not improbable that the privation of direct solar light—as in the gorges of mountains, or in deep dells—may diminish the excitability of the frame so much, as to render them salutary retreats for certain classes of valetudinarians; and we may thus, perhaps, explain the diminution in the frequency of the pulse, which is said to have been found to occur in such situations, and which is often referred to other influences.

In the infancy of anthropology it was affirmed, that the great diversity of colour in the different races of mankind is mainly ascribable to the difference in the intensity of the solar rays;—and, that the sun is capable, within certain limits, of modifying the colour, is indisputable. The difference between one, who has been for some time exposed to a tropical sun, and his brethren of the more temperate climes, is a matter of universal observation. It is asserted, too, that the southern Asiatic women of the Arab race, when confined within the walls of the seraglio, are as white as the fairest Europeans. There are, many exceptions, however, to the notion which has prevailed, that there is an exact ratio between the heat of the climate and the blackness of the skin; and Tourtelle, Londe, and others err greatly, when they state, that the negro race is not found beyond the limits of the torrid zone. (See the Author's *Human Physiology*, 5th edit. ii. 598, Philad. 1844.) On our own continent, none have ever been met with, except what have been imported; and these, after repeated descents, have still retained their original character; but negroes have been found in Australia, under a climate as cold as that of Washington. Were we, however, to admit this effect of climate, it would seem, that the coloration ought rather to be ascribed to a chemical effect of the calorific, than of the luminous rays of the sun.

The experiments of Edwards (*Op. citat.* p. 211,) exhibit that light is necessary for the full development of many animals, and it is probable that its privation may give occasion, with other causes, to the deviations in form observed in children in confined, and dark situations. This applies especially to those in large manufacturing establishments, who are often misshapen, and unhealthy. When the subject was brought before the British parliament some years ago, by Sir Robert Peel, Mr. Owen, of New Lanark, stated, that although the children employed in his manufactory were extremely well fed, clothed, and lodged; looked fresh, and to a superficial observer were healthy, yet their limbs were generally deformed; their growth stunted, and they were incapable of making much progress in the first rudiments of education. The extensive experience of Mr. Owen corresponds with that of numerous other observant individuals, and was corroborated by Sir Astley Cooper on the same inquiry,—who stated, that the result of confinement is not only to stunt the growth, but to produce deformity. How striking indeed is the contrast between the pale, deformed being, brought up in this manner, and the ruddy native of country situations, who is accustomed to spend the greater part of his time in the open air, and to take adequate exercise; and how rare is it for us to meet with deformities under the latter circumstances!

It is proper, however, to remark that, of late, many distinguished individuals have maintained that these evils are dependent rather upon *town* than upon *factory* influence; upon *domestic* rather than upon *industrial* relations; and have maintained, that no peculiar evils to health and life attach necessarily to manufacturing pursuits (Dr. A. Ure, *Philosophy of Manufactures*, Lond. 1835; and *British and Foreign Medical Review*, April 1843.) Hereafter, the lethiferous agency of ill-conditioned localities and occupations in large towns will be strikingly illustrated.

Privation of light disposes to rest and inactivity, hence the necessity of keeping animals, which we are desirous of fattening, excluded from its stimulation;—quietness, and the absence of all excitement preventing the loss by exhalation, which would otherwise take place, and disposing to obesity. To completely exclude the light in these cases, the ancients not only kept their fowls in dark places, but barbarously stitched up the eyes.

In occupations, in which intense or continued light is made to fall on the eye, as in engraving, watchmaking, &c. mischief is done to the organ by the over excitation, and hence such artisans are liable to amaurosis, cataract, &c.

The electrical condition of the atmosphere and of the animal body has, been considered by many writers, to be intimately connected with animal health; and certainly the feelings are, at times, much affected by this circumstance.

Death even results, if we are so situate as to be connected with the discharge from a sufficiently charged electrical cloud. Many persons, too, exhibit a manifest difference in the performance of their functions when the air is highly electric, and are apt to suffer considerably from headachs, and from pains of various kinds to which they may be subject.

This is not the place to treat of the general laws and phenomena of the electric fluid, the consideration of which belongs to works on physics—in its more restricted signification. We may remark, however, that it is probable all living bodies develope electricity, although it may be to a less degree than we witness in certain inorganic substances. We find, at least, in them all the conditions, which in inorganic bodies are accompanied by electrical phenomena;—such as the evaporation of liquids; changes in the state of aggregation; and alterations of composition—as in the acts of assimilation, respiration, nutrition, and secretion. Different experiments on living bodies likewise favour this conjecture. M. Pouillet asserts, that he observed a disengagement of electricity during the germination of plants; and he presumes, that plants develope electricity when they exhale carbonic acid; as this gas gives indications of electricity at the moment of its formation. The action of vegetables upon the air is, indeed, in his opinion, one of the principal sources of atmospheric electricity.

In living animals, we have the very best evidences, derived from experiment, of the disengagement of "*electricity by contact,*" or "*galvanic*" or "*animal electricity.*" When nerves and muscles, previously exposed, are brought into contact, contractions or convulsions immediately occur in the muscles. This was first observed by Galvani, and the experiment has been repeated by numerous, and trusty observers. Aldini asserts, that he not only observed convulsions produced by the muscles and nerves of the same frog when brought into contact, but when the nerves of one frog were made to touch the muscles of another; and even when he connected the nerves of a frog with the muscular flesh on the neck of a recently killed ox. These experiments—and the cases of the different electrical animals might be also adduced—show, that a constant development of electricity is going on within the human frame, which may be variously modified by the condition of the atmospheric electricity. If the air be very dry and insulating, whilst the clouds are high, and at a great distance from the earth, all electrical communication between the earth, the living bodies attached to it, and the clouds is intercepted, and no electrical phenomena are manifested. Under such circumstances, partly owing perhaps to these electrical conditions, and partly also to the favourable barometric, thermometric, and hygrometric conditions, the individual feels full of energy and elasticity. On the other hand, if the air be charged with moisture, it becomes a good conductor of electricity, and there is a more free communication between the earth and the clouds. If the communication be immediate, or very extensive, the equilibrium of electricity takes place insensibly, and without any apparent phenomena, except that a degree of languor and lassitude is experienced unconnected with muscular action or disease. If, again, the communication be not sufficiently complete, or not sufficiently extensive proportionally to the electric charge in the clouds, the equilibrium is established by violent explosions, which give occasion to thunder, and lightning; and if an animal be situate in the line of passage of the electric fluid, it may experience such a shock as will destroy it.

Independently of the electricity, which is communicated by conduction, bodies are affected by induction, in such manner that if a cloud, highly charged with electricity, approaches the earth within the requisite distance, the earth becomes charged with opposite electricity; and as the animal body is affected by electricity in a manner analogous to other material objects, it participates in the condition of the earth, and it is in this way that much of the uneasiness, ascribed to electricity, is produced in those, who are particularly liable to be affected when the air is sultry, and thunderous.

We have said, that if a person be situate in the line of passage of the electric fluid, during a thunder storm, he may be instantaneously killed. It does not follow, however, that he must be in the line of passage from the cloud to the earth. If the cloud, which is discharging its electricity, be very extensive, a large surface of the earth is imbued with the opposite electricity, and it will occasionally happen, that a *return shock* will take place, at the extremity of the cloud farthest distant from that which is discharging its electricity to the earth. In other words, at one extremity, the cloud may be discharging itself to the earth, and at the other the earth may be giving off its electricity to the cloud; and, if the animal body be situate in either of these lines of passage, its vitality may be extinguished.

It is not improbable but that the varying conditions of the atmosphere, as regards its electricity, may, in conjunction with the other states that have been considered, be connected with the prevalence of particular diseases, which affect districts of country during certain years, and seasons, and not during others. We shall see hereafter, however, that our knowledge of epidemic diseases, or of those which, in the present state of science, we refer to modifications of the " constitutio aeris," is extremely limited. Dr. Foster, —who, in his various essays on atmospheric phenomena, has much that is interesting and logical, with much that is fanciful,—is of opinion, " that it is not the heat, nor cold, nor dampness, nor drought of the air, which is chiefly concerned in producing disorders, nor the sudden transitions from one to another of those states: but that it is some inexplicable peculiarity in its electric state." The pain, felt in limbs which have been formerly broken, previous to a change of weather, and the disturbed state of the stomach of many persons, before and during thunder-storms, are sufficient, he thinks, to warrant such a conjecture. It may be so; but we do not see why the diminished pressure of the air, in these cases, with its altered hygrometric condition, might not explain the indispositions to which he alludes, as well as those other pains, and aches, which are proverbial, as indicating some change of the weather, when the air has been previously dry, and dense;—such as rheumatic pains, toothache, shooting and tenderness of corns, &c.

A recent writer (Dr. James Johnson, *Treatise on derangement of the liver*, &c. Amer. edit p. 198)—too exclusively, we think—refers the uneasy feelings, occasionally experienced on the approach of a storm, to barometric changes. " On many constitutions," he observes, " and particularly on people denominated *nervous*, certain barometrical changes in the atmosphere have a remarkable effect. Thus, when the glass is very low, the wind southerly, and a storm impending, such a sense of sinking, weakness, tremor and dejection is often felt by valetudinarians, that they are quite miserable till the equilibrium of the atmosphere is restored, when all their morbid feelings vanish into air, thin air.' "

Man furnishes fewer prognostics of atmospheric changes than animals, and we can scarcely refer their habits, under such circumstances, to mere electrical differences in the atmosphere. When the swallow, for example, which, in all ages, has been regarded as a weather guide, flies low, and skims backward and forward over the surface of the earth and the waters, prior to falling weather, it is probable that the altered density of the aerial regions, in which it is accustomed to fly, renders its progress less ready, and agreeable, or, at all events, different, and accordingly it seeks the lower and denser strata. But, howsoever we may account for the circumstance, and difficult, nay impracticable, as it may be to explain it in most cases, it seems certain, that animals, even many of the very lowest tribes, can appreciate differences in the condition of the atmosphere, which make little or no impression upon the frame of man.

## SECTION III.

Changes in the air by respiration—black hole at Calcutta—black assize of Oxford, &c.—effects of carbonic acid gas—carburetted hydrogen—sulphuretted hydrogen—animal and vegetable exhalations—endemic, epidemic, and other influences—malaria—its nature not known—does not arise from vegetable putrefaction singly—nor from animal putrefaction singly—nor from aqueous decomposition singly—nor from all these combined—conflicting opinions upon the subject—nature of the emanations, that cause other endemic diseases, likewise unknown—our ignorance of the origin of epidemic, and contagious diseases.

We have yet to speak of various admixtures to which the air is liable, and which modify materially its action upon the animal economy, as well as of different chemical changes, that may be effected in it by natural agencies.

It has been already remarked, that the essential constituents of atmospheric air are *oxygen* and *azote*, in the proportion of one part of the former to four of the latter; and that, in addition, carbonic acid is always contained in it. The proportions of oxygen and azote have been found the same, wherever the air has been taken; and this uniformity has led to the conclusion, that as there are many processes, which consume the oxygen, there must be some natural agency, by which a quantity of oxygen is produced equal to that consumed. The only source, however, by which oxygen is known to be supplied is the process of vegetation. A healthy plant absorbs carbonic acid under the influence of light, appropriates the carbon to its necessities, and gives off the oxygen with which it was combined: this is the process of nutrition. Throughout the twenty-four hours respiration is going on, by which oxygen is taken from the air, and carbonic acid given off. Experiments, however, show, that plants, in the twenty-four hours, yield more oxygen than they consume. It is difficult to look to this as the main cause of equilibrium between the oxygen and azote, as it would be more than compensated, in many cases, by the great consumption of oxygen, and formation of carbonic acid, during the respiration of animals. Its influence could, indeed, extend to a trifling distance only, yet the uniformity in the proportions of oxygen and azote in the air has been found to prevail in the most elevated regions, and in countries, whose arid sands never admit of vegetation.

The gas which is most essential to respiration, is oxygen,—hence called *vital air:* azote appears to be a simple diluent, proving fatal, when respired, *negatively*,—that is, by excluding oxygen; whilst carbonic acid singly is completely irrespirable, killing more speedily than azote, and apparently by exciting spasmodic contraction of the glottis, and suffocation. Sir Humphry Davy found that air was still irrespirable, when it contained three-fifths of its volume of carbonic acid.

In the respiration of animals the oxygen largely disappears, and carbonic acid, of pretty nearly equal volume, takes its place; in other words, the vital portion of the air is abstracted, and an equal volume of air, which is altogether irrespirable, is added to the azote. We can hence readily understand why, if an animal be confined in a small portion of atmospheric air, it can exist so long as there is oxygen enough to support it, and so long as the deadly agencies of the carbonic acid and azote are not powerful enough to destroy. The bad effects of confined air might, therefore, be mainly, if not wholly, ascribed to the presence of an undue quantity of carbonic acid, and of uncombined azote, left after the disappearance of the oxygen. Such is one view of the matter; but those physiologists, who believe, that the air is taken into the pulmonary vessels and that its oxygen disappears in the course of circulation, whilst carbonic acid is formed in the system, and merely given off at the lungs,—a view, which, as has been elsewhere shown, (*Human Physiology*, 5th edit. ii. 53, Philad. 1844,) is the most philosophical— would ascribe the phenomena mainly to the deleterious agency of the carbonic acid, and in a slight degree to the azote, which appears to be exhaled from the lungs.

The physiologist has not unfrequently observed the effects produced on animals by restricting them to a confined space, and watching the phenomena of death as they gradually supervened. Instances, too, have ocasionally occurred where man himself has expired from this cause, as in a diving bell, when the air could not be renewed; but the most melancholy example was witnessed in the, since celebrated, Black Hole at Calcutta—a place of confinement 18 feet by 18, or containing 324 square feet, in which one hundred and forty-six persons were shut up, when Fort William was taken, in 1756, by Surajah Dowla, Nabob of Bengal. The room allowed to each person a space of $26\frac{1}{2}$ inches by 12 inches, which was just sufficient to hold them without pressing violently on each other. To this dungeon there was but one small grated window, and the weather being very sultry, the air within could neither circulate nor be changed. In less than an hour, many of the prisoners were attacked with extreme difficulty of breathing; several were delirious, and the place was filled with incoherent ravings, in which the cry for water was predominant. This was handed to them by the sentinels, but without the effect of allaying their thirst. In less than four hours many were suffocated, or died in violent delirium. In an hour more, the survivors, except those at the grate, were frantic, and outrageous. At length, most of them became insensible; and, eleven hours from the time they were imprisoned, of the one hundred and forty-six that entered, twenty-three only came out alive, and these were in a "highly putrid fever," from which, however, by fresh air, and proper attention they gradually recovered. A similar instance happened in London, in 1742. Twenty persons were forced into a part of Saint Martin's round-house, called *the hole*, during the night, and several died.

The carbonic acid gas, given off during respiration, is heavier than atmospheric air, and, consequently, accumulates near the ground, where ventilation is impracticable, and it can thus be understood, that where the only aperture into the chamber is by the roof, or by a window high above the ground, the lower strata of the air may become irrespirable for some time before the upper. How horrible must have been the condition of the wretched negroes in the slave ships, when that infamous traffic was in full vigour—would to God we could say, that it no longer exists!—and how easy to anticipate the dreadful mortality that befel them, especially when crossing the hot, and still seas, in what have been called the *Horse latitudes!*

Jail fevers, hospital fevers, camp fevers, owe their origin to the deteriorated air of these places;—deteriorated by the formation of carbonic acid gas, with the various animal exhalations and excretions, with which the neighbourhood of the body must be necessarily imbued, where thorough ventilation is impracticable. The *Black Assize* of Oxford, in July 1577, exhibits the concentrated character of these pestiferous emanations as strongly as any fact in history. It received its name from the great mortality produced in court by the effluvia from a prisoner brought to the bar after having been for some time confined in a small dungeon. On one side of the culprit was an open window, and almost all the judges, counsel, jury, and others, who were placed to the lee of the prisoner, were attacked with putrid fever, and many died. At Exeter, in 1586, and at Taunton, in 1730, from similar causes the same thing occurred; and, in 1750, the contagious jail fever, introduced into the court, destroyed two judges, the Lord Mayor, and several of the spectators.

Carbonic acid gas accumulates wherever combustion is going on; but it is the accumulation from brasiers of charcoal, where ventilation is impeded, that has been most deleterious. Many individuals have perished during the night from this cause, and it was the method adopted by the younger Berthollet to rid himself of a disagreeable existence, in which he succeeded. In crowded apartments, artificially heated and well lighted, inconvenience,—hurried respiration, and circulation, giddiness, &c.—are not unfrequently experienced from the presence of the gas. The lights burn dimly; the healthy and the strong feel oppressed, whilst the more feeble and delicate swoon; but owing to the facility with which the air of our apartments is changed, it cannot often happen that it is so much deteriorated as to occasion fatal results, or even serious inconvenience. Yet, as has been suggested by Dr. Hodgkin, (*Lectures on the means of promoting and preserving health*, Lond. 1835) the constant and frequent application of the cause cannot fail to produce injurious effects, and it is not improbable, that the unhealthy appearance of the poor who have large families crowded together in small and ill-contrived chambers, and more especially the sickly state of their children, originate, in part in its agency. Carbonic acid is the fixed air, given off during the vinous fermentation; and in the large vats of the English porter brewers, sufficient of the gas is very often contained at the bottom to destroy those who venture down. It is usual to pass a lighted candle to the bottom, and if it continue to burn, the descent may be made with safety;—carbonic acid not supporting combustion. In like manner, it is met with in deep wells, and the same plan is adopted to discover, whether the air will allow of combustion, and respiration; but many a workman has fallen a victim to his want of attention to this precautionary measure. This gas also constitutes the *choke-damp* of the coal mines, in contra-distinction to the *fire-damp*, which consists of carburetted hydrogen. Carbonic acid is likewise extricated in lime-kilns, by the agency of heat, which drives it off from the limestone or carbonate of lime, and the public prints have detailed many cases in which life has been lost, owing to the poor benighted traveller having lain down to rest in the warm, but destructive, atmosphere around one of these furnaces.

Persons affected by this gas feel great heaviness, or pain in the head; singing in the ears; disposition to sleep; excessive loss of voluntary power; difficulty of breathing; palpitation, and suspension of respiration, and circulation. These are the symptoms when the gas is diluted so as to be respirable, but when concentrated it causes immediate suffocation.

Carburetted hydrogen, we have said, constitutes the *fire-damp*, formerly so fatal to miners by its extensive explosions; now, however, rendered not only comparatively harmless, but inservient to the advantage of the miner, by the important discovery of the *safety lamp* by Sir Humphry Davy,—one of the proudest gifts of science to humanity. When this gas is largely diluted with atmospheric air it occasions giddiness, and sickness, with diminished vascular, and nervous power. In an undiluted state it can scarcely be respired. It is not in this way, however, that its deleterious agency has been usually manifested. Even when mixed with atmospheric air, in such quantity as to admit of respiration, it is susceptible of ignition, and in its explosions has involved the lives of almost all exposed to it. The gas, which is used to light the streets, and shops of various towns, consists of carburetted hydrogen, and if care be not taken to shut it off carefully it may accumulate in a chamber in such quantity as to ignite on the approach of a lighted body. Such cases have occurred. There is not much danger, however, of its acting injuriously by respiration, as it can be detected by the olfactory organs long before it accumulates in the necessary quantity to produce mischief.

It has been frequently observed, that nightmen, on descending into the pits of privies, have been attacked with serious indisposition on breaking the crust, and not a few have perished;—suddenly seized as if a weight held them down, and dying in convulsions. The experiments of Thénard and Dupuytren first showed the deleterious gas, in this case, to be *sulphuretted hydrogen,*—ammoniacal gas never being in quantity sufficient to produce much mischief, and at the farthest exciting a pungent uneasiness in the eyes, nose, and throat, with occasional inflammation of those parts.

Sulphuretted hydrogen is an extremely deleterious gas, killing instantly when respired in a pure state, and it is so powerfully penetrant that it is sufficient to place an animal in a bag containing the gas, without any approaching the mouth, for it to act fatally. Even when mixed with a considerable portion of air it may prove destructive. Dr. Paris refers to the case of a chemist of his acquaintance who was suddenly deprived of sense, as he stood over a pneumatic trough in which he was collecting the gas; and from the experiments of Thénard and Dupuytren it would seem, that air containing a thousandth part kills birds immediately. A dog perished in air containing $\frac{1}{100}$ part, and a horse in air containing $\frac{1}{150}$th. When breathed in a more diluted state, it produces powerfully sedative effects, the pulse being rendered extremely small and weak; the contractility of the muscular organs considerably enfeebled, with stupor, and more or less suspension of the cerebral functions; and if the person recover, he gains his strength very tardily. Fortunately, we possess, in chlorine and the chlorinated preparations, agents capable of acting chemically on this substance, and of completely removing all deleterious agency. There is, consequently, no reason why injurious consequences should result from the requisite operation of emptying privies, which is an extensive business in many large towns, especially in such as are not well provided with water, and common sewers.

The air is apt, also, to be loaded with *emanations* from animal and vegetable substances in a state of decomposition; and there are many trades—as those of the gutspinner, the hartshorn manufacturer, the dealer in cat's and dog's meat, technically called a *knacker*—which are carried on in putridity; but we shall endeavour to show, that the admixture of such emanations with the air does not affect public salubrity to such an extent as might be imagined, although the nervous, and the delicate, before they become accustomed to the offensive odours, may be more or less disagreeably impressed. The same may be said of butcheries, dissecting rooms, and cemeteries.

All these, unpleasant odours, it may be remarked, are equally destroyed by chlorine and the chlorinated preparations, for the employment of which, as disinfecting agents, we are indebted to M. Labarraque—a skilful pharmacien of Paris—who gained a prize, offered by the *Society for the encouragement of National Industry, of Paris*, about twenty years ago, for any process, that could render the manufacture of catguts less offensive.

In many occupations, too, the air is apt to be vitiated by mineral emanations, and in others, minute particles—animal, vegetable, or mineral—are mixed with it, enter the lungs, and occasion the peculiar effects of those substances on the system, or irritate the lungs in a chemical, or mechanical manner,—but the consideration of their effects on health will fall more properly under another head.

We have yet to consider those conditions of the air,—totally inappreciable by eudiometric researches,—which give occasion to epidemic, endemic, and contagious diseases, and on which, unfortunately, the information we possess does not enable us to pronounce very definitely. We have many facts, however, which manifest how little we do know of the matter; and, next perhaps in importance to positive knowledge, is the being enabled to feel the want of certain information, which we are compelled to experience on so many topics. If the philosophic inquirer will cast his eyes over the multitude of "facts," as they have been called, which have descended from one generation and individual to another without examination, he will be astonished at the number that rest upon no certain basis, and one of the greatest gifts, that could be offered to science, would be the careful separation of the established from the uncertain,—the true from the false,—the grain from the chaff, instead of the perpetual straining after insignificant originality, which so much characterises the efforts, and the publications of the present period in the various departments of science.

The medical profession generally have adopted three terms to express their leading ideas of the causes of diseases that affect large portions of a community, and are manifestly connected with the air or locality. Those causes, which seem to be seated wholly in the atmosphere—in the "constitutio aeris"—and affect a more or less considerable extent of country, unconnected apparently with locality, are said to be *epidemic;* those that are connected with locality only, are called *endemic;* and such as are produced by some emanation from an individual labouring under a similar disease are said to be *contagious*:—the diseases resulting from those causes being termed, respectively—*epidemic, endemic,* and *contagious.*

It will be obvious, that these causes may not act singly in all cases; but may be, and frequently are, combined: for instance, there may be some condition of the locality, connected with a favouring state of the atmosphere, which may occasion one place to be insalubrious, whilst others, in the immediate vicinity, are entirely healthy. Of this, malignant cholera affords a striking example, which attacked several of the towns of the United States, and elsewhere, in the most virulent manner; whilst others, and some of these, to all appearance, similarly circumstanced, wholly escaped. The locality, which seemed to favour its visitation, was the confined air of towns, and these towns situate on the seas or rivers. On this continent, Quebec, Montreal, Albany, New York, Philadelphia, Baltimore, Washington, Richmond, Cincinnati, New Orleans, &c. suffered largely; yet Fredericksburg on the Rappahannock, and Lynchburg on the James,—and similar instances of immunity in other States might be adduced,—had scarcely a case. This complaint, then, required a combination of local and atmospheric causes to induce it; in other words, the causes were of an *endemico-epidemic* character. Perhaps, the requisite union of local and atmospheric causes may never again meet in those places, and the scourge may not reappear.

We frequently see the most salubrious districts desolated by malignant fever, by a complaint, perhaps not previously known there, and possibly destined never again to return, because the precise endemico-epidemic influence may be wanting. The University of Virginia is situate in a district of country, which is proverbially healthy, and the Institution is admirably planned for thorough ventilation; yet, in the winter and spring of 1829, a malignant typhoid affection appeared there, continued for two or three months, and disappeared, without leaving the slighest trace of its existence; and, what is singular, scarcely a case occurred without the precincts,—the town of Charlottesville, not more than a mile distant, being, during the whole period, perfectly healthy.

The beautiful, and elevated coast of Long Island, in the neighbourhood of the Narrows, which enjoys the constant and invigorating sea-breeze, in the summer and autumn of 1828, was so subject to intermittent, and remittent fever, that few families or members of a family escaped; yet scarcely a case of intermittent had occurred in that salubrious region for upwards of forty years previously. The combination of atmospheric and local causes, necessary for producing these diseases, somewhat resembles that required in certain complex locks, where two numbers, out of a great many must come together before the lock can be opened. In all other conjunctions, it remains secure.

Again:—there may be a constitution of the atmosphere favourable for the extension of a disease which is unquestionably contagious, or the causes of the extensive spread of such disease may be of an *epidemico-contagious* character. Small-pox is contagious. It is rarely produced in any other manner than by an emanation from one labouring under it: yet, prior to the introduction of inoculation, it was not always committing its ravages in the same locality, but visited it after the lapse perhaps of years; and accordingly it was an objection, strongly-urged against the practice of inoculation, that it was the means of keeping the contagion always present, so that more persons actually died of small-pox, after the introduction of inoculation, than before, although the mortality from the disease, in those who were inoculated, was amazingly diminished.

In all cases of endemic, epidemic, or contagious diseases, and in all combinations of these, there must be some modification of the atmospheric condition; but such modification has, in every instance, escaped the researches of the chemist. Julia, a writer on marshy miasmata, affirms, that he sixty times subjected to examination the air of the marshes of Cercle, near Narbonne; of the pond of Pudre, near Sigéan; of Salces and Salanque, in Roussillon; of Capestang, not far from Béziers, and of the different marshes on the coast of Cette; yet in all cases he found only the same constituent principles as are contained in the purest atmospheric air. Séguin, again, examined the infectious air of an hospital, the odour of which was intolerable, yet he could discover no appreciable deficiency of oxygen, or other peculiarity of composition; and Professor Woodhouse, of the University of Pennsylvania, on examining the air from the gallery of a crowded theatre, was not more successful. These failures, however, do no more than indicate the imperfect condition of chemical analysis: that certain agents are there is sufficiently shown by their effects, and the day may yet arrive when we may be enabled to detect them.

It has been frequently affirmed as a general truth, that the great difference of one country from another, in point of salubrity, consists in the greater or less proportion of soil which exhales noxious effluvia. The comparative unhealthiness of most low, swampy situations is well known. We have too many instances in our own country, and in every part of it, for any one to be ignorant of this. The unhealthiness is assigned, and doubtless with truth, to some emanation, of the nature of which we are ignorant, that takes place from such soils, and to which the names *marsh poison*, *marshy miasm*, and, with the Italians, *malaria*, and *aria cattiva*, have been appropriated. It is the great exciting cause of endemic fever—intermittent and remittent—and if we are to credit recent writers of prolific imagination, of almost all diseases that exhibit a periodical character, or what has been termed periodicity. Dr. Macculloch enumerates fever, apoplexy, lethargy, coma, paralysis, epilepsy, hysteria, asthma, palpitation, mania, hypochondriasis, dyspepsia, nervous disorders, atrophy, hepatitis, rheumatism, dysentery, pellagra, goître, tic douloureux, and the whole tribe of neuralgic complaints.

But we meet with diseases, that are usually produced by marshy miasms, in particular districts far remote from marshes, and on elevated regions where it is impossible to conceive that any marshy miasms can exist. From recent statistical reports of the British army in every part of the globe it has been inferred, that although the vicinity of marshy or swampy ground appears to favour the development of malaria, it does not necessarily prevail in such localities, nor are they by any means essential either to its existence or operation. In many elevated parts of the Maremma district in Italy,—a tract reaching from Leghorn to Terracina, lying near the sea, and varying in breadth from thirty to forty miles,—intermittents and remittents prevail to a most destructive extent; and as these elevations are generally of volcanic formation, it has been inferred, that although malaria ordinarily escapes from marshes, it may be the product of volcanic soils also. This may be so; but it does not solve the question. It is, indeed, one involved in much obscurity, as will be seen presently, when we examine the hypotheses that have been entertained upon the subject. We see this malaria making its appearance in the vicinity of our towns, and in situations where it was previously unknown. We observe it, as in the case of the Narrows, encroaching upon parts of our coast where it had before rarely appeared, driving the inhabitants from their possessions, and spreading desolation and terror through districts previously esteemed salubrious. We observe it, also, dissipated by human ingenuity, yet capriciously returning to the same haunts after the lapse of years. The Island of Portsea, in England, on which Portsmouth is situate, was entirely freed, several years ago, from ague by draining; but, of late, there has been a return of the endemic, not only in the best drained places, but in localities where it had never been known within the memory of man. (See an article, by the author, in the *American Quarterly Review*, vol. viii. p. 392.) The causes of these changes are utterly inappreciable; but that they depend upon peculiar emanations from the locality, or are geological in their character, seems obvious. On the whole subject of endemic disease our real information is scanty; our false facts are numerous, and unhappily our theories erroneous, or too often unwarrantable. In the obscurity of the subject the speculatist has had ample space for hypothesis; and hence the various phantasies which have been indulged, not only regarding the causes that give rise to malarious emanations, but the precise character of malaria itself. One affirms it to be azote; another, carbonic acid; another, hydrogen; another, carburetted hydrogen; and a fifth sulphuretted hydrogen; the evidence being alike in all, and in all unsatisfactory. A flocculent organic matter is said to have been found in the air over malarious ground, but this has thrown no light on the subject.

Leaving, for the present, these suppositions, let us inquire into the causes that have been assigned for the production of those terrestrial emanations, which do unquestionably take place in marshy, and certain other districts, and to which the term *malaria* has been given;—an investigation, which will demonstrate how little is really known of the matter, and how erroneous are many of the positions, which, by those who have not given due attention to the subject, are looked upon as canonical.

By some writers on malaria, it has been ascribed to vegetable putrefaction; by others, to aqueous or to animal putrefaction, or to

## TERRESTRIAL EMANATIONS. 69

different combinations of these; but we shall attempt to show, that there is no positive—no historical evidence—that any one, or any combination, of these varieties of putrefaction does ever occasion, even in marshy districts where the poison exists in the greatest abundance, malarious or miasmatic disease.

In the *first* place, it may, we think, be laid down as incontrovertible,—that *we have no satisfactory proof, that malaria arises from vegetable putrefaction singly,*—by which term is meant the humid decay of vegetables.

The reasons, which probably led to the belief in its originating from vegetable decomposition, were—the universal prevalence of the vegetable kingdom, and the difficulty of discovering any other adequate cause. It was known, too, that when vegetables undergo decomposition, the air is frequently impregnated with disagreeable odours, and also that certain gases are exhaled under such circumstances, which, when respired singly, are unfavourable to animal existence. But that malaria must be something more than the mere product of vegetable decomposition is shown by numerous facts. It has been found in many cases most virulent, and abundant, on the driest surfaces: often where vegetation has *never*, apparently, existed nor could exist, as in the steep ravine of a dried water course. Dr. Ferguson, who had extensive experience in this matter during the war in Spain, as well as in many of the British West India Islands, and who is, withal, a philosophic observer,—bent upon the discovery of truth, and determined to discard error by whomsoever supported, but whose observations have been lightly regarded and misrepresented or misunderstood by those, who adhere to old opinions,—has given some striking instances, in a paper on *Marsh Poison*, read before the Royal Society of Edinburgh, in the year 1820. (See also, Boott's *Life of Armstrong*, vol. i. p. 555.)

The first time he observed any extensive " epidemic intermittent" in the army was in 1794, when, after a very hot and dry summer, the British troops, in the month of August, took up the encampments of Rosendaal and Oosterhout in South Holland. The soil, in both places, was a level plain of sand, with a perfectly dry surface, where no vegetation existed, nor could exist, but stunted heath plants. On digging, it was universally found to be percolated with water to within a few inches of the surface, which, so far from being putrid, was perfectly potable in all the wells of the camp.

Again, on their advance to Talavera, the British army had to march through a very dry country, and, in the hottest weather, fought that celebrated battle, which was followed by a retreat into the plains of Estremadura, along the course of the Guadiana river, at a time, when the country was so arid, for want of rain, that the Guadiana itself and all the smaller streams had, in fact, ceased to be streams, and were no more than lines of detached pools, in the courses that had formerly been rivers; yet the soldiers suffered from remittent fevers of such destructive malignity, that the enemy and all Europe believed the British host was extirpated. For the accuracy of this description, a recent writer (Dr. Brown, in *Cyclopædia of Practical Medicine*, Art. *Malaria and miasma*. Amer. edit. by the author, Philad. 1844) asserts, that he can vouch from personal observation; and he adds, "he has repeatedly observed, that cases of fever and ague abounded in parts of Estremadura, so remote from the Guadiana or any stream, that no influence from visible water or dampness could be supposed to have a share in their production."

Many similar topographical illustrations of Spain, of great interest, are adduced by Dr. Ferguson, from all of which he legitimately deduces,—that, in the most unhealthy parts of Spain, we may in vain, towards the close of summer, look for lakes, marshes, ditches, pools, or even vegetation; and that Spain, generally speaking, though as prolific of endemic fever as Walcheren, is beyond all doubt one of the driest countries in Europe, and it is not till it has again been made one of the wettest by the periodical rains, with its vegetation and aquatic weeds restored, that it can be called healthy, or even habitable with any degree of safety. In another part of his communication, Dr. Ferguson observes, that malaria is never found in savannahs or plains that have been flooded in the rainy season, till their surface has been thoroughly exsiccated, vegetation burnt up, and its putrefaction rendered as impossible as the putrefaction of an Egyptian mummy: and again, he states, that in the months of June, and July, the British army marched through the singularly dry, rocky, and elevated country on the confines of Portugal, the weather having been previously so hot, for several weeks, as to dry up the mountain streams. In some of the hilly ravines, that had lately been water-courses, several regiments took up their bivouac, for the sake of being near the stagnant pools of water that were still left among the rocks. Many men were seized with intermittent fever.

Can any thing demonstrate more clearly, that vegetable decomposition singly could not, in these instances, have produced fevers, notwithstanding, unequivocally *malarious*? Yet we are surprised to find one individual, (Eberle, *Treatise on the Practice of Medicine*, vol. i. p. 42,) who on almost all subjects exhibits unusual good sense,—remark, in alluding to the last of the examples quoted from Dr. Ferguson, that " half dried ravines, and stagnant pools of water are precisely the conditions most favourable to the emission of miasmata from vegetable, and animal decomposition." Can Dr. Eberle mean to affirm, that in the steep, rocky ravines, which had a short time previously been water courses, and which had become dry under the solar heat, and in the detached pools left in the course of these streams, sufficient vegetable matter could have existed to account for the malignant fevers observed there? The rocky beds exhibited at no time any vegetation: from whence then, except from the air,—as in the case of the conferva or river weed, which makes its appearance on water when exposed to the air,—could the vegetable matter have been obtained; and can we suppose for a moment, that it could exist, from this source, in quantity sufficient to produce, even when united with " animal decomposition"—the existence of which is equally supposititious—endemic fever?

The following remarks of Dr. Eberle will show how imperfectly he accounts for the cases—impregnable in our view—referred to by Dr. Ferguson. " It may be observed, that in every instance adduced by Dr. Ferguson in proof that the extrication of miasmata does not depend on the *humid* decay of vegetable, and animal matter, the soil from which the miasmata were emitted had been previously thoroughly saturated with water, during the rainy season, and moisture must, therefore, have existed in sufficient abundance a short distance under the *surface* of the soil, however parched the latter may have been. Under such circumstances, misamata might be abundantly sent forth, without any obvious humidity, and vegetable decomposition on the surface; for the vegetable and animal remains, collected during the rainy season, must have been gradually decomposed during the drying process, and left, in part at least, mingled with the portions of the soil on the surface. In this state, then, the slow evaporation of the humidity under the surface, in passing up into the air, would dissolve the putrid but dry particles of animal and vegetable remains, and convey them in the form of an effluvium into the circumambient atmosphere."

Dr. Eberle could scarcely design this as a sufficient explanation of the case to which he has particularly referred—of the steep ravine of a dried water course—where there could be no moisture in sufficient abundance beneath the surface of the rock, and, as we have attempted to show, little, if any, vegetable matter. In the examples given by Dr. Ferguson, the soil was particularly free from all evidence of vegetable growth, and in many of the situations such growth could not have existed; yet endemic fever, such as is known to be produced by malaria, prevailed, and in some instances to a frightful extent. It is impossible, therefore, to refer the disease to vegetable decomposition. Indeed, the very period of the year in which malarious fevers occur opposes the view of their being occasioned by the humid decay of vegetables. In summer, especially at the commencement, the plant is more succulent, and all other circumstances are equally favourable to decomposition; yet malaria is given off in greatest abundance in the autumn, when the waters, if the district be marshy, have been more or less evaporated, vegetation completely destroyed by desiccation, and putrefaction rendered almost impossible.

But, it has been said, a considerable degree of humidity is especially favourable, and even essential to the evolution of miasmata, as is evidenced by the circumstance, that marshes, stagnant pools, and the oozy shores of rivers, have been found, in all ages, and in all countries, the most insalubrious portions of the earth during hot seasons. The facts do not seem to us to establish the position. Such situations, doubtless, are often insalubrious, but not, we think, from the cause assigned. If the marsh be submerged, so as to add to the humidity, and if the stagnant pool, the oozy shores of the river, or mill-ponds have none of their water drained off, so that no particle of the bottom becomes exposed to the solar heat, we have no reason for believing that they will give off miasmata. One of the modes for obviating the insalubrity of marshy lands, which do not admit of draining, is to completely submerge them, to prevent the solar rays from acting upon a soil, which has been previously under water, and the remedy is complete. Beecher has related several cases in which this plan was successfully adopted, and Empedocles is said to have delivered the Salentini from the dangerous exhalations, to which they were subject, by conducting into their marshes two neighbouring streams.

Our knowledge on all this matter seems to be limited to the fact, that in particular climates, and under certain unknown and inappreciable circumstances, the bottoms of our stagnant pools, mill-ponds, marshes, &c. are miasmatic—a knowledge which we acquire by lamentable experience, and by that alone—that the soil becomes more or less exposed by the evaporation of the water in summer and autumn; and during the heats of the latter season more especially, it gives off the mysterious, subtile and pestiferous agent, which we call *malaria*.

Again, if vegetable decomposition singly were capable of producing malarious diseases, in the cases already given where no sensible evidence of vegetable matter existed, how much more strongly ought we to be exposed to them in situations, where the vegetable kingdom flourishes in the utmost exuberance, and where the decomposition in question must be perpetually going on in spite of every effort to the contrary. In country situations, we ought to be in the *foyers* of malarious emanations; as the very grass around us is suffered to go through its stages of growth, and decay without interference; whilst the settlers of the forest are surrounded with dead vegetable matter, necessarily undergoing more or less decomposition. In the West India sugar ships, the drainings of the sugar, mixed with the bilge water of the hold create a stench that is absolutely suffocating to those unaccustomed to it, yet it is denied that malaria and malarious diseases are generated even from this combination. (Ferguson, *loc. cit.*)

The *Tarro*—a species of arum—the roots of which are extensively used as food by nearly all the Polynesians, requires to be cultivated in shallow fresh water, and, where natural marshes do not occur, they are constructed artificially by the natives. In such situations, it is common to find their towns in all islands within the tropics, in the Pacific ocean, standing in the midst of, or surrounded by, "tarro patches;" suffering from musquetoes, and sometimes from the stench of stagnant water. Such places were visited by the officers and scientific corps of the late Exploring Expedition, at the Friendly, Society, Fejee, Samoan, and Sandwich groups of islands, without a case of intermittent fever occurring either among the natives or foreigners; and without the latter suffering from the marshy atmosphere, although they were frequently exposed to it both day and night. Most commonly, they suffered from the violent heat of the tropical sun all day on their shore journeys, and slept in open huts in the vicinity of the tarro patches at night. On the other hand, on the arrival of the Expedition on the North West Coast of America, a party was detached to the interior, and remained on the Wallamette river about a month, at a place near which there was no marshy ground that could lead to the supposition, that the intermittents from which they all suffered could have originated in it. Both the earth and the atmosphere were remarkably dry. (See a letter to the author from T. R. Peale Esq., Geologist to the Exploring Expedition, in *Med. Examiner*, Nov. 25, 1843, p. 269.)

The belief in the vegetable origin of malaria is extensive, and prevailed early, having been transferred, without due examination, from one writer to another, until it has been regarded as established; accordingly, when malarious disease arises, all eyes are directed to the vegetable kingdom, and if a harmless heap of vegetable matter be discovered, it is esteemed sufficient to account for the whole mischief. Some years ago, endemic fever attacked a whole family without any assignable cause; the physician, however, on looking by accident into the cellar, found a quantity of shingles, and this discovery was esteemed sufficient to explain everything. A more harmless occupant could scarcely have been met with; yet, being vegetable, it was held to be a satisfactory cause of the endemic; and the inference was accordingly drawn, that shingles ought not to be kept in such situations.

Perhaps the error has originated in the loose mode in which many medical writers have expressed themselves on the subject of vegetable decomposition. By almost all, the putrefaction or decomposition of the succulent vegetable is alone contemplated; some, however, have presumed, that vegetable matter, in any form, may undergo putrefaction or decomposition, and give off exhalations capable of inducing disease. Were this the case, we should be constantly exposed, in our ordinary habitations, to insalubrious exhalations, and ever liable to malarious disease. Every house, covered with shingles, every wooden dwelling, especially if surrounded by dead trees, and in the woods, and *à fortiori*, every collection of such wooden dwellings, ought to be a constant prey to them. This is fortunately not the case, and the reason seems sufficiently obvious. The shingles, of which a roof is constructed, and the additional covering of flat roofs,—and these remarks apply equally to the blocks, of which wooden pavements are constructed, —are deprived of their succulency, and reduced nearly to the state of Lignin or woody fibre, in which, as every chemist knows, nothing like the putrefaction of the succulent vegetable can take place. But if we suppose for an instant, that such a covering *could* give off malaria, how minute must be that emanation at any one period, which requires a series of years for the destructive decomposition of the substance exhaling it; and if, as has been attempted to be shown, the rapid putrefaction of the succulent vegetable be incapable of inducing malarious disease, how much more inadequate must that slow decomposition be, which has to operate on the woody fibre! The fever, which prevailed at the University of Virginia in the year 1829, was ascribed by some to the decay of the pine roofs covering the different buildings. The idea was regarded by the author at the time as preposterous; and the fact of no solitary instance of the endemic having occurred since that period, although the extent of decay is necessarily greater now than it was then, is some evidence of its inaccuracy.

In the author's view of the subject, it is requisite, first of all, to prove that vegetable matter does, *in any case*, give rise to malaria, before we go into the investigation of the particular vegetables or form of vegetable matter, which in a state of decomposition, exhale it in the greatest abundance.

In the second place; *we have no satisfactory proof that malaria ever arises from animal putrefaction singly*. M. Londe, (*Traité élémentaire d'Hygiène*) asserts, that butchers are indebted for their florid tint, and the high colouration of their tissues, to the "emanations from the blood, and palpitating flesh of animals;" —these emanations possessing, in his opinion, no deleterious property so long as they are not in a state of putrefaction. But the rubicund visage may, we think, be better explained by the constant use of animal food—too frequently tempered with fermented liquors—than by the cause assigned by M. Londe. We believe, however, fully with him, that these emanations are entirely innocuous. But we go farther, when we affirm, that malarious disease is probably never produced from animal putrefaction, and rarely disease of any kind. Putrescent animal food is eaten, and yet not habitually—for it might be properly urged that custom may render that wholesome, which, without the agency of this " second nature," might have been far otherwise—by many of the nations of the earth. The Greenlander, and Kamtschadale devour putrid flesh with as keen a relish as the European or Europeo-American finds in his greatest dainties. The southern Asiatic revels in putridity, and even amongst some of the civilized nations game is preferred in a state of incipient putrefaction, and when the odour is repulsively offensive, yet no malarious disease is induced.

The author of this volume has practised to some extent in the vicinity of the workshops of the " knackers," whose occupation is to convert the dead horse to various useful purposes,—cats' and dogs' meat, bones for the distillation of hartshorn, &c. &c.—and although the atmosphere is intolerably fetid to the casual visiter, neither the workmen nor the families around are liable to malarious, or to any disorders, which can be fairly referred to this cause. In the year 1828, a committee was appointed, in Paris, to inquire into the circumstances connected with the knacker's operations. Every one, examined by the committee, agreed, that they were most offensive and disgusting, but no one that they were unwholesome. It was even inferred, that they were conducive to health. All the men, women, and children, concerned in the works, had unvarying health, were remarkably well in appearance, and strong in body. The workmen commonly attained old age, and were generally free from the usual infirmities that accompany it. Sixty, seventy, and even eighty were common ages. Persons, living close to the places, or going thither daily, shared these advantages with the workmen. During the time that an epidemic fever was in full force at two neighbouring places, not one of the workmen in the establishment of Montfaucon was affected by it; and during the prevalence of epidemic cholera in Paris, the workmen in the *chantiers* were remarkably exempt from disease. Fewer patients were admitted into the Hospital Saint Louis, which is situate in the district of the *chantiers d'équarrisage,* than into any other hospital of the French metropolis. (Parent Duchatelet, *Hygiène Publique,* Paris, 1836.) Nor did it seem that this freedom from disease applied altogether to the men that were habituated to the works; for when, from press of business, new workmen were taken into the establishment, they did not suffer in health from the exhalations. It is affirmed, in the same statement, that above two hundred exhumations are made yearly at Paris, about three or four months after death; yet not a single case of disease, that could be ascribed to putrid emanations, has been observed.

Reference has already been made to the offensive nature of the business of the gutspinner, and to the reward, which was bestowed upon M. Labarraque of Paris for his valuable discovery of the disinfecting power of chlorine and the chlorinated preparations, by which the process has been rendered comparatively devoid of offensiveness. That accurate observer remarked, that although the gutspinners, prior to his discovery, lived in a continually putrid atmosphere, arising from macerated intestines, they enjoyed remarkable health. Again, the tainted air of the dissecting room is breathed, month after month, and for many months, by hundreds of students in different parts of the globe, yet no endemic fever is generated. M. Londe remarks, that in a single scholastic year of the *Faculté de médecine* of Paris, one thousand six hundred subjects of both sexes, and of all ages, were dissected by five hundred students, who passed five or six hours daily in the dissecting rooms, all of which were cold and damp, and consequently predisposing strongly to disease, yet not one suffered.

Parent Duchatelet (*Op. cit.*) unhesitatingly expresses his conviction, from ample observations, that there is no ground for the belief that dissecting rooms are *foyers* of morbific emanation. In support of this position, he adduces numerous facts, and the decided opinions of MM. Lallemand, Desault, Dubois, Dupuytren, Boyer, and many others; and as regards the influence of dissecting rooms on the health of students and persons attached to, and employed in them, his testimony is no less unequivocal. He states,—and he brings the testimony of M. Andral, Mr. Lawrence and others, in confirmation,—that there is no species of disease to which they are subject from exposure to the cadaveric emanations;—that gastroenteritis, meningitis, and typhoid fevers are very frequent, according to M. Andral, among the students during the first year of their stay in Paris, but that these diseases depend so little upon the mere circumstance of dissecting and remaining in the dissecting rooms, that they are more common among those who have not begun to dissect. Desault was in the habit of expressing his firm belief that the air of the dissecting rooms had saved him from attacks of epidemic and other diseases, of which those hospital physicians and surgeons who seldom or never dissected, appeared to be much more susceptible than he.

In stating the opinion, that putrefaction singly does not occasion malarious disease, it is not meant to affirm, that air, highly charged with putrid miasms, may not, in certain individuals and circumstances, powerfully impress the nervous system, so as to induce syncope, and high nervous and other disorder, or that when such miasms are absorbed from the lungs, in a concentrated state, they may not excite putrid or other disorders; or dispose the frame to unhealthy erysipelatous affections. On the contrary, experiment seems to have shown, that they are deleterious when injected into the blood; and cases are detailed in which, when exhaled from the dead body, they have excited serious mischief in those exposed to their action. According to Baron Percy, a Doctor Chambon was required by the Dean of the *Faculté de médecine* of Paris, to demonstrate the liver and its appendages before the " Faculty," on applying for his license. The decomposition of the subject, given him for the demonstration, was so far advanced, that Chambon drew the attention of the Dean to it, but he was required to go on. One of the four candidates, Corion, struck by the putrid emanations, which escaped from the body as soon as it was opened, fainted, was carried home, and died in seventy hours: another—the celebrated Fourcroy—was attacked with a burning exanthematous eruption; and two others, Laguerenne and Dufresnoy, remained a long time feeble, and the latter never completely recovered. "As for Chambon," says M. Londe, "indignant at the obstinacy of the Dean, he remained firm in his place; finished his lecture in the midst of the commissioners, who inundated their handkerchiefs with essences, and doubtless owed his safety to his cerebral excitement, which, during the night, after a slight febrile attack, gave occasion to a profuse cutaneous exhalation." Yet this case is almost unique; and all the experience of the author leads him to the inference, that such examples form the exception, not the rule. A few years ago, Dr. Maxwell Wood, of the United States Navy, furnished the author with the history of some cases of endemico-epidemic fever, which, by those who regard animal decomposition as the cause of such affections, will be invoked to establish that view of the question; and if it do not prove this, it will be admitted, that it affords ample reason for the belief, that vegetable decomposition could have had no agency in the causation.*

* It would appear from recent British journals, (April, 1844) that Mr. Chadwick, in the supplement to his valuable *Sanitary Reports*, which relates to "Interments in Cities," has brought forward much testimony to establish, that cadaveric emanations are more frequently noxious than they would appear to be from the statements in the text. The Author has not been able as yet to obtain a copy of this report. In their main inferences, however, there cannot be any very marked difference between Mr. Chadwick and himself. The great object of the Author has been to show, that putrefaction singly does not occasion malarious disease in the technical sense of the term; yet he has freely admitted, that air, charged with putrid miasmata, or with products of animal decomposition arising from bodies confined in a small space, as in the case of private vaults when first opened, may be decidedly morbific; and hence, several years ago, (*American Medical Intelligencer*, July 1, 1837.) when speaking of "Rural Cemeteries" he thus expressed himself. "The possibility of such evils is highly favourable to the view now everywhere prevalent—that the cemeteries of large towns should be at some distance from the inhabited portions. Even were we to set aside hygienic considerations, there are others, which come home forcibly to the minds of all. In every age it has been the custom, with mankind generally, to regard the depositories of the dead as objects of veneration. In ancient Rome, the place was held religious where a dead body, or any portion of it, had been buried; and the violation of the tomb was punished by fine, the loss of a hand, working in the mines, banishment, or death. Even in the savage Tonga Islands, the cemeteries are accounted so sacred, that if the deadliest enemies should meet there, they must refrain from acts of hostility. Yet, occasionally in a civilized age, and in countries unquestionably enlightened, in the ordinary acceptation of the term, the sanctuary of the grave is needlessly violated, and political anarchy, religious bigotry, infidelity, or what is esteemed the spirit of improvement, but which is too often the thirst after lucre, have subverted sensibilities which are ordinarily held sacred. How often has it happened, in the progress of our own city, (Philadelphia) to its present population, that places of worship have been disposed of and their cemeteries desecrated; and ashes, which at the period when they were deposited there, it was presumed, would ever remain free from violation, been exhumed and scattered to the winds. These and other considerations have given rise to the beautiful cemete-

The cases occurred in a small coral neck, of twelve acres extent, called Indian Key, at the southern extremity of Florida. Its surface, with the exception of a few insulated trees, presents a naked, white, clean exposure of carbonate of lime, and there is not on the Key a natural receptacle for water as large as a wash-hand basin,—rain being collected in cisterns for the use of the inhabitants, who number from 50 to 60. The houses, which have all been erected upon the plan of a single proprietor, are neat, new, one story cottages, separate from each other, raised two or three feet from the ground on stone supports, and ranged around the island, facing the ocean, with a large open space behind them; the breezes from the sea having a clear sweep over the Key, and through all the buildings. There is nothing to generate vegetable miasmata, and the place is remarkably free from disease. Thirteen men, in charge of an officer, were quartered in two of these cottages. Some weeks afterwards, Dr. Wood found the officer and one of the men under violent febrile disease. Subsequently, two others were attacked. Three of these cases proved fatal, under excessive encephalic disturbance. The other men, with their baggage, were removed on board ship; but, amongst them, several cases appeared, marked by cerebral oppression, nervous agitation, and but little disposition to reaction; intense pain in the head, back and limbs; the skin and conjunctiva assuming from the third to the fifth day a very yellow tinge. The disease likewise exhibited itself amongst those who had simply visited the houses on shore, and, in these cases, it presented a different type, the tendency to reaction being greater, and the grade of fever much higher. All the phenomena of the

ries of Père la Chaise near Paris, of Mount Auburn near Boston, and of Laurel Hill near Philadelphia. The preceding remarks, have, indeed, been suggested by a recent visit to the last of these. Situate at a convenient distance from the city of Philadelphia, yet so far from it as to almost preclude the possibility of future molestation in the progressive improvement of the city, or from other causes; on a sylvan eminence immediately skirting the Schuylkill, and commanding a beautiful view of that romantic river; embellished in a manner most creditable to the taste and liberality of spirit of the respectable individuals under whose management it has been projected, and carried into successful execution,—it is indeed a hallowed place, where affection may delight to deposite the remains of those on whom it has doated—

————' a port of rest from troublous toyle,
The world's sweet Inn from paine and wearisome turmoyle.'"

disease—Dr. Wood remarks—were such as he has seen resulting from the influence of "marsh miasmata," in its various degrees of action, from the condition of overpowering congestion, seen in the *cold plague* of the Mississippi, to the symptoms marking the yellow fever of the southern states and the West Indies. An attentive examination of the houses, although it indicated a want of cleanliness, showed no accumulation of decomposed vegetables any where; but there was an oppressive, animal, jail-like smell, which seemed to emanate from the houses themselves. There had been much and continued intemperance amongst the men, and part of a barrel of spoiled salt beef, which was very offensive, had been covered with fresh brine, and served out as the men's rations. This beef was stowed in one of the out-houses, and had been just consumed when Dr. Wood arrived at the Key.

These were all the facts that could be collected during the researches into the cause of the disease. The points in this singular endemico-epidemic, which were striking, are:—the entire absence of general or local vegetable miasmata; the concentration of the poison, as seen in the prostration of the powers of life; the very short exposure to its influence required to generate the disease; and its insulation, there being no case among the inhabitants of the Key, although the neighbouring cottages were occupied." (*Amer. Med. Intelligencer,* for Jan. 15th, 1840.)

It is probable, that during the decomposition of animal substances—of certain of them at least—morbid poisons are formed, which, when they enter the system, are capable of exciting local, or general disorder. It would seem, from the cases on record, that when wounds have been received by the dissector, on opening those that have died of malignant inflammation of the peritoneum, diffusive inflammation has more frequently followed the cut than when the wound has been received in the dissection of bodies, that had died of other affections. It is known, too, that this kind of diffusive inflammation supervenes occasionally, upon wounds, inflicted in eviscerating or "drawing" certain animals. The author has been consulted in several such cases produced by drawing the English hare. It appears, moreover, from the report of the Parisian committee to which reference has been made, that a morbid poison of this kind is more apt to be generated by some animals than by others. On making inquiries of the tradesmen, to whom the horses' skins were sent by the knackers, the committee learned, that the workmen, who had to handle them when very putrescent, had no fear, and never suffered injury. Horses' skins were never found to affect them, but in this they differed from the skins of oxen, cows, and especially sheep, "which did sometimes occasion injury, though not so often as usually supposed." In the public prints for September, 1824, the death of a person at South Dedham, Massachusetts, was announced, which was ascribed to poisonous matter received into his system from an ox, which died out of a drove, and which he, with some others, was engaged in skinning. All those, who were concerned with him, were more or less affected, and one was dangerously ill.

Admitting then, that putrefactive miasmata may be—and they unquestionably are, under certain circumstances—morbific, the facts exhibit, that the diseases, produced by them, are not such as are attributed to malaria, but resemble somewhat, in their nature, the exhalations themselves.

In the third place, *we have no satisfactory proof, that malaria is produced by aqueous decomposition.* The bilge water, in the holds of ships, is at times insupportably offensive, yet endemic disease is not generated from this cause. It is, indeed, a common observation with sailors, that "a leaky ship is a healthy ship." The British ships of war, when about to proceed on a long voyage, lay in a stock of water, generally from the Thames, which is loaded with animal, and vegetable matter. The quantity taken in is at times so great as to constitute many floorings, or tiers of barrels, close to which the sailors sleep with impunity, although the water is disgustingly putrid, and could scarcely fail to affect them, if it contained any seeds of disease. In some ships, again, the water is kept in large tanks, over which the crew sleep in safety. They, who have never seen the water of the Thames, can have but little idea of its impure condition, yet it is preferred on a long voyage, inasmuch as it has the property of self-purification. After it has been for some time in the casks or tanks, the animal and vegetable substances contained in it become putrid, and so much gas is disengaged, that it may be readily inflamed on the surface of the water; the solid and insoluble parts are then deposited, and the water becomes comparatively pure, and potable. In this case, then, we have a combination of animal and vegetable decomposition, with humidity, and under the most favourable circumstances for generating malaria, yet no evidence of malaria is discoverable.

Dr. Ferguson has adduced a similar example occurring on land. At Lisbon, and throughout Portugal, there can be no garden without water; but the garden is almost every thing to a Portuguese family. All classes of the inhabitants endeavour to preserve it, particularly in Lisbon, for which purpose they have very large stone reservoirs of water that are filled by pipes from the public aqueducts, when water is abundant; but these supplies are always cut off in the summer. The water, consequently, being most precious, is husbanded with the utmost care for three months of absolute drought of the summer season. It falls, of course, into the most concentrated state of foulness and putridity, diminishing and evaporating, day after day, till it subsides into a thick, green, vegetable scum, or a dried crust. In the confined gardens of Lisbon particularly, these reservoirs may be seen in this state close to the houses, close even to the sleeping places of the household, in the atmosphere of which they literally live and breathe; yet no one ever heard or dreamed of fever being generated amongst them from such a source, although the most ignorant native is well aware, that were he only to cross the river, and sleep on the sandy shores of the Alentejo, where a particle of water, at that season, had not been seen for months, and where water, being absorbed into the sand as soon as it fell, was never known to be *putrid*, he would run the greatest risk of being seized with remittent fever.

It appears to be manifest, then, that malaria requires for its production something more than animal, or vegetable decomposition, or humidity, singly or combined; and if the cases already brought forward were insufficient to prove the fact, the innocency of the dung-hill, and of the animal and vegetable refuse in every extensive farm yard would establish it,—the salubrity of such situations being proverbial; yet where could there be, in the autumnal season,—under the idea of malaria being the product of animal and vegetable decomposition,—circumstances more favourable for the generation of such miasmata. After a shower of rain, the solar heat, which is always necessary, as the emanations are not produced in the cooler months, acts upon the commingled materials which are in a state of great humidity, yet not the slightest evidence of malaria exists, *unless the district is itself malarious.* In other words, where malarious diseases do not prevail nothing is better established than that the combination of animal, and vegetable decomposition, which we have instanced, does not induce them; nay, it is probable, that where the soil is truly malarious, such a layer may even diminish the amount of mischief. It is well known, that the low, crowded, and abominably filthy quarter of the Jews on the banks of the Tiber, near the foot of the Roman Capitol, is almost exempt from malaria; and this has been ascribed to its sheltered site, and inconceivably dense population. Hygienic writers would say, *à priori,* that this kind of locality is most favourable to the prevalence of malarious disease. Such is not, however, the fact. It would appear, indeed, that any thing, which prevents the solar rays from beaming upon a malarious soil, may diminish the amount of emanations from it; and hence we can understand why, as a general principle, population and malaria are in an inverse ratio in any locality. It is worthy, moreover, of remark, that in the "*Local Reports on the sanitary condition of the labouring population of England, in consequence of an inquiry directed to be made by the Poor Law Commissioners,*" presented to both houses of parliament in July 1842, although numerous medical reporters ascribe the origin of typhus to animal or vegetable decomposition or to both combined, the Author does not observe that one of them refers intermittents to this cause, except in situations *known* to be malarious, or in other words where those fevers had prevailed previously. Most of the reporters lay great stress upon the influence of the effluvia from animal and vegetable remains in stagnant pools, &c., in the production of typhus, and one reporter states, that "in every case he could trace the origin of the disease to miasmata arising from stagnant pools of water containing vegetable matter in a state of decomposition, and situate in the immediate neighbourhood of the dwelling houses of the deceased individuals." Yet it may admit of great question, whether the typhus could be properly referred to such miasmata.

Of the harmlessness of a combination of aqueous and vegetable putrefaction, the case of the sugar ship, before referred to, is sufficient. It has, however, been repeatedly asserted, (Brown, *loc. citat.*)

that the steeping of hemp, which is frequently done in stagnant pools, is an unhealthy process, and the Italians have accordingly issued ordinances to prevent it; but these ordinances,—as Dr. Ferguson has correctly remarked,—have overlooked the leading primary causes, which are seated in the stagnant pool, the autumnal season, and the miasmatic or malarious soil around, and have had their attention directed to a concomitant circumstance of little or no importance. We have reason for believing, that where the soil is not markedly malarious—no operation of the kind will render it so ; and in the vicinity of the University of Virginia, we know, that the growth and preparation of hemp are largely undertaken on the extensive farm of a friend of the author, without there being the least reason to ascribe the production of malaria to the process. It is only in malarious localities, that its insalubrious character has been apparent, and in such localities the pools, necessary for steeping it, are certainly more abundantly favourable to the development of miasmata.

Similar remarks apply to the preparation of indigo. It is the product of hot countries—where malaria is known to prevail to a greater or less extent. The plant succeeds best on newly cleared lands, on account of their moisture : it requires protection against high winds, and irrigation in time of drought; but every effort is made by the manufacturer to prevent the fermentation, which is necessary for the formation of the indigo, from proceeding too far, for if *putrefaction* be permitted, the product is spoiled.

Again, in order that miasmata may arise in marshy districts, it is necessary, that there shall be an elevation of temperature, sufficient to evaporate more or less of the water, and to expose the bottom to the solar heat; the marsh must, in other words, cease to be a marsh, before the surface can become the source of disease. It is the part, which is thus exposed, that alone gives off malaria, and the same may be said of the lake, and stagnant pond. The mode of cultivating the land in some of the departments of France,—Basse Bresse, Brenne, Sologne, and Dombes, consists in forming it alternately into ponds, and submitting it to tillage. It is kept in the state of pond for eighteen months, or two years, at the expiration of which time the water is made to run into a neighbouring field; the land is recultivated for one or two years, and, afterwards, is again formed into a pond. The consequence of this system is, that the whole country is rendered almost uninhabitable: the labourer enters upon the land, as soon as the water has been drained off, to put it into a state of culture, and imbibes the miasmata in full concentration. The mortality is excessive, amounting, according to Fodéré, to one half the labourers.* But the ponds are not thus unhealthy until more or less drained, or evaporated. The ditcher, too, may pursue his vocation in malarious districts with impunity, until the water is more or less absorbed, or evaporated, but so soon as an extensive drying, and dried surface is exposed, the place becomes insalubrious. A striking instance of the increase of malaria after draining, is given by M. Rigaud Delile. At the time of the erection of the bridge of Felice, in order to unite all the waters of the river, Sextus V. was obliged to divert a branch of the Tiber, which passed behind the hills of Magliano, leaving to time the task of filling up the old bed. Half the population perished. In one single convent of nuns containing sixty-nine sisters, including novices, sixty-three died in two years.

Some authors have maintained, that malaria does not exist as a specific poison, and several of the Italian writers, in particular, have ascribed the phenomena, attributed to it, to the influence of sudden alternations of temperature, humidity of the atmosphere, irregularities of living, &c. These causes are, however, insufficient to account for the appearance of malarious diseases in certain localities, without invoking exhalations from the soil. They may act as predisponents, but the development of the disease must be excited by malaria, and need not necessarily be excited, unless such predisposition exists. This view is strongly corroborated by the observation of Sir James Clark, (*Op. citat.* p. 228.) who had extensive experience of malarious diseases, and localities, during a long residence in Italy.

"It may be stated as a general rule, that houses in confined, shaded situations, with damp courts or gardens, or standing water close to them, are unhealthy in every climate and season; but especially in a country subject to intermitting fevers, and during summer and autumn. In our own country, nothing is more com-

* See an article on *malaria*, by the Author, in the *London Quarterly Review*, vol. xxx. p. 134. This was written in the year 1823, and the Author's subsequent experience in both hemispheres has fully confirmed the views there expressed.

mon than to see houses built in very unhealthy situations, a few hundred yards distant only from a good one. Again, houses in places otherwise unexceptionable, are often so closely overhung with trees, as to be rendered far less healthy residences than they otherwise would be. Thick and lofty trees close to a house tend to maintain the air in a state of humidity, by preventing its free circulation, and by obstructing the free admission of the sun's rays. Trees growing against the walls of houses, and shrubs in confined places near dwellings, are injurious also, as favouring humidity; at a proper distance, on the other hand, trees are favourable to health. On this principle it may be understood how the inhabitants of one house suffer from rheumatism, headach, dyspepsia, nervous affections, and other consequences of living in a confined humid atmosphere, while their nearest neighbours, whose houses are more openly situated, enjoy good health; and even how one side of a large building, fully exposed to the sun and to a free circulation of air, may be healthy, while the other side overlooking damp, shaded courts or gardens, is unhealthy.* The exemption of the central parts of a large town from these fevers is partly explained by the dryness of the atmosphere which prevails there, and the comparative equality of temperature. Humid, confined situations, subject to great alternations of temperature between day and night, are the most dangerous. Of all the physical qualities of the air, humidity is the most injurious to human life; and, therefore, in selecting situations for building, particular regard should be had to the circumstances which are calculated to obviate humidity either in the soil or atmosphere, in every climate. Dryness, with a free circulation of air, and a full exposure to the sun, are the material things to be attended to in choosing a residence. A person may, I believe, sleep with perfect safety in the centre of the Pontine marshes by having his room kept well heated by a fire during the night."

What then is this malaria, arising so frequently from marshy situations as to be called *marsh poison*, but emanating also, at times, from soils far distant from any marshy lands; affecting the whole of our country below tide water, and more or less unknown in many of

* Quibus etiam in locis (quod sane mirum) brevissimi intervalli discrimine, hic aliquantum salubris existimatur aer; illic contra noxius et damnabilis. Baglivi, De Prax. Med., Lib. i., cap. xv.

our mountain regions; occurring in certain localities in spite of every care, and not producible in others by any process with which we are acquainted? We have endeavoured to prove, that it is not caused, so far as we know, by any ordinary kind of decomposition; that it is not animal in its nature, nor vegetable, nor compounded of both, but that in marshy, and stagnant situations it seems to require, that the bottom, previously submerged, should be exposed to the solar heat. Dr. Ferguson, indeed, considers that a highly advanced stage of the drying process is necessary for its production; and he adds, that in the present state of our knowledge, we can no more tell what that precise stage may be, or what that poison actually is, the development of which must be ever varying, according to circumstances of temperature, moisture, elevation, perflation, aspect, texture, and depth of soil, than we can define and describe those vapours that generate typhus fever, small pox, and other diseases.

Such is the negative opinion of Dr. Ferguson with regard to the origin of malaria. On the other hand M. Julia ascribes it to a union of *animal* and *vegetable putrefaction*, but expresses his total ignorance of the nature of the emanation. Dr. Macculloch maintains, that putrefaction, in the proper sense of the term, is not necessary, but that the stage or mode of *vegetable decomposition*, required for the production of the malaria, is different from that which generates a fetid gas. Others have supposed the miasm to be animalcular, and others again, that it is produced by animalcular putrefaction. Lastly, Dr. James Johnson, in a work already cited—thinks that we are pretty safe in concluding, that, " generally speaking, it is the product of animal and vegetable decomposition by means of heat and moisture." Yet, in another page of his work, when speaking of *pellagra*—a singular nervous affection, endemic in the Lombardo-Venetian plains—he expresses himself in a manner, which would seem to show that he by no means esteemed it " safe" to deduce any such conclusion; for he wisely observes;—" The cause of this frightful endemic pellagra has engaged the pens of many learned doctors. But it is just as inscrutable as the causes of hepatitis on the coast of Coromandel, elephantiasis in Malabar, beriberi in Ceylon, Barbadoes leg in the Antilles, goître among the Alps, the plica in Poland, cretinism in the Vallais, or *malaria* in the Campagna di Roma. It is an emanation from the soil; but whether conveyed in the air we breathe, the food we eat, or the water we drink, is unknown. If this, or any of the endemics, which I have mentioned, depended on the filth or dirty habits of the people, we ought to have similar complaints in Sion, or the Jews' Quarter in Rome, the narrow lanes of Naples, and the stinking alleys of all Italian towns, and cities. But such is not the case. The Jews' Quarter in Rome is the dirtiest and the healthiest spot in that famous city. The inhabitants of Fondi, Itri, and other wretched villages in the Neapolitan dominions are eaten up with dirt, starvation, and malaria; but no pallagra, no elephantiasis, no goître, no cretinism is to be seen. The inevitable, and the rational inference is, that each country, where peculiar or endemic maladies prevail, produces them from some hidden source, which human knowledge has not yet been able to penetrate."

Such inference, we would unhesitatingly say, is applicable to malaria as we have been considering it; and this is strikingly confirmed by the discrepancies in the opinions of writers. Can we then, in the state of ignorance that envelopes us, fix positively, or even with any thing like probability, upon any cause, or combination of causes, of any kind, likely to give origin to those emanations? It has been already asserted, that we are uninformed regarding the nature of the emanations from even the most unhealthy situations, where we *know*, from the results, that such emanations exist. They have utterly defied the art of the chemical analyst. They cannot consist of hydrogen, or of carburetted, or sulphuretted, or phosphuretted hydrogen, for no such adventitious gases have been detected by the chemist, which they could readily have been, if present; nor has there been found any additional quantity of carbonic acid gas, or azote.—The revival of the ancient theory of animalcules scarcely requires a comment. It sufficiently shows the obscurity, that environs the subject. Of late, the notion of sulphuretted hydrogen being the essence of malaria has been revived under a more imposing, but not less fallacious, form. Professor Daniell, of King's College, London, found that water—sent to him from certain unhealthy localities on the coast of Africa, where pernicious intermittent and remittent fevers prevail—contained sulphuretted hydrogen (*Lond. Med. Gazette*, July 16, and July 23, 1841) and he thence inferred, that it might be the great febrific agent. A similar view, as the result of experiments on the air of malarious regions in this country, has been more recently maintained by Dr. Daniel P. Gardner, (*American Journal of the Medical Sciences*, April 1843.) But supposing the presence of sulphuretted hydrogen to be a fact, it alone would be obviously insufficient to account for the phenomena, inasmuch as in situations in which sulphuretted hydrogen exists to a much greater extent, these malarious fevers are wholly unknown. The view of Professor Daniell has, however, been completely overthrown by Dr. McWilliam, the senior medical officer in the disastrous expedition to the Niger during the years 1841-2, who has shown most satisfactorily (*Medical History of the Expedition to the Niger*, &c., Lond. 1843) that no such gas as free sulphuretted hydrogen is found in the waters of the Niger, and that what was detected in the specimens sent to England, and examined by Professor Daniell, originated in the decomposition of the contents of the bottles. Yet, on the slender evidence afforded by such examination, Professor Daniell inferred, that no vessel should be allowed to cast anchor or linger in sulphuretted [?] waters." " But, if paramount duty," he adds, " should oppose itself to such a course, we have a certain remedy to propose. You have seen how instantly chlorine destroys the gas. Chlorine and sulphuretted hydrogen cannot co-exist together. Plentiful fumigations of chlorine would therefore infallibly prevent the deleterious effects; and the antidote is at once cheap, and incapable, under proper management, to produce any injurious effects to counterbalance its advantages." Accordingly, at Professor Daniell's suggestion, ships, proceeding to the Niger, were provided with ample means for the disengagement of chlorine; but lamentably fatal experience has destroyed at once the hypothesis of Professor Daniell as to the nature of the pestiferous emanations, and the means for destroying them. (See the Author's *Practice of Medicine*, 2nd edit., ii. 422, Philad. 1844.)

Such is our ignorance of the nature and causes of the malaria, which emanates from marshy lands more especially—of that which gives rise to remittent, and intermittent fevers. But, although unacquainted with it in these particulars, we do know some of the laws by which it is governed. It is carried up in the air during the day along with aqueous vapour; and, during the night, by reason of its greater specific gravity than that of atmospheric air, it is in greatest concentration near the surface of the earth; hence, the inhabitants of the ground floor of any habitation are more exposed to its morbific agency than those who occupy the upper stories. The wall of the wing of the hospital at Padua, where the clinical wards are situate, is washed by a branch of the sluggish Brenta, and it has frequently happened, that the windows of these wards, which are about sixteen feet above the surface of the water, having been carelessly left open until too late an hour, several of the patients have been attacked with intermittent fevers—in some instances of the pernicious kind. This has never occurred in the women's wards, which are immediately over those of the men, though there is no reason to believe, that more care was taken in shutting the windows of those apartments than of the former. It was also remarked by the British medical officers, during the expedition, in 1809, to Walcheren, that those who slept in the upper stories of houses were less liable to the endemic disease, and had it in a milder form, than those who slept on the ground floors. The testimony of the natives was in favour of the correctness of this observation; and Dr. Ferguson, when one of the principal medical officers of the British army in St. Domingo, remarked, that two thirds more men were taken ill on the ground floors than in the upper stories. It would seem, consequently, that, in order to ensure, as far as practicable, the salubrity of dwellings in unhealthy situations, they should be raised on arches, or the lower story be suffered to be wholly uninhabited.

Again, owing to the greater specific gravity of malarious emanations, it may be understood, that a high wall, or barricade may completely fence in the more virulent emanations, and preserve the inhabitants of the vicinity free from disease. The intervention of woods, too, may form a screen to impede the wafting of miasmata by the winds; and perhaps this may have been a reason, why the ancients consecrated the woods, in the vicinity of Rome, to Neptune, in order to secure them from the axe. In the distresses, however, in which the great expenditure of Pius VI. involved the Holy See, a large district of these woods was sold, and cut: and to this event, Sir Charles Morgan thinks, may, with some reason, be attributed an increase of danger to the unprotected city.

The good effects of the intervention of woods, or rather the evils resulting from cutting them, under the circumstances mentioned, are strongly exemplified by M. Rigaud Delile, several of whose observations were collected in the environs of Rome, the Pomptine marshes, &c. Of these we shall adduce only the two following. Near St. Stephano, on Mount Argentel, a convent is situate which was famed for the salubrity of its air; but since the forests, which surrounded it, have been cleared, it has become unhealthy. At Velletri, near the Pomptine marshes, the cutting of an intermediate wood occasioned immediately, and for three successive years, fevers and other diseases, which committed great ravages. The same effect was observed from a similar cause near Campo Salino; and analogous examples might be adduced from Volney, Lancisi, and others. Allusion has already been made to the oft observed phenomenon, that the inhabitants of elevated regions in the vicinity of marshy lands are occasionally affected by malarious disease, when those, on the same level as the marsh, may be unaffected.

Again, it may be understood, that the health of a locality may be often connected with the winds that prevail during the latter part of summer, and in autumn. In this country, they are chiefly from the southward, or have what the sailors term *southing* in them. These winds are warm, and, when from the east, are moist at the same time. Inhabitants of the northern shores of our rivers that exhale malaria, or to the northward of any malarious locality, may, therefore, be expected to suffer more than those to the south of such localities; and this is *cæteris paribus,* the fact.

Of the nature, and causes of the malaria, which gives rise to other endemic diseases,—plague, goître, cretinism, elephantiasis, beriberi, pellagra, &c.—we know, if possible, less than we do of the marsh poison. The plague, it is well known, has its great nidus at Grand Cairo. That city is at once its birth place, and cradle. It has been attempted to account for the pestilence there by the crowded population, poverty, filth, narrow streets, hot climate, and the filth of the canals. But most, if not all, these elements are present in other cities, where plague does not exist, and has rarely, if ever, been known to exist. The Jews' Quarter at Rome, and other situations in France, and Italy,—some of which have been referred to in the extract from Dr. Johnson's work on " *Change of Air,*"—appear to possess the requisite materials, yet there is no plague. Lisbon, too, has been immortalized for dirt, and for every evil entailed upon a crowded city, by long continued municipal apathy and neglect, yet there is no plague. All may recollect the description of that noisome metropolis by Byron:—

> "But whoso entereth within this town,
> That sheening far celestial seems to be,
> Disconsolate will wander up and down
> Mid many things unsightly to strange ee:
> For hut and palace show like filthily,
> The dingy denizens are rear'd in dirt:
> Ne personage of high or mean degree
> Doth care for cleanness of surtout and shirt,
> Though shent with Egyp'ts plague, unkempt, unwash'd, unhurt."

Something more than dirt is required to produce these endemic maladies, but all that we know of the invisible enemy seems to be, that it consists of some peculiar terrestrial emanation of which we know nothing. At one period, not a doubt was entertained, that goitre or swelled neck was occasioned by drinking snow water, which had descended from the summits of lofty mountains,—at the base of which the disease was endemic,—into the valleys. The discovery, that the affection is common at the foot of lofty mountains in every region of the globe, and in countries where no snow is perceptible, at length exploded the vulgar belief.

It would be ludicrous, but humiliating, to refer to the absurd conceits, that have been indulged to account for the various endemic diseases to which allusion has been made. One, by no means the least amusing to an inhabitant of the United States, is, that pellagra is produced by eating Indian corn. Before the opinion had been hazarded, and it has been so in full gravity, it might have been useful to inquire whether the disease had ever been met with on this side of the Atlantic.

Unfortunately, our ignorance is not restricted to endemic disease. We know no more of the "constitution of the atmosphere," which gives occasion to epidemics,—the *influenza* or epidemic catarrh, for example, which frequently visits us,—than we do of the cause of the incessant vicissitudes that occur in the atmosphere itself; nor can we afford the slightest satisfactory explanation for those endemico-epidemics, which so frequently affect districts previously healthy. The anxieties, the fears, the interests, the prejudices, and the superstitions of individuals are active on such occasions to suggest a cause, but it is extremely doubtful, whether any adequate cause has in any instance been discovered. It has fallen to the lot of the author to witness many examples of endemico-epidemic disease in situations, which were previously, and subsequently, amongst the most salubrious; but, in every instance, on the most scrutinizing investigation, no satisfactory cause was discoverable. Many, it is true, were suggested, but most of the suggestions were founded in medical or physical error, and in the natural credulity of mankind. In the year 1816, the town of Havre, and several other places in Normandy were affected by epidemic cholera morbus putting on pretty nearly the same symptoms as are induced by some varieties of poison. The public mind was much agitated, and many persons were persuaded, that the disease was occasioned by oysters, which had been obtained from a new bed, formed at Havre in earth recently excavated in the moat of the old castle. So much excitement prevailed, that Messrs. Chaussier and Vauquelin were sent to Havre by the *Faculté de Médecine* of Paris to report on the causes. These gentlemen found the oysters perfectly sound, that the symptoms were merely those of an accidental epidemic, and that the whole of the excitement had originated in jealousy towards the new establishment. The result confirmed the accuracy of their report.

On epidemics, as on endemics the discrepancy of writers sufficiently exhibits the want of fixed ideas. Whilst some refer them to excessive atmospheric heat, others have ascribed similar affections to cold. Dryness, and moisture, and opposite states of electricity have also been invoked to account for the same phenomena. Nor are our ideas more fixed with regard to the circumstances, that favour the spread of contagious diseases, and to the constituents of any emanation from the subject of any contagious disease, small pox, measles, &c.—active as such emanations unquestionably are. On all these topics we are in the state of old Gobbo;—

"More than sand-blind, high gravel-blind."

## SECTION IV.

Powerful influence of locality on man—comparative salubrity of different soils—comparative mortality of different countries—mortality, and longevity of the counties of England and Wales—mortality, and longevity not always in a like ratio—longevity in different counties of Virginia—insalubrity of great towns—comparative mortality of different cities—the human species, especially the young, require a pure air—great improvement in the value of life—salutary effects of change of air—effect of winds—action of the heavenly bodies on man.

THE various facts, to which reference has been made, exhibit the powerful influence of situation on the health of mankind, and a wider inspection instructs the anthropologist, that the whole physical, and moral condition of man is modified by climate, or locality, so that we may at once distinguish the Esquimaux from the American Indian to the south; the Asiatic from the European; the German from the French, &c. &c. Nay, the physiognomy is so much changed by endemico-epidemic influences, that we are enabled, in our legislative halls, to discover at a glance the resident of the unhealthy districts of the low country from the more ruddy inhabitants of the mountain region.

It has been already remarked, that we are totally unacquainted with the precise causes, that give occasion to the production of malaria, as well as with its nature. We can from experience, however, form some judgment on entering particular districts, whether the miasms, that excite malarious fevers, are likely to emanate from them; and yet in other countries, unquestionably malarious—as in many districts of Italy—there may be no manifest physical circumstances that could enable us to entertain the slightest judgment as to their degree of insalubrity.

Marshy districts are the *foyers* of disease in almost all countries. This we know from experience. In the same manner we learn, that the deltas of large rivers are formed of a soil apt to teem with malarious emanations. Those of the Nile and the Po are proverbial, as well as the unhealthy islands of Walcheren, and the others constituting Zeeland, which seem to have been formed by the accumulation of the *detritus* carried down to the German ocean by the Rhine and the Scheldt. We could pronounce, too, that the city of New Orleans might be liable to malarious disease, from its climate, and the peculiarity of its locality. Its temperature is elevated; the surface of the city is several feet below the level of the Mississippi at high water, and the adjacent country is low and marshy. But further than as regards marshy lands, or stagnant pools, our judgment of localities does not extend. Some of the most smiling portions of Italy are not the less desolated by the fitful malaria.

> "In florid beauty, groves, and fields appear,
> Man seems the only growth that dwindles here."

"Let us," observes a modern writer—Dr. Macculloch—"turn to Italy; the fairest portions of this fair land are a prey to this invisible enemy; its fragrant breezes are poison; the dews of its summer evenings are death. The banks of the refreshing streams, its rich and flowery meadows, the borders of its glassy lakes; the luxuriant plains of its overflowing agriculture; the valley where its aromatic shrubs regale the eye and perfume the air—these are the chosen seats of this plague, the throne of malaria. Death here walks hand in hand with the sources of life, sparing none; the labourer reaps his harvest but to die, or he wanders amidst the luxuriance of vegetation and wealth, the ghost of man, a sufferer from his cradle to his impending grave; aged in childhood, and laying down in misery that life, which was but one disease. He is even driven from some of the richest portions of this fertile yet unhappy country; and the traveller contemplates at a distance deserts, but deserts of vegetable wealth, which man dares not approach,—or he dies."

What but lamentable experience could teach us, that countries possessing all that could delight the eye, and teeming with those products of the earth that minister so largely to the sustenance and comfort of man, should be, at the same time, exhaling a bane, capable of rendering all those advantages nugatory!

The state of the Maremma district resembles, in these respects, many situations in our country, where malaria exists to such an extent as to render them uninhabitable. Who could pronounce, except instructed by experience, that the verdant banks of many of our streams should be liable to this noxious exhalation! On many parts of the elevated banks of the Schuylkill, and Delaware, villas were erected at a time when intermittents were scarcely known in those localities; but, of late years, many of them have been abandoned owing to their insalubrity. In the case of the Narrows, of which we have already spoken, refreshed by a constant sea-breeze, and devoid of malarious diseases for perhaps forty years, the most fatal affections of this kind appeared for a season; committed extensive ravages, especially amongst the poor— and too often intemperate—labourers, employed at the time in the erection of Fort Hamilton, and in the following year, part of which the Author spent at the Narrows, all was again salubrity. Yet no difference was perceptible in the locality.

It has been imagined, by some, that the character of the soil of a district may aid us in determining whether it be liable to malarious exhalations; but we can deduce imperfect inferences only from this circumstance, except in the case of the soils of bogs, marshes, &c. which *cæteris paribus* are the most likely to be morbific. The sandy and calcareous soils are usually regarded as most salubrious; and, as a general principle, this is true; but a slight stratum of these soils may, in certain cases, cover the surface, and the character of the substratum may enter as an important element into our calculations as to the salubrity of a district where such soils occupy the surface.

Next to the soil of marshes and turbaries, Fodéré places the argillaceous or clayey, " because it retains the water, which ferments there, and undergoes decomposition." The value of this theory of aqueous decomposition has been already inquired into: we are prepared also to contest the facts on which the view of Fodéré rests. It certainly cannot be maintained by any one, who has inspected the soils of malarious regions, that the clayey soil is most insalubrious next to the marshy, and turfy. Some of the most healthy districts are formed of this soil, and on the other hand, as we have previously seen, some of the most unhealthy are sandy. The district of Virginia, which runs along the south-west mountains, particularly that in Albemarle and Orange, has its soil chiefly composed of red clay; yet it is eminent for its salubrity. It is but little affected with diseases that have been looked upon as miasmatic, and always presents unusual instances of longevity, although, as will be seen presently, salubrity and longevity may not always go hand in hand. In this mountain range is the former seat of Ex-President Jefferson—the patriot and philosopher—who died in his eighty-fourth year; and his no less distinguished successor, Mr. Madison, died at a yet more advanced a geat the foot of the same mountain chain.

The vicinity of large masses of water, lakes, rivers, or the sea, is regarded, by most writers, to be healthy; and in certain countries, and districts such is the case, but on this continent the exceptions are almost as numerous as the rule. Fodéré affirms, that such situations are ordinarily healthy, unless there is an admixture of salt, and fresh water, remaining in a state of stagnation on the bank; but these again are circumstances, that seem to mock our acquaintance with the causes of terrestrial emanations. In certain insalubrious districts, such stagnant admixture of salt and fresh water does certainly exist; but in others, the water is entirely fresh, and in all cases the real cause is probably seated in the malarious soil forming the banks of the stream or the vicinity; but of the nature of which soil, as we have before attempted to show, we absolutely know nothing. It *may* require an admixture of argillaceous earth. It *may* require animal, and vegetable remains. It *may* be a gaseous emanation. It *may*, as Fodéré thinks, resemble the product of organic decomposition. All these are possibilities; but requiring substantiation, and in which the negative evidence preponderates, we think, largely over the positive.

The following communications will sufficiently show how little we know of the precise localities that may exhale the most pestilential malaria excepting by the results. After having promulged to his class views similar to those contained in the preceding pages in the winter of 1843, the Author received the following letter from Dr. J. S. Whittle of the United States Navy, in reference, it will be observed, to the severe endemic experienced by the party to which Mr. Peale was attached on the banks of the Wallamette river. (See page. 74.)

*Philadelphia, January*, 18*th*, 1843.

Sir,—Your remarks on the subject of Malaria, [in a lecture] a few afternoons since, bring to my mind, in a manner more forcible than they were ever presented to it before, some circumstances which came under my observation in the year 1841. Late in the month of July of that year, I was put in medical charge of a party of about forty persons, who were about making a journey from Fort Van Couver, on the Columbia river, to the mouth of the Rio Sacramiento, in Upper California. After we had proceeded about one hundred and thirty miles, and had reached the banks of the Wallamette, opposite the American Missionary settlement, counter-orders reached us, and we were detained, encamped immediately on the bank of this river, for a month or nearly so. During this time, almost the whole party were attacked with intermittent fever, generally assuming the tertian type; and, in a few instances, the quotidian. I was called also to several cases in the neighbouring country. Through this region runs the Wallamette, a rapid stream two hundred yards wide. The shores are thickly covered with a fine growth of pine and other trees, and the undergrowth is rich and luxuriant. A very short distance from the river, the country is prairie (hill and dale,) with occasional groves and narrow strips of oak; and here there is no undergrowth (except a high grass, which does not rot in summer, but is perfectly cured, there being no rain,) the surface being as clean as if attended to with the most constant care. The climate is very peculiar. In midsummer, when we were there, the thermometer frequently ranged from 80° to 85° F. in the shade, and, notwithstanding this great degree of diurnal heat, there was often frost; and sometimes ice an eighth of an inch in thickness at night. The whole river-region was enveloped in a thick fog every morning,—so thick sometimes, that it was impossible to see a man twenty steps off. The weather was perfectly clear almost the whole time;—there not being rain, enough to wet the skin during the month. The soil is generally light, and gravelly. We lived in tents *immediately* on the bank of the river, sleeping on the ground from which we were only separated by a blanket or bearskin. The missionaries and other whites, living on the river in houses, were affected with the malady, but not to so great an extent as ourselves; and numbers of the Indians had it also. It was equally prevalent on the *upper* part of the Columbia, where the whites in the employ of the Hudson's Bay Co., and the Indian inhabitants suffered largely. But, in the settlement at the mouth of the Columbia, near the sea, I was informed, that the inhabitants were entirely free from it, as were those few settlers, who lived in the upper country at a distance from the large water-courses. In some districts, the Indians have died by hundreds. This is probably, in part at least, owing to their mode of treatment, which consists in heating themselves in a vapour-bath and then plunging suddenly into the river. I have seen the bones of a whole village occupying one common grave! It is as fatal among them as cholera. *The Indians say, and some white men, who had been there a number of years, concur with them, that they were strangers to the disease till the whites came there to inhabit. And one or two of the oldest white settlers, men who have lived there thirty years or more, attribute its appearance, without hesitation, to the turning up of the soil for agricultural purposes. They say, that in any of their river regions, the sticking of a plough or hoe into the ground is followed by ague, at certain seasons of the year, as invariably as the thunderclap succeeds a flash of lightning.* These are the statements of people who are, of course, entirely ignorant of the principles of medicine or philosophy; but in a matter of mere fact, their observation is, probably, as much to be relied upon, as that of persons of much more cultivated minds, especially when we consider, that they can have no theory to support, and are consequently free from the very strong prejudices and fallacies of reasoning, which so frequently arise from this source. What staggers my belief on this subject, however, is, that the quantity of cultivated ground seems to me to be too small to produce such direful and wide spread effects,—the country being very sparsely inhabited by whites, and the aborigines not cultivating it at all.

If what I have related possess any interest, I hope that circumstance may serve as an apology for my having troubled you so much. With great respect, I am, Sir, your very obt. servant,

J. S. WHITTLE,
Asst. Surgeon, U. S. Navy.

To Professor Robley Dunglison.

The above letter was published in the *Medical Examiner* for Nov. 25, 1843; along with that of Mr. Peale, already referred to, as valuable contributions to the history of malaria " a terrestrial or geological phenomena," as the author designated it, " always of deep interest to the profession." At the same time he published the following extract of a letter, dated Fort Macomb, Middle Florida, Jany. 11, 1842, from Dr. R. S. Holmes. U. S. A., formerly a pupil of his class, to Dr. James R. Spear, of Pittsburg, which signally comfirms the views above expressed.

"My post of which I have the sole medical command, has been long known as the most unhealthy in Florida: so much so that it is always abandoned about the first of May, and not re-occupied until September. What influence makes it bear such a character I cannot imagine. A full and rapid stream, of about one hundred yards in width, called the Swanne flows by it. The river is navigable for steamboats fifty miles above this; is very deep; has not a single weed or decayed vegetable in it, and flows at the rate of three miles an hour. Its banks are formed of light granular disintegrating limestone. The country around is dry and thickly covered by a profuse growth of tall pines: there is not a marsh within five miles of us, and even then one that scarcely deserves such a title: there is not a greater undergrowth of vegetable matter than I have seen about the most healthy ports in Florida; and the dry sand, which covers the whole country like a mantle, absorbs water like a sponge. I am inclined to think the geological nature of the banks of the river has something to do with the malaria so prevalent here. I can conceive of nothing else! the situation is high, and a perfectly dry one; yet I have scarcely ever less than twenty on my sick list from sixty-six men: probably twenty more in the company are so debilitated with disease that they are unfit for active duty in the field."

When we cast our eye over the published statistical accounts of the mortality of various countries, we observe the greatest difference; and although the bills of mortality may be kept with less accuracy in some countries than in others, they may be esteemed, in all, sufficiently accurate to enable us to draw some inference with regard to comparative salubrity. Dr. Bisset Hawkins (*Elements of Medical Statistics*, p. 31, Lond. 1829,) who founds his statements on "instructive returns, from nearly all the counties, cities, and hospitals on the continent," gives the average mortality of the Pays du Vaud, as 1 in 49; of Sweden and Holland, 1 in 48; of Russia, 1 in 41; of France, 1 in 40; of Austria, 1 in 38; of Prussia, and Naples, 1 in 33 to 35, and of South America, 1 in 30. The same rate of mortality as that of France is assigned by Mr. Bristed to the United States; but we know not on what authority: there can, indeed, be none. The census, taken every ten years throughout the United States, has hitherto been deficient in that instructive piece of information to the physician, and the statesman. A writer in the *American Almanac*, on as little foundation, estimated the mortality of the United States, many years ago, to be 1 in 50. The Author prepared a table of the comparative mortality, and longevity of the different counties of England and Wales, from the "Abstract of the Answers and Returns, made pursuant to an act passed in the first year of George IV. entitled—"An act for taking an account of the population of Great Britain, and of the increase or diminution thereof." The 'Abstract' was prepared by Mr. Rickman, who was appointed by the secretary of state for the home department to digest, and reduce into order, the population returns, and by the privy council to arrange the Parish Register Returns; and, although the estimates may be occasionally erroneous, yet as a comparative view they may afford a satisfactory approximation to the truth, as the same system of enumeration, and of parish register abstracts was adopted throughout.

MORTALITY OF COUNTRIES. 103

## ENGLAND.

| COUNTIES. | MORTALITY. One burial to | LONGEVITY. Proportion of those from 90 to 100 years old, in 20,000. | Proportion of those, 100 years and upwards, in 20,000. |
|---|---|---|---|
| Bedford, | 62 | 6.71 | 0.23 |
| Berks, | 58 | 11.46 | 0.48 |
| Buckingham, | 56 | 9.41 | |
| Cambridge, | 58 | 4.71 | |
| Chester, | 55 | 9.53 | 0.15 |
| Cornwall, | 71 | 10.09 | 0.32 |
| Cumberland, | 58 | 18.42 | 1.01 |
| Derby, | 63 | 9.48 | 0.10 |
| Devon, | 61 | 12.10 | 0.19 |
| Dorset, | 66 | 18.72 | |
| Durham, | 55 | 21.79 | 1.88 |
| Essex, | 59 | 7.76 | 0.22 |
| Gloucester, | 64 | 10.55 | 0.25 |
| Hereford, | 63 | 15.95 | 0.78 |
| Hertford, | 58 | 5.94 | 0.32 |
| Huntingdon, | 63 | 8.35 | |
| Kent, | 50 | 7.76 | 0.34 |
| Lancaster, | 55 | 6.72 | 0.31 |
| Leicester, | 59 | 7.23 | 0.35 |
| Lincoln, | 62 | 11.11 | 0.36 |
| Middlesex, | 47 | 6.04 | 0.54 |
| Monmouth, | 70 | 17.46 | 0.87 |
| Norfolk, | 61 | 14.21 | 0.48 |
| Northampton, | 58 | 6.96 | 0.13 |
| Northumberland, | 58 | 24.70 | 1.09 |
| Nottingham, | 58 | 8.70 | |
| Oxford, | 61 | 10.66 | 0.16 |
| Rutland, | 62 | 13.00 | |
| Salop, | 58 | 12.69 | 0.32 |
| Somerset, | 63 | 9.64 | 0.06 |
| Southampton, | 58 | 9.82 | 0.21 |
| Stafford, | 56 | 10.30 | 0.37 |
| Suffolk, | 67 | 11.45 | 0.15 |
| Surrey, | 52 | 9.40 | 0.35 |
| Sussex, | 72 | 6.87 | 0.19 |

| COUNTIES. | MORTALITY. | LONGEVITY. | |
|---|---|---|---|
| Warwick, | . 52 | . . 9.07 | . . 0.48 |
| Westmoreland, . | . 58 | . . 10.09 | . . 0.39 |
| Wilts, . . . | . 66 | . . 9.97 | . . 0.10 |
| Worcester, | . 56 | . . 10.13 | . . 0.51 |
| York, East Riding, | . 57 | . . 8.60 | . . 0.42 |
| —— North Riding, | . . 63 | . . 20.48 | . . 0.83 |
| —— West Riding, | . 61 | . . 7.43 | . . 0.09 |
| Average . . | . 57 | . . 9.90 | . . 0.34 |
| WALES. | | | |
| Anglesey, . . | . 83 | . . 9.58 | |
| Brecon, . . | . 67 | . . 21.44 | . . 1.40 |
| Cardigan, . . | . 70 | . . 14.49 | . . 1.03 |
| Carmarthen, . | . 67 | . . 20.19 | . . 0.64 |
| Carnarvon, . . | . 69 | . . 16.92 | . . 0.34 |
| Denbigh, . . | . 62 | . . 21.53 | |
| Flint, . . . | . 64 | . . 14.30 | |
| Glamorgan, . | . 69 | . . 17.93 | . . 0.83 |
| Merioneth, . . | . 67 | . . 20.73 | . . 0.35 |
| Montgomery, . | . 65 | . . 14.81 | . . 1.51 |
| Pembroke, . . | . 83 | . . 26.88 | |
| Radnor, . . | . 64 | . . 16.90 | |
| Average, . . | . 69 | . . 17.97 | . . 0·50 |

These tables afford some singular and inexplicable results. It appears, that the mean annual mortality of England and Wales was, at the time, 1 in 58, and that there was a surprising difference in the mortality of the different counties,—varying from 1 in 47 (Middlesex,) to 1 in 83 (Anglesey and Pembroke.) In the first edition of this work, the Author thought it probable, that the mortality throughout the country was greater than 1 in 58, inasmuch as it was so much less than the rate in the despotic countries of Europe, where the estimates, it might be presumed, were at the time, kept with greater regularity,—but this he stated as a mere surmise. The reports of the Registrar-General have confirmed this surmise. From the "*Fourth annual Report of the Registrar-General of Births, Deaths and Marriages, in England,*" (London 1842 p. 6,) we extract the following table, which shows that the mean mortality of four years was 1 in 45.

## PROPORTION OF BIRTHS, MARRIAGES, AND DEATHS TO POPULATION.

| | Annual proportion of marriages, births, and deaths to a population of 100. | | | Numbers living out of which one marriage, birth or death occurred. | | |
|---|---|---|---|---|---|---|
| | Marriages, | Births, | Deaths. | 1 Marriage in | 1 Birth in | 1 Death in |
| July 1, 1840, 41 | .772 | 3.189 | 2.248 | 129 | 31 | 44 |
| 1839, 40 | .796 | 3.213 | 2.242 | 126 | 31 | 45 |
| 1838, 39 | .786 | 3.119 | 2.148 | 127 | 32 | 47 |
| 1837, 38 | " | " | 2.247 | " | " | 44 |
| | .785 | 3.174 | 2.221 | 127 | 32 | 45 |

From an experience of many situations in this country as well as in England, the Author may express a doubt, whether the climate, in many of our mountain districts, do not equal, if not exceed, the mean of England, although we have no positive data to guide us. The mortality may, indeed, be greatly less than 1 in 45. Yet when the Author was about to leave Great Britain, to occupy the station for which he had been selected in the University of Virginia, a Life Insurance Company, of which he was a member, declined continuing the insurance, unless the premium was doubled,—a requisition which compelled him to sacrifice the policy; and a brother Professor, who desired to effect an Assurance at another office, was told, that they must decline insuring the life of any resident of a country in which the rivers froze over in a single night! Again in an essay on *malaria and miasma*, (Dr. Brown, *Cyclopædia of Practical Medicine*, Amer. edit., by the Author, Philad. 1844,) we have the following exaggerated representation. "In the marshy districts of certain countries,—for example, Egypt, Georgia, and Virginia, the extreme term of life is stated to be forty; whilst we learn from Dr. Jackson, that at Petersburgh, in the latter country, a native, and permanent inhabitant rarely reaches the age of twenty-eight!" Yet, there are many situations in the United States, which are as healthy probably as any in the world, whilst the rate of mortality of Philadelphia is less than than that of almost any European city, whose medical statistics have been taken.

It would appear from the first of the tables, that the healthiest counties in England, or those at least in which the mortality is lowest, are Sussex, Cornwall, and Monmouth in England; and Anglesey, Pembroke, and Cardigan in Wales,—Anglesey, and Pembroke having the lowest recorded rate of mortality in Europe, or perhaps in the world. Middlesex, Kent, Surrey, and Warwick exhibit the greatest mortality in the table. The table shows, also, what was before mentioned, that there is no exact ratio between the mortality, and the longevity of a district. This discrepancy has been noticed by Hufeland, and other writers on Hygiène. As a general rule, the proportionate mortality will be greater where the duration of life is less; and this fact is strikingly exemplified in some of the very insalubrious regions of France, which are cultivated by the system of ponds, explained in an earlier section. The picture, given by Fodéré of the physical and moral abjection that characterizes the inhabitants of these pestiferous localities, is, indeed, deplorable.—" From his earliest infancy, man begins to experience the sad effects of this unhappy country. He is scarcely weaned, before his complexion becomes sallow, and his eyes assume a bilious tint. He falls away; his growth is arrested; his viscera become engorged; and he attains with difficulty his seventh year. If he clears this term, he does not live; he vegetates; he continues doughy, obstructed, cacochymous, bloated, hydropic,—liable to malignant putrid fevers, to interminable autumnal fevers, to passive hemorrhages, and to ulcers of the legs extremely difficult of cure. In perpetual strife with all these diseases, which frequently attack him at once, so that he may be almost regarded as in a protracted agony, the inhabitant of Brenne attains the age of twenty or thirty years, when nature begins to retrograde; the faculties sink, and the age of fifty years is commonly his final term. In this manner several generations rapidly pass away. The population, however, maintains pretty nearly an equilibrium. They marry early and repeatedly. It is not uncommon to find men and women, thirty or forty years of age, married for the third or fourth time. The three brothers Dupont, one of whom is a widower, have married fifteen women amongst them. The certainty of finding vacant habitations and lands to let attracts foreign families. Day labourers, and hired servants proceed thither, marry and settle; and in this way the problem is solved,—why so inhospitable a country is not depopulated." (*Traité de Médecine Légale et d'Hygiène Publique*, tom. v. p. 166.)

Thus it is everywhere.—The most fertile soil is situate in the river bottoms, and these are apt to be the very localities in which malarious diseases prevail.

More recent enumerations, in regard to the mortality of different counties and divisions of England, do not exactly accord with those of the Abstract, but they sufficiently show the wide difference that exists between them. The following table is from the "*Fourth Report of the Registrar-General*" (p. 14, Lond. 1842.)

Relative mortality showing the annual number of deaths among 100,000 females living in each of the three years ending 30th June 1839, 1840 and 1841.

| Divisions. | Counties. | 1839, | 1840, | 1841, | Mean. |
|---|---|---|---|---|---|
| North-western, | Chester, Lancaster, | 2.541 | 2.847 | 2.622 | 2.670 |
| Metropolitan, | Middlesex (part of,) Surrey (part of,) Kent (part of,) | 2.376 | 2.256 | 2.384 | 2.339 |
| York, | York, | 2.162 | 2.276 | 2.229 | 2.222 |
| North Midland, | Leicester, Rutland, Lincoln, Nottingham, Derby, | 1.910 | 2.274 | 2.185 | 2.123 |
| | ENGLAND, | 2.055 | 2.157 | 2.171 | 2.113 |
| Western, | Gloucester, Hereford, Salop, Worcester, Stafford, Warwick, | 1.971 | 2.077 | 2.183 | 2.074 |
| South Midland, | Middlesex (part of,) Herts, Bucks, Oxford, Northampton, Huntingdon, Bedford, Cambridge, | 1.978 | 2.067 | 2.137 | 2.061 |
| Northern, | Durham, Northumberland, Cumberland, Westmoreland, | 1.879 | 2.097 | 2.151 | 2.042 |
| Eastern, | Essex, Suffolk, Norfolk, | 1.991 | 1.906 | 2.047 | 1.981 |
| Welsh, | Wales, Monmouthshire, | 1.860 | 1.982 | 1.963 | 1.935 |
| South-eastern, | Surrey (part of,) Kent (part of,) Sussex, Hants, Berks, | 1.771 | 1.814 | 1.841 | 1.809 |
| South-western, | Wilts, Dorset, Devon, Cornwall, Somerset, | 1.763 | 1.787 | 1.847 | 1.799 |

It has been already remarked, that the census of the United States does not enable us to judge of the mortality of the different States, but with all its inacuracies and imperfections it sufficiently indicates the truth of the position laid down,—that the mortality of a district, and the longevity of its inhabitants do not always preserve the same ratio. Northumberland, Durham, and the North Riding of Yorkshire, which are the counties, in England, most favourable to longevity, are not those in which the mortality is least; and the same general remark applies to Wales. By the same census, it appears, that the maximum longevity in Scotland was found to be in Ross and Cromarty, in which the proportion of persons aged from ninety to one hundred, was **34.39 in 20.000**; and of those aged one hundred and upwards, 9.22. In the shires of Inverness, and Argyle, the proportion of individuals, aged from ninety to one hundred, was 32.49, and 29.84, respectively, in 20.000. All these are mountainous districts.

The following table drawn up from the census of 1830, exhibits the longevity of different counties of Virginia,—Middlesex, Lancaster, and Princess Ann lying on the Chesapeake, and extremely subject to malarious disease. Perhaps they are unhealthy as any in the state. The county of Dinwiddie forms the border between the upper and lower country,—a part being below tide water, and a part above. The town of Petersburg lies within this county but it is not comprised in the estimate. The counties of Albemarle, Orange, and Culpeper lie at the base of the Blue Ridge, and are regarded as eminently salubrious. The table also contains the number of aged persons in Eastern and Western Virginia ;—that is in Virginia east, and west of the Blue Ridge ;—the former being the chief slaveholding portion, and of course comprising the whole of the lower country—the proverbially insalubrious. To these estimates are added the ratio of the aged—free, and enslaved—throughout the whole of the United States.

| | LONGEVITY. | | | | |
|---|---|---|---|---|---|
| | Proportion in 20,000. | | | | |
| | FREE. | | | | SLAVES. |
| | Above 70 and under 80. | Above 80 and under 90. | Above 90 and under 100 | 100 and upwards. | 100 and upwards. |
| Middlesex, | ...107 . | None. | None. | None. | ..18.7 ... |
| Lancaster, | ..141.6. | ...20.2 .. | None. | None. | ....7.38 . |
| Princess Ann, | ....60.3 | ...16 ..... | ....8........ | ...4........ | ..24.3 ... |
| Dinwiddie, | ..223.5. | ...75.8.... | ..11.3.... | ...3.8..... | ....2.66 . |
| Albemarle | ..254.4... | ...88 ...... | ..17.2.... | | ....3·4.... |
| Orange, | ..306.6... | ...96 ..... | ....9.13... | | ...20....... |
| Culpeper, | ..202.5... | ...63.1.... | ..11.6..., | ...1.66... | ..10.5.... |
| EASTERN VIRGINIA, | ..224.8... | ...63.5... | ..11.7 .... | ...1.43 .. | ..12.3.... |
| WESTERN VIRGINIA, | ..207 ..... | ...63.5... | ....9.5.... | ..1.7..... | ....7.8.... |
| UNITED STATES, | ..220.6 . | ...63.5... | ....8.67.. | ...1.02... | ..14.1.... |

The table exhibits the correctness of a remark, before made,—that in very unhealthy districts the rate of longevity may be low. This is strikingly evinced in the cases of Middlesex, and Lancaster; yet Princess Ann—a very malarious county—has more than the average proportion—free and slaves—above one hundred; and Dinwiddie, which is largely a prey to malarious disease, is above the average, as regards the free population,—below it, in the case of the enslaved. It is somewhat singular, too, that the proportion of slaves above one hundred, should be largest in one of the most unhealthy counties of the table. Throughout the United States the number of coloured persons, who are reported to attain the age of one hundred and upwards, bears a large ratio to the whites. It is obviously a matter of more difficulty to arrive at correct information regarding the precise ages of the enslaved than of the free; but the error, if any exist, can hardly amount to the difference established by the census; in which the proportion of slaves, that reach the age of one hundred and upwards, is to that of the free, in the ratio of 14. 1 to 1.02. This estimate, coupled with the unquestionable fact, that the slaves in the principal slave-holding states double their number in something less than twenty-eight years, is a sufficient answer to Hufeland, who, without the possibility of having data to guide him, affirms, that " the most terrific mortality reigns amongst the negro slaves of America, and amongst foundlings: a fifth or a sixth of the former dying every year,—that is nearly as much as the most horrible plague could destroy"!

We have said, that Middlesex, Kent, Surrey, and Warwick, exhibit the greatest mortality in the British " Population Abstract." This is, doubtless, owing to London, and its suburbs being situate in the first three; Birmingham in the last. Great towns have, indeed, been regarded as the " graves of mankind," and, even at the present day, when, by well adapted regulations, their salubrity has been surprisingly augmented, the mortality is much greater than in the rural districts. Fodéré affirms, that the tables of the probabilities of life indicate, that the value of life is one-third greater in non-marshy districts than in large cities; and Hufeland infers, that the mortality in cities may be estimated at 1 in 25 or 30; whilst in the country it is not more than 1 in 40 or 50. In Belgium, according to M. Quetelet (*Sur l' Homme.*, &c. or the English translation—

*A Treatise on Man*, &c. p. 27, Edinburgh, 1842) the following are the results of late inquiries—

|  | Population. | Average number of Deaths. | 1 Death to |
|---|---|---|---|
| Cities | 998.118 | 27.026 | 36.9 Inhabitants. |
| Country | 3.066.091 | 65.265 | 46.9 |

In a most valuable contribution to Hygiène lately made to both houses of Parliament by the direction of the Queen of Great Britain (*Report to her Majesty's principal Secretary of State for the Home Department from the Poor Law Commissioners, on an inquiry into the Sanitary Condition of the Labouring Population of Great Britain*, &c. &c., p. 157, Lond. 1842,) we have returns of the average ages of death amongst the different classes of people in Manchester and Rutlandshire, which strikingly exhibit the difference between the amount of civic and rural mortality.

|  | Average Age of Death | |
|---|---|---|
|  | In Manchester. Years. | In Rutlandshire. Years. |
| Professional persons and gentry, and their families . . . . | 38 | 52 |
| Tradesmen and their families (in Rutlandshire, farmers and graziers are included with shopkeepers) . . . . . | 20 | 41 |
| Mechanics, labourers and their families . . . . . | 17 | 38 |

The following table exhibits the same result as regards England (Mr. Farr, in *Third Annual Report of the Registrar-General of Births, Deaths, and Marriages in England*, p. 98, Lond. 1841.)

|  | Area in square miles. | Estimated population Jan. 1, 1839. | Deaths registered in two years. | Inhabitants to one square mile. | Annual mortality per cent. |
|---|---|---|---|---|---|
| County distr. | 17.254 | 3,359.323 | 129.628 | 206 | 1.821 |
| Town distr. | .747 | 3,769.002 | 197.474 | 5045 | 2.620 |

From the same report it appears, that the diseases chiefly incidental to childhood are twice as fatal in the town districts as they are in the country.

|  | Deaths in 1.000.000 living in the | |
|---|---|---|
|  | Country. | Towns. |
| By Hydrocephalus, Cephalitis | 419 | 1071 |
| Convulsions, Teething | 942 | 2586 |
| Pneumonia | 905 | 2028 |
| Small-pox, Measles, Scarlatina, Hooping-cough, Croup | 1999 | 4004 |

The deaths by several diseases of old age, were almost as numerous in the towns as in the country: asthma—probably not always nervous asthma—is, however, an exception.

|  | Deaths in 1.000.000 living in the | |
|---|---|---|
|  | Country. | Towns. |
| Old Age | 2446 | 1922 |
| Paralysis | 333 | 334 |
| Apoplexy | 374 | 409 |
| Asthma | 182 | 645 |

These are mere approximations. The fact of the much greater salubrity of rural than of town existence is, however, unquestionable.

The following has been given as the comparative annual mortality of some of the chief cities of this country, and of Europe.

| | | |  | | |
|---|---|---|---|---|---|
| Philadelphia, | - - | 1 in 45-68 | Geneva, | - - | 1 in 43. |
| Glasgow, | - - | 1 in 44. | Boston, | - - | 1 in 41.26 |
| Manchester, | - - | 1 in 44. | Baltimore, | - - | 1 in 41. |
| London, | - - | 1 in 40. | Nice & Palermo, | - | 1 in 31. |
| New York, | - - | 1 in 37.83 | Madrid, | - - | 1 in 29. |
| St. Petersburg, | - - | 1 in 37. | Naples, | - - | 1 in 28. |
| Charleston, | - - | 1 in 36.50 | Brussels, | - - | 1 in 26. |
| Leghorn, | - - | 1 in 35 | Rome, | - - | 1 in 25. |
| Berlin, | - - | 1 in 34. | Amsterdam, | - | 1 in 24. |
| Saint Louis, | - - | 1 in 33. | Vienna, | - - | 1 in 22½. |
| Paris, Lyons, Strasburg, and Barcelona, | - - | 1 in 32. | | | |

It is extremely doubtful, whether we ought to deduce any positive or relative inferences from such tables, unless we knew that the same mode of computation was always adopted. The mortality of the different towns of this country, with the exception of Baltimore, is given on the authority of the *Journal of Health*, (vol. i. p. 271,) which professes to have obtained it from "authentic documents." Its statement, however, respecting Baltimore, is erroneous, as the Author discovered on investigation; and it is equally probable, that some of the others are not more to be relied on. The population of Baltimore, in the year 1830—when the paragraph was published in the *Journal of Health*—was 80,990, according to the United States' census, and the number of interments, according to the published report, was 2,086. Of these 112 were stillborn; so if we include the stillborn, the deaths were in proportion to the population, as 1 to 38.82; and, if we reject them, as 1 to 41; yet the mortality of the city is stated, in the "Journal," as high as 1 in 35.44. The mortality of Saint Louis is on the authority of a recent writer. (V. J. Fourgeaud, *Saint Louis, Med. and Surg. Journ.*, March 15, 1844.)

The greater degree of mortality assigned to cities not very remote from each other, as to New York,—and it probably applies to Baltimore to a less degree,—over that of Philadelphia, may be partly accounted for by the greater influx of emigrants to those towns, most of whom belong to the lower classes of society; and of these a large proportion, especially of the emigrants from Ireland, are in the deepest indigence, exposed consequently to every privation, and too many of them grossly intemperate.

But how are we to explain the great difference between the mortality of the town and that of the country? The probability seems to be, that it is chiefly owing to the confined, and deteriorated atmosphere of the town acting in a manner directly unfavourable to human life; in other words, as a deleterious agent,—a morbid poison. All living bodies, when crowded together, deteriorate the air so much as to render it unfit for the maintenance of the healthy function. If animals be kept crowded together in ill-ventilated apartments, they speedily sicken. Fowls become attacked with pep, and sheep with a disease peculiar to them if they be too closely folded. The strongest support, however, of the view, that looks upon this

> "Nauseous mass
> Of all obscene, corrupt, offensive things,"

as a morbid poison, is the astonishing mortality in towns amongst children under five years of age. Of 4.629 deaths amongst the labouring classes in Manchester, in the year 1840, the proportion at different ages was as follows:—

| | | |
|---|---|---|
| Under five years of age | - - - | 2.649 or 1 in $1\frac{7}{10}$ |
| Above 5 and under 10 | - - - | 215 or 1 in 22 |
| Above 10 and under 15 | - - - | 107 or 1 in 43 |
| Above 15 and under 20 | - - - | 135 or 1 in 34 |

From the mode in which the London bills of mortality were formerly kept, they could not be depended upon as registers of individual diseases: they were not drawn up by medical practitioners, but by the parish clerks on the report of two old women in every parish, called *searchers*. Still they may be esteemed sufficiently accurate as registers of ages. At the present day, however, an admirable system prevails: registers are regularly kept as accurately as circumstances permit, and are published at stated periods by the Registrar-General; from whom we have already had some most valuable reports.

In the following table, formed from the London bills for a single year, the proportion of deaths, at different periods of life, is stated. The whole number of deaths amounted to 23,525.

| *Of these there died.* | | *Per cent.* |
|---|---|---|
| Under 2 years, | 6,710 | or 28.52 |
| Between 2 and 5, | 2,347 | or 9.97 |
| " 5 and 10, | 1,019 | or 4.33 |
| " 10 and 20, | 949 | or 4.03 |
| " 20 and 30, | 1,563 | or 6.64 |
| " 30 and 40, | 1,902 | or 8.08 |
| " 40 and 50, | 2,093 | or 8.89 |
| " 50 and 60, | 2,094 | or 8.89 |
| " 60 and 70, | 2,153 | or 9.15 |
| " 70 and 80, | 1,843 | or 7.83 |
| " 80 and 90, | 749 | or 3.18 |
| " 90 and 100, | 95 | or 0.40 |
| " 101, | 1 | or 0.0042 |
| " 108, | 2 | or 0.0084. |

On the 23.525, consequently, 9,057 or about 38.5 per cent. died under five years of age. Yet great as this proportion is, it was much more considerable at the commencement of the last century. In Paris, during the year 1818, the number of deaths amounted to 22,421, whereof 3,942, or 17.58 per cent. were children under the age of one year; and 5,576 or 24.86 per cent. died before the expiration of the second. In Philadelphia, during a period of twenty years, ending January 1st, 1827, the proportion of deaths of children, under a year old, to the whole number, was rather more than a fifth; and of those from birth to two years rather less than a third. The deaths of children under two years of age were as 1 to 11 of the whole number of children.

The following table exhibits the proportion of deaths at different ages, compared with the total number of deaths, in the city of Philadelphia and the Liberties, on an average of ten years, from 1821 to 1830 inclusive, on the authority of Dr. Gouverneur Emerson, (*American Journal of the Medical Sciences*, for November, 1831,) who has published some valuable remarks on the medical statistics of Philadelphia; and in Baltimore, from the average of returns by the Health Office, for the years 1829, 1830, 1831, and 1833, as deduced by the Author—the year 1832, during which the cholera committed its ravages in the city, being rejected. In both, the stillborn are excluded.

| AGES. | PHILADELPHIA. | BALTIMORE. |
|---|---|---|
| Under 1 year | 22.7 | 24.11 |
| From 1 to 2 years | 8.6 | 8.55 |
| " 2 to 5 " | 7.3 | 11.18 |
| " 5 to 10 " | 4 | 5. |
| " 10 to 20 " | 5 | 6.3 |
| " 20 to 30 " | 12 | 9.87 |
| " 30 to 40 " | 12 | 10.58 |
| " 40 to 50 " | 10 | 8.88 |
| " 50 to 60 " | 7.2 | 5.78 |
| " 60 to 70 " | 5 | 4.5 |
| " 70 to 80 " | 3.5 | 3. |
| " 80 to 90 " | 1.9 | 1.67 |
| " 90 to 100 " | 0.5 | 0.26 |
| " 100 to 110 " | 0.09 | 0.18 |
| " 110 to 120 " | 0.013 | |

The cholera infantum is the scourge of our cities during the summer months, whilst in country situations it is comparatively rare. Dr. Rush, asserted, that he never knew but one instance of an infant being affected with the disease, which had been carried into the country to avoid it; and it is always found to prevail most in crowded alleys, and in the filthiest and impurest habitations.

"By far the greatest proportion of the annual sickness and mortality of ordinary seasons," says Dr. Emerson, "is furnished by the narrow, and confined alleys and courts, existing in various parts of the town (Philadelphia.) The low terms upon which the small houses and rooms in such places can be obtained, causes them to be literally crowded with a class of population, for the most part negligent of cleanliness, and it can occasion no surprise, that there should be a great disparity between the proportions of sickness and mortality among these, compared with that which takes place in the portion living in larger dwellings, having a freer circulation of air. The difference just mentioned, though sufficiently obvious in adults, is most lamentably conspicuous among children. Notwithstanding the great numbers of these which die annually of cholera, we feel ourselves warranted in asserting, that deaths from this disease are rare in houses with large and well-aired apartments. To one who, in the capacity of physician to a dispensary or other charity, has been engaged in the arduous duties of attending the poor in their uncomfortable abodes, evidences of our assertions must be abundantly familiar. The numerous instances wherein the mercenary calculations of individuals have tempted them to put up nests of contracted tenements in courts or alleys admitting but little air, and yet subjected to the full influence of heat, has often induced us to wish that there could be some public regulations by which the evil might be checked. Mankind have inhabited cities long enough to know from severe experience, that there are certain limits to the denseness of population which, when passed, always lead to disease and mortality." To remedy this source of mischief, Dr. Emerson judiciously suggests, that a law should be passed by which the undue crowding of population might be prevented, and the number, and size of dwellings be duly regulated. "There are at present," he adds, "municipal regulations intended as a protection against conflagration, by designating the materials of which houses shall be constructed; and if such precautions be deemed so important when property is the consideration, of how much more consequence would be those for the preservation of health and life."

Such a law would doubtless be productive of incalculable advantage. Perhaps one of the most signal blessings that ever befel the metropolis of Great Britain was the great fire in 1666, immediately succeeding the plague of the year before. The conflagration destroyed the narrow streets—so narrow that it was practicable to shake hands from the attic windows of opposite sides of the streets—gave occasion to a better system of ventilation and medical police, and was thus a more efficient agent than any quarantine regulations in preventing the recurrence of the plague, which has not visited London since that period.

It would appear that the young of the animal creation in general, but especially of the human species, require the respiration of pure air, otherwise they are apt to perish. Some curious experiments were instituted by the illustrious Jenner, and since his time by his biographer—Dr. Baron—which indicate, that if young animals be deprived of their open range, and especially if the character of their nourishment be modified, a foundation is laid for disorganization, and death. Dr. Baron placed a family of young rabbits in a confined situation, and fed them with coarse green food—such as cabbage and grass. They were perfectly healthy when put up. In about a month one of them died: the primary step of disorganization was evinced by a number of transparent vesicles, studded over the external surface of the liver. In another, which died nine days after, the disease had advanced to the formation of tubercles on the liver. The liver of a third, which died four days later still, had nearly lost its true structure, so universally was it pervaded with tubercles. Two days subsequently, a fourth died: many hydatids were attached to the lower surface of the liver. At this time Dr. Baron removed three young rabbits from the place where their companions had died to another situation, dry and clean, and to their proper, and accustomed food. The lives of these three were obviously saved by the change. He obtained similar results from experiments, of the same nature, performed on other animals.

There is some difficulty, however, in arriving at positive and satisfactory deductions from these experiments. How are we to determine, whether the confined and deteriorated air, or the loss of the ordinary free range, or of accustomed food, or all combined, produced the baneful effects? and this perplexity occurs, when we attempt to appreciate the effect of city air on the annual influx of residents from the country;—whether, for example, we are to refer the deaths to the new circumstances of diet, and exercise under

## GREATER SALUBRITY OF COUNTRIES. 117

which the stranger may be presumed to have been placed, or to the positive insalubrity of the

> "Chaos of eternal smoke
> And volatile corruption from the dead,
> The dying, sick'ning, and the living world."

But none of those difficulties environ us in investigating the causes of the excessive mortality of infants in cities, compared with that in the country. From the earliest moment of existence they have respired the same medium, and have been subjected to no changes. We are, consequently, forced to the conclusion, that the air of cities is unfavourable to their existence, and we can understand how it may be, to a certain extent, detrimental to the adult likewise.

A great change for the better has occurred, in modern times—in the salubrity not only of cities but of countries generally. Without going back to more ancient periods, we may affirm, that within the last century particularly, the value of life has gone on progressively, and rapidly improving. The experience of the United States would, we are satisfied, exhibit the truth of this assertion, were the requisite data attainable. The census, established from time to time in England, affords us, however, information of an unquestionable character. The first actual enumeration of the inhabitants was made in the year 1801. It gave to England, and Wales a population of 9,168,000, and a mortality of 204,434, or 1 in 44.8. The second was made in 1811. The population was then 10,502,900, and the mortality 1 in 50; the third which was made in 1821, gave a population of 12,218,500, and a mortality of 1 in 58, (See page 104.)

Again, in France, the annual deaths, were in 1781, 1 in 29; in 1802, 1 in 30; and in 1823, 1 in 40; and in Sweden, the mortality has decreased from 1 in 35 (1755 to 1775) to 1 in 48.

A like improvement has taken place in the health of most cities—"those sepulchres of the dead and hospitals of the living." The annual mortality of London, in 1700, was 1 in 25; in 1751, 1 in 21; and in 1801, and the four years preceding, 1 in 35; in 1811, 1 in 38; in 1821, 1 in 40:—the value of life having doubled in London within the last eighty years. In Paris, about the middle of the last century, the mortality was 1 in 25; a few years ago, about 1 in 32; and it has been estimated, that in the 14th century it was 1 in 16 or 17. Berlin improved in salubrity during 60 or 70 years, from 1 in 28, to 1 in 34. The mortality in Manchester, about the middle of the last century was 1 in 25; in 1770, 1 in 28; forty years afterwards—in 1811—the annual deaths had diminished to 1 in 44; and in 1821 they seem to have been still fewer, although the population has quadrupled within the sixty years through which the deaths have so diminished. In the middle of last century, the mortality of Vienna was rated at 1 in 20. It has not, however, improved in the same ratio as some of the other European cities; according to recent calculations it was even 1 in 22.5, or about twice the proportion of Philadelphia, or Glasgow. This is ascribed to the faulty political and municipal arrangements for which Austria is almost proverbial. One city only seems to have retrograded, owing, perhaps, to declining commerce, and political vicissitudes. In 1777, the ratio of deaths at Amsterdam was 1 in 27, a period at which it was one of the healthiest and most prosperous cities of Europe. The deaths were lately 1 in 24; and the city is one of the least healthy and flourishing seaports. It is difficult indeed, to conceive how it could be otherwise than unhealthy, seated, as it is, on a malarious soil in common with almost every other city of Holland. At Geneva, good bills of mortality have been kept since 1549, and the results are in the highest degree gratifying to the philanthropist. It seems, that at the time of the Reformation half the children born did not reach six years of age. In the seventeenth century, the probability of life was about $11\frac{1}{2}$ years: in the eighteenth century it increased to above 27 years. The probability of life to a citizen of Geneva has consequently become five times greater in the space of about three hundred years.

The following table has been formed by Mr. Edward Mallet,

|  | Years, Months and Days. | | | Proportionate rate of increase as compared with the end of 16th century. |
|---|---|---|---|---|
| Towards the end of the 16th century the probabilities of life, were to every individual born— | 8 | 7 | 26. | 100. |
| In the 17th century. | 13. | 3. | 16. | 153 or 53 per cent. |
| 1701-1750 | 27. | 9. | 13. | 321 or 221 |
| 1750-1800 | 31. | 3. | 5. | 361 or 261 |
| 1801-1813 | 40. | 8. | 0. | 470 or 370 |
| 1814-1833 | 45. | 0. | 29. | 521 or 421 |

from the Genevese registers. (*Sanitary Report from the Poor Law Commissioners*, p. 175, Lond. 1842.)

Other satisfactory data, to the same purport, are contained in the work of Dr. Bissett Hawkins, to which reference has already been made; and the British Insurance offices afford similar evidence. It was found in 1800, by Mr. Morgan the actuary, that the deaths, which had occurred among 83,000 persons insured during thirty years in the *London Equitable*, were only in the proportion of 2 to 3 of what had been anticipated; that is,

Between the ages of 10 and 20 . . as . . 1 to 2
                20 " 30 . . as . . 1 to 2
                30 " 40 . . as . . 3 to 5
                40 " 50 . . as . . 3 to 5
                50 " 60 . . as . . 5 to 7
                60 " 80 . . as . . 4 to 5

a fact, which exhibits the immense profit, that must have been derived by such establishments, almost all of which are founded on old Northampton bills of mortality; and were continued when manifestly inapplicable to the existing order of things. The following table, in which the rates of mortality according to the Carlisle and Northampton bills, and the experience of the Equitable Society, are ranged in parallel columns will show this more strikingly than words.

| | | | ACCORDING TO THE | | |
|---|---|---|---|---|---|
| Out of | Who attain the age of | There die before the age of | Carlisle table. | Experience of the Equitable Society. | Northampton table. |
| PERSONS. | YEARS. | YEARS. | PERSONS. | PERSONS. | PERSONS. |
| 6,460 | 10 | 20 | 370 | 309 | 618 |
| 6.090 | 20 | 30 | 448 | 443 | 886 |
| 5.642 | 30 | 40 | 567 | 579 | 965 |
| 5,075 | 40 | 50 | 678 | 652 | 1,086 |
| 4,397 | 50 | 60 | 754 | 900 | 1,260 |
| 3.643 | 60 | 80 | 2,690 | 2.244 | 2,805 |

Mr. Babbage, one of the most distinguished mathematicians of the age, pronounced, a few years ago, the Northampton tables to be erroneous throughout a large part in the proportion of 2 to 1. It will be evident, therefore, that the annual premium, which was *equitable* at the commencement even of the present century, must be far otherwise now. Many years ago, Mr. Finlayson drew up the following table, to exhibit the improvement in the value of life that had taken place between two corresponding periods of the seventeenth and eighteenth centuries; and if it had been calculated for the present time the results would have been still more remarkable, as vaccination has been chiefly introduced since the commencement of the present century. This alone, if pushed to the extent of exterminating small-pox, Mr. Milne conceives, would diminish the mortality from 1 in 40 to 1 in 43.5, or nearly 9 per cent.

| Ages. | Mean duration of Life, reckoning from 1693 | 1789. | So that the increase of Vitality was in the inverse ratio of 100 to |
|---|---|---|---|
| YEARS. | YEARS. | YEARS. | |
| 5 | 41.05 | 51.20 | 125 |
| 10 | 38.93 | 48.28 | 124 |
| 20 | 31.91 | 41.33 | 130 |
| 30 | 27.57 | 36.09 | 131 |
| 40 | 22.67 | 29.70 | 131 |
| 50 | 17.31 | 22.57 | 130 |
| 60 | 12.29 | 15.52 | 126 |
| 70 | 7.44 | 10.39 | 140 |

The following table from the *Fourth Annual Report of the Registrar-General* of England (p. 20, Lond. 1842) is illustrative of the same subject.

Comparative table of the Annual Mortality per cent. in England, in the Metropolis, and in Manchester; with the mortality on which the Northampton, Swedish and Carlisle Tables were calculated.

| Age. | Mortality—mean of Males and Females. | | | | Mortality of the entire Population. | | |
|---|---|---|---|---|---|---|---|
| | England 4 years 1838-41 | Metropolis. | | Manchester and Salford 4 years 1838-41 | Northampton | 21 years 1755-75 Sweden. | 9 years 1779-87 Carlisle. |
| | | 4 years. | 1 year 1841. | | | | |
| 0—5 | 6.607 | 9.118 | 8.238 | 13.171 | 14.729 | 9.009 | 8.228 |
| 5—10 | .935 | 1.291 | 1.024 | 1.540 | 1.947 | 1.416 | 1.023 |
| 10—15 | .550 | .502 | .431 | .664 ⎱ | .990 | .709 | .585 |
| 15—20 | .776 | .657 | .595 | .913 ⎰ | | | |
| 20—30 | .981 | .912 | .850 | 1.192 | 1.321 | .918 | .754 |
| 30—40 | 1.148 | 1.399 | 1.255 | 1.654 | 1.772 | 1.220 | 1.059 |
| 40—50 | 1.433 | 2.041 | 1.809 | 2.339 | 2.375 | 1.741 | 1.434 |
| 50—60 | 2.139 | 3.284 | 3.016 | 3.493 | 3.183 | 2.641 | 1.827 |
| 60—70 | 4.049 | 5.890 | 5.609 | 6.187 | 4.950 | 4.809 | 4.125 |
| 70—80 | 8.737 | 11.665 | 11.472 | 12.180 | 10.195 | 10.232 | 8.299 |
| 80—90 | 19.083 | 22.519 | 21.563 | 21.062 | 20.467 | 20.777 | 17.563 |
| 90—100 | 34.758 | 31.496 | 34.346 | 40.008 | 39.620 | | |
| 100 and upwards | 45.245 | 53.481 | 43.703 | 77.757 | | 39.410 | 28.444 |
| All ages. | 2.227 | 2.676 | 2.437 | 3.438 | 4.055 | 2.890 | 2.500 |

It is not easy to assign exact causes for the great improvement, which has taken place in the salubrity of many countries, within the last century. It may be with probability referred to the more ample supply of food, clothing, and fuel; better habits; greater attention to cleanliness and ventilation, and improved medical practice. The Island of Great Britain has been exempt, for upwards of a century and a half, from those wide-spreading epidemic, and contagious diseases, which had, from time to time, scattered gloom, and desolation over the whole country. Some more efficient causes of exemption must exist than the quarantine regulations. These probably lie in the intrinsic circumstances, just referred to. The surprising diminution in the mortality, within the last thirty years, is doubtless to be ascribed, in part, to the introduction of vaccination. There is, however, one cause peculiarly interesting to this community, and on which we must briefly touch, in closing our observations on this topic. It is an old and prevalent opinion, that poverty is conducive to longevity; and that health is enjoyed to a greater extent among the poorer classes of society than among the rich. The very opposite is the fact. Wherever accurate statistical information has been obtained, it has been clearly shown, that where misery prevails, *there* will be found the largest share of mortality.

According to M. Villermé, (*Tableau de l'Etat Physique et Morale des Ouvriers employés dans les Manufactures de Coton, de Laine et de Soie*, ii. 245, Paris, 1840) in the city of Amiens, men of the age of from 20 to 21 have been most frequently found unfit for military service, owing to stature, constitution and health, when they belonged to the poorer or manufacturing class (*class ouvrière de la fabrique*.) To obtain 100 men fit for military service, 193 conscripts were required of the easy, and 343 of the poorer classes.

He has ascertained, moreover, that whenever the people have suffered from any cause, the deaths have increased correspondently; the births have decreased, and the mean duration of life has been shortened; whilst in times of prosperity the results have been directly opposite. The inferences he draws from his investigations are; *First*, that the mortality in France, and, consequently, the mean duration of life, is very different among those in easy circumstances from what it is among the poor, and destitute. *Secondly*, that this difference is so great, that in some of the wealthy departments, such as Calvados, Orne, and Sarthe, the deaths are only 1 in 50; whereas among the inhabitants of the 12th *Arrondissement* of Paris,—in which, according to M. D'Arcet, (*Amélioration du Régime alimentaire des Hôpitaux*, p. 16. Paris, 1844,) of 83.000 persons, 16.732 are registered poor,—the proportion is 1 in 24 and a fraction. In the first *Arrondissement* of that city, they amount to 1 in 41. In Philadelphia, when the deaths amongst the whites, according to Dr. Emerson, were 1 in 42.3; amongst the blacks, they were 1 in 21.7; and in the Sanitary Report of the Poor Law Commissioners of Great Britain, (p. 153, Lond. 1842,) it is stated, that in one district of the same town, the mortality was only 1 in every 57 of the population; whilst in another it was 1 in every 28. But the operation of noxious influences connected with locality is more signally shown in the following table, by Mr. Farr, of the mean annual mortality of females, in twelve metropolitan districts, during the two years and a half ending December 31st, 1839.

| Districts. | Annual Deaths, 1 in |
|---|---|
| Hackney | 57.87 |
| St. George, Hanover Square | 57.05 |
| Camberwell | 55.34 |
| Islington | 50.03 |
| Rotherhithe | 38.58 |
| Clerkenwell | 38.54 |
| St. Luke | 38.49 |
| Greenwich | 38.42 |
| St. George, Southwark | 33.77 |
| East and West London | 33.50 |
| St. Giles and St. George | 33.46 |
| Whitechapel | 28.15 |

The conservative tendency of easy circumstances is likewise evinced, in the inferior degree of mortality and disease among persons insured at the various life offices. We have stated, that in the Equitable life office Mr. Morgan found, that the actual deaths, which had occurred among eighty-three thousand persons insured, during thirty years, were in the proportion of only 2 to 3 of what had been anticipated; and in this case the mortality among the women was still less than among the men. The annual average of deaths among the persons insured at the Equitable, from 1800 to 1820, was only about 1 in 81.5. Of one thousand members of the University club, only thirty-five died in three years, which is a still lower rate, being about 1 in 86 annually. Of ten thousand pupils, who, in different years, passed through Pestalozzi's institution in Switzerland, it is asserted that not one died during his residence there.

What gratifying prospects are afforded by these estimates to the population of this Union! Blessed, as we are, with a government whose sole object must be the happiness, and prosperity of the States, and where oppression is impossible; with equal laws, and an extent and capability of country such that none need perish through want; but, on the contrary, where each, with due temperance and industry, may enjoy affluence, compared with the wretched lower classes of many portions of the old world! "So intimate a connexion,"—says Dr. Hawkins, (*Op. cit.* p. 232,) from whom some of these facts have been taken,—" subsists between political changes and the public health, that wherever feudal distinctions have been abolished, wherever the artisan or peasant has been released from arbitrary enactments, there, also, the life of the lower classes has acquired a new vigour; and it is certain, that even bodily strength, and the power of enduring hardships are divided among the nations of the earth in a proportion relative to their prosperity and civilization." And he judiciously adds—" If political and moral circumstances actually possess so preponderant an influence on the production of disease, and on the guidance of its fatality, it seems to be incumbent on our profession to study their progress, and to profit by their results. A peculiar set of diseases appears to belong to every age, and it may be almost affirmed, that there is also a mode of treatment adapted to every age. But the science of medicine, purified from obsolete mysteries, no longer idly promises to extend existence beyond the term originally assigned to it, and only endeavours to conduct the feeble and the unfortunate in safety to the natural boundaries of their present being. And altogether we must conclude, that the causes which shorten life are generally those which render it miserable; and that wherever a people enjoys a higher degree of prosperity, of rational freedom, and of moral dignity, there also will a greater number of individuals reap the full harvest of their years."

Such are some of the multitude of data, which exhibit the powerful influence, that country, or locality exerts on human health. We have said, that the mode in which its agency is exerted is altogether beyond our appreciation. It acts in a similar manner to those influences, that occasion the various endemic diseases to which reference has been made; that develope a widely spreading pestilence at times in the most healthy districts; and that cause the general salubrity of such districts. It would have to be appreciated by the same process of investigation, which should indicate to us why marshy districts produce ague; why the same districts, when drained, should be found to have experienced an increase in the number of consumptive cases, and why, as in the case of Portsea, these same districts, still continuing drained, should have a recurrence of ague after the lapse of a considerable period; why, again, consumption is comparatively unfrequent in the torrid zone, and acute diseases rarely experienced in Australia. How are we to account for the great difference in the mortality of counties, situate so close to each other as some of those in England and Wales, and for the surprising preponderance of Wales in point of salubrity? It cannot be presumed, that the Cambrians are better acquainted with the means of preserving health than their English neighbours; or that even if better acquainted, they are less prone to commit those excesses, which have been regarded as the great causes of diminished health in particular situations.

We may conclude, then, that a great and ever-acting cause of the difference of salubrity of countries is seated in the locality; that is, in the earth that forms them, and in the air, that circulates above them; and although we may be able to slightly modify the condition of the former, and improve the circulation of the latter, we can rarely succeed in annihilating either of those influences.

We have before alluded to the principal notions, entertained by certain writers on the subject of medium temperature, and endeavoured to show, that it is neither well adapted for vegetable nor animal existence. It is probable, indeed, as was then remarked, that the different barometric, thermometric, hygrometric, electric, and other vicissitudes, when within due bounds, are actually conducive to health. Who, that has breathed the deteriorated air of the crowded city—less subject, certainly, to thermometric vicissitudes than that of the country, and deficient in the intensity of light to which the rural resident is perpetually exposed—has not experienced the cheerful, invigorating effects of a short visit to the pure air of the country, where all the physical circumstances of the atmosphere, which are susceptible of modification, are changed? What is this but a vicissitude? Yet how advantageous the results! The spirits are exhilarated; nervous depression, produced by monotony, rapidly disappears, with the ills dependent thereon; and all is buoyancy, and elasticity, where languor, and lassitude before predominated; the civic etiolation or blanching, marked upon the countenance, vanishes; and the ruddiness of rude health usurps its place; the appetite becomes augmented, and the powers of nutrition are largely increased,—as indicated by the increase of weight, which follows a sojourn of even a week or two in a pure salubrious region. "On the continent (of Europe,)" observes a recent writer, whose remarks are applicable, perhaps to an equal extent to our cities—"the beneficial effects of change of air are duly estimated; and the inhabitants of this country (England,) and more especially of this metropolis (London,) are now becoming fully sensible of its value. The vast increase in the size of our watering places, of late years, and the deserted state of London during several months, are sufficient proofs, not to mention others, of the increasing conviction among the public in general, that, for the preservation of health, it is necessary, from time to time, to change the relaxing, I may say, deteriorating air of London, for the more pure and invigorating air of the country. This, indeed, is the best, if not the only remedy for that terrible malady which preys upon the vitals, and stamps its hues upon the countenance of almost every permanent resident in this great city, and which may be justly termed the *Cachexia Londinensis*. When the extent of benefits, which may be derived from this remedy, both on the physical and moral constitution, is duly estimated, no person, whose circumstances permit him to avail himself of it, will fail to do so." (Sir James Clark, *The Sanative Influence of Climate*, &c. p. 3, Lond. 1841.)

A great deal of this effect is caused simply by *change of air*, or by the altered feelings and functions, produced by a modification in different atmospheric influences; so that the change from a better to a worse air has even been found serviceable. In Edinburgh, the inhabitants of the most airy parts of the New Town frequently send their children, when labouring under hooping-cough, to the Cowgate—a filthy street, which runs at right angles under one of the largest thoroughfares in the Old Town, and in which, at a certain hour of the night, the inhabitants eject all the offensive accumulations from their houses, to be washed away by the water of the reservoirs let on for the purpose.

In all diseases, in which the affection appears to be kept up, in some measure, by habit, and especially in those that implicate the nervous system, the beneficial effects of change of air are proverbial, and are acquiesced in by all observers. There is one writer, indeed, more distinguished for the quaintness of his style, and the eccentricity of his notions, than for the profoundness of his hygienic precepts, who has inculcated a contrary doctrine. "Well then," he remarks, "in nine cases out of ten, to change the atmosphere we have been long accustomed to is as unadvisable as a change in the food we have been long used to; unless other circumstances make it so, than the mere change of place:"—and again, "the opulent individual, who has been long indulged with a home comfortably arranged to his own humour, must beware of leaving it during any indisposition; it would be almost as desperate a procedure as to eject an oyster from his shell." (Kitchener, *Directions for invigorating and prolonging life*, &c. p. 108. New York edition, 1831.)

The multitudes of valetudinarians, who annually leave their habitations to visit the watering places of this country, and of Europe, and who return to their homes in the enjoyment of health, and full of confidence in the virtues of the waters near which they may have resided, and of which they may or may not have partaken, furnish satisfactory replies to these musings. It is probable, indeed, that a great portion of the salutary effects, ascribed to the waters, is dependent upon change of air, and other extraneous circumstances. Long before the citizen of one of our Atlantic towns reaches the Alleghany springs of Virginia, he has an earnest of the advantages he is about to derive from change of air; and many a valetudinarian finds himself almost restored during the journey, fatiguing as it is, through the mountain regions, which have to be crossed before he reaches the White Sulphur, in Green-Brier county. There is a large mass, too, of individuals, who cannot drink that water with impunity, and who consequently are indebted for their improvement chiefly to change of air, but somewhat also to varied scenery and society, absence from cares of business, and to greater regularity of living, perhaps, than they have been accustomed to. In making these observations, we do not mean to affirm, that mineral waters, as in the case of the valuable spring in question, may not occasionally be important agents in the cure of disease; but, taking invalids in general, we are satisfied that more is dependent upon change of air than upon the administration of the waters. The inhabitant of one of the Atlantic cities, and of most of the districts to the east of the Blue Ridge, removes from a hot atmosphere to one which is comparatively cool, and where all the diseases, that are common to hot and malarious climates, are extremely unfrequent, and many of them unknown. The advantage is obvious. He escapes the diseases, which might have attacked him had he remained through the summer in his accustomed locality; and hence the wealthy families of lower Virginia are in the habit of spending those months in the mountain regions, in which they are especially liable to disease in their own malarious districts.

We can thus understand the reputation acquired by the inert Bath, and Matlock waters of England, the latter of which has scarcely any solid ingredient; and yet what crowds flock to these agreeable watering places;—to the former for the perpetual amusements, that keep the mind engaged, and cause it to react beneficially on the corporeal or mental malady; to the latter for the enjoyment of the beauties of nature for which Derbyshire is so celebrated. It is obvious, that were such waters bottled and sent to a distance, so that the invalid might drink them at his own habitation, the charm would be dissolved. The garnitures—more important in this case than the dish—would be wanting, and the banquet would be vapid, and without enjoyment, or benefit. Less than twenty years ago, amidst the bubbles, that were engaging the minds, and money of the English public, it was proposed to carry sea-water by pipes to London, in order that the citizens might have the advantage of sea-bathing, without the inconvenience of going many miles after it. Had the scheme been carried into effect, the benefits from metropolitan sea-bathing would not have exhibited themselves in any respect comparable to those of the same agent employed at Brighton or Margate.

It would seem, therefore, that a mere change of the physical circumstances of the atmosphere, in which we are habitually placed, is advantageous to the economy, and that the vital forces act with increased energy whenever we leave a locality to which we have been long accustomed, and where the functions are executed under the influence of unvaried excitants, and pass to one differing essentially from it. Nor is it always necessary, as we have seen, that this difference should be extensive. Sir James Clark, (*Op. cit.* p. 315) remarks, that notwithstanding the uniformity of temperature, which prevails among many of the West India Islands, the effect of a change from one to another is often very remarkable in improving the health,—a fact frequently observed, on a large scale, among the British troops stationed in the West Indies; and he considers, that one of the most powerful means of diminishing the sickness among the troops in that climate would be to remove them frequently from one healthy island to another. We shall see, hereafter, that a similar mutation is indispensable in our aliments,—where we may have been accustomed to variety,—and that if we be restricted to one only, however nutritious and wholesome it may appear intrinsically to be, sickness is apt to be induced.

Discrimination is, of course, necessary in prescribing change of air as a curative agent. It is inadmissible during the existence of acute affections in general, but when the violence of the disease has passed away, and when the inflammation—especially if of the mucous textures—has become chronic, we have no means to which we can have recourse, that are calculated to exert a more beneficial influence, under proper precautions, than a modification of the atmospheric influences surrounding the patient. Hence it is, that travelling, which combines change of air with proper exercise, is so salutary in chronic irritation of the mucous membrane of the intestines, and of the bronchia. Many of the cases, indeed, that have been looked upon as phthisis removed by this course, have been chronic bronchitis. When the patient,—as Sir James Clark (Art. *Change of Air*, in *Cyclopædia of Practical Medicine.* Amer. edit. Philad. 1844,) properly remarks,—in treating of the utility of change of air during convalescence, and the remark is equally appropriate to the states of disease just mentioned—resides in a crowded city, or other confined situation, the change is more urgently called for, and, under such circumstances, many cases of severe disease occur, complete restoration from which is not effected without its agency. The person, deprived of the benefit of such a measure, attains only to a degree of health inferior to that which he enjoyed before the occurrence of his disease; and the remainder of his life is often little better than a state of improved convalescence.

It is in such cases, that the inhabitants of our cities, convalescent from acute diseases, or labouring under chronic affections, kept up, as it were by habit, find so much advantage from a trip to our mountain regions, especially to the Trans-Alleghany Springs, where, as we have seen, every thing around them is modified: advantage is soon and signally apparent.

Of the good effects of change of air in hooping-cough, mention has already been made. These are most strikingly exemplified when it is had recourse to after the disease has continued for some time, and the febrile symptoms. which so often attend the first period, have passed away. The change from one room of the house to another appears to be salutary, and even, as we have before seen, from a pure air to one that is less so.

In every form of impaired digestive function, change of air can be employed with advantage, and when combined with travelling exercise, the benefits are marked. A recent writer, Dr. James Johnson, (*Op. cit.*) in pointing out the decided and obvious influence of travelling on the digestive function, and, through it, on the constitution at large, goes so far as to affirm his positive belief, that the most inveterate dyspepsia—where no organic disease has taken place—would be completely removed, by a journey of two or three thousand miles through Switzerland, Germany, or any other country, conducted on the principle of combining active with passive exercise in the open air, in such proportions as would suit the individual constitution, and the previous habits of life.

In states of the uterine system connected with atony, the exciting influence of new atmospheric conditions, new scenes, and occupations, are amongst our most valuable resources; and in dysmenorrhœa, become inveterate by habit, these influences will occasionally break in upon the morbid catenation; and if the female should marry, or, being married, should be fortunate enough to pass one period without suffering, she may become pregnant, and the resulting gestation may completely remove the mischief, by eradicating the morbid habit.

In most of the diseases affecting the nervous system, and especially in those often characterized by great mobility, and irritability,—epilepsy, chorea, hypochondriasis, &c.—the new impressions, excited by change of air, society, and scenery, are strikingly useful, especially if the diseases have been connected with a sedentary life in a confined situation. In all such cases, as Sir James Clark has observed, this is a remedy for which we have no adequate substitute. " But change of air," as the same writer judiciously adds, " is not more valuable as a remedy in the cure of disease, and its consequences, than as a preventive of disease, more especially in childhood and youth. At this tender and susceptible period of life, the rapid influence of the atmosphere in which we live, in deteriorating or improving the health, is very remarkable; a change of a few weeks from the country to a large town being often sufficient to change the ruddy, healthy child, into a pale, sickly-looking creature, and *vice versâ.* The comparative influence of a town and country air on the health of children is seen in a striking manner in the families of the higher ranks of society, who spend a considerable part of every year in town. Children should never be reared in large towns, when this can be avoided; and, when unavoidable, they should be sent, during a part at least of every summer, into the country, which, indeed, is the proper place for children, until their system has acquired sufficient strength to resist the injurious effects of city life. When they cannot have this advantage, we consider it the duty of the medical attendants of families to urge a temporary annual residence in the country, as essential to the health of children more particularly those who are delicate. How many neglect this invaluable means of improving the health of their offspring, who have it in their power, and would willingly adopt it, were they aware of its importance! So strongly, indeed, are we impressed with the value of this measure, from ample observation, that we consider parents resident in towns, who have the means of giving their family the advantage of country air, and neglect it, deficient in one of their chief duties. To young females, who, by the habits of society, are much more confined to the house than boys, a temporary annual residence in the country becomes a measure of still greater importance, and should be continued at least to the full period of their growth. We have reason to believe, that the advantages of country air to the young, and delicate, are not sufficiently appreciated by the profession, and we are therefore anxious to call their attention to it, that they may use their influence with the public, upon whose minds, if they succeed in impressing the full value of pure air, they will be the means of contributing greatly to the health of the rising generation." Such has long been the Author's impression, and for years he has acted upon it wherever it has been practicable. Independently of the signal benefits derived, by the young especially, from simple change of atmospheric influences, the large proportion of children who die under the age of two years, in towns, compared with the country, sufficiently exhibits, as we have before observed—that the air of towns acts upon them deleteriously, and hence the necessity for moving them into the country, —during the heats of summer, especially,—when the infantile mortality is greatest.

Analogous to the effect of change of air, produced by travelling, is that occasioned by those extensive displacements of large masses of air, that constitute winds. The primary effect of these is to remove all stagnant air, and to replace it by that which is more pure; and, accordingly, where endemic diseases have prevailed in a district, the occurrence of a high wind has been regarded as a favourable event, under the expectation, that the morbific emanations might be dispersed by it, and the endemic be in this manner arrested. Under such circumstances, the ventilation, thus forcibly effected, is doubtless advantageous; but as it does not remove the condition of the soil that gives rise to the noxious emanations, the good effects are only temporary.

It is manifest, that the impression made by any wind upon the human body must depend greatly upon the character of the air as to heat, dryness, and electricity, or according as it is modified, or not, by noxious emanations. If the wind be extremely cold, like the north-west wind of this continent during winter, it rapidly robs the system of its caloric, by fresh portions coming in contact with the body in rapid succession. In Parry's voyages to the Arctic regions, no more inconvenience was felt when the temperature was —51° Fahr. in calm weather, than when it was at 0 Fahr. during a breeze.

The character of the *Tramontana of* Italy, the *Maestro* or *Mistral* of Provence, and the *Bize* of Switzerland, resembles that of our north-west wind. "The Tramontane," says Dr. Johnson, (*Op. citat.* p. 296,) " comes down from the Alps, or Apennines, with such a voracious appetite for caloric, that it sucks the vital heat from every pore,—shrivels up the surface of the body,—impels the tide of the circulation with great violence, upon the internal organs, and endangers the lungs or whatever other structure happens to be the weakest in the living machine."

If the wind be cold and damp, like the east wind of England and of this country or our north-east wind, the system is liable to all the irregular action of capillaries, apt to be induced by cold, and dampness. It is the blast, too, which is felt most sensibly by the aguish, and by the convalescent from malarious, and other maladies. On the other hand, if it be hot, and damp, like the relaxing and oppressive *Sirocco* of Sicily and Italy, the nervous energy is impaired, or exhausted as it were; and all mental, and corporeal power appears to be annihilated. This enervating blast is supposed, by some, to be the same as the dread Simoom, tempered by its passage across the water, but loaded with watery vapours from the Mediterranean.

Of the dry Harmattan, of Africa, we have already spoken. It resembles the Chamseen, or Khamseen, a south-west wind which blows three or four days, between July 15, and August 15, in Egypt, Arabia, and on the Persian Gulph.

The notion of the influence, exerted by the sun, moon, and the various celestial luminaries on the animal body, has nearly expired with astrology. There are still some, however, who regard certain healthy functions, which are distinguished by *Periodicity*, or by their regular supervention after determinate intervals, to the sun, or the moon—according to the interval that may elapse between the accessions. Menstruation is one of these functions. As its recurrence corresponds to a revolution of the moon around the earth, it has been presumed, that it may be connected with lunar influence; but before this solution can be received, it must be shown, that the effect of lunar attraction is different in the various relative positions of the moon and earth. There is no day in the month, in which numerous females do not commence this function; and whilst it is beginning with some, it is at its height or decline with others. The hypothesis of lunar influence, must, therefore, be rejected.

Dr. Foster, in his work "*On Atmospheric Phenomena*," is one of the latest writers who have dwelt on the effect of the different phases of the moon on human health; and his remarks exhibit the loose kind of evidence on which the belief rests. "There is yet," says he, " another extremely curious circumstance about the effect of the place of the moon. It is well known to physicians that there are periods of greater and lesser irritability in the human body; and that, at the irritable periods, many diseases occur to which the patient may be predisposed : now it seems, by the result of long continued observation, that these periods of irritability oftener occur about the new and the full of the moon, than about the quarters. Every body almost must know from his own experience, that he gets up in the morning on particular days less disposed to be pleased, and with more general irritability than usual; these days also happen nearer to the times of the full moon, or of the new moon, than that of either quadrature. To bring this observation into a smaller compass, and to confirm it by future remarks, I have proposed to meteorologists to divide the lunar revolution into four equal parts or weeks, in the middle of each of which one of the changes of the moon shall take place. By doing this, we shall find the greater proportion of headaches, and nervous diseases of many kinds, to occur in those weeks, in the middle of which the opposition and conjunction of the moon shall take place. Moreover, the sudden occurrence of east winds, so obnoxious to nervous persons, seems to me to produce more sudden effects when they occur near to the conjunction or opposition of the moon."—Now, there is not an affirmation in this extract but requires confirmation; and we can with far more propriety appeal to the universal " experience" of those physicians, who are not wedded to the notion of lunar influence, in the very cases alluded to by Dr. Foster, to negative the positions he has assumed.

Not many years ago, it would have been esteemed culpably skeptical to disbelieve in the effect, imagined to be produced by the full moon on the insane, or as they have been termed—from this very belief in lunar influence—*Lunatics*. The notion has even been incorporated into the legal definition of this deplorable condition. "A Lunatic," says Sir Wm. Blackstone, "is, indeed, properly one that hath lucid intervals, sometimes enjoying his senses, and sometimes not, and that *frequently depending upon the changes of the moon.*" Yet it has been most unequivocally established, by careful and accurate observation in large insane establishments, that if the light of the full moon be excluded, the patients are no more liable to exacerbations in their disorder at these, than at other periods. Dr. Haslam—a well known writer on insanity—affirms, that he kept an exact register of cases for more than two years, but without finding in any instance, that the aberrations of the intellect corresponded with, or were influenced by, the vicissitudes of the moon. The results of the observations of Dr. Woodward, at the Massachusetts Insane Hospital, and of the Author at the Philadelphia Hospital, correspond with those of Haslam; and M. Esquirol—the distinguished physician to La Salpêtrière—states, that he cannot confirm the long prevalent opinion regarding lunar influence. The insane he found certainly to be more agitated about the full moon, but so they are about the break of day every morning. He therefore properly conceives, that light is the cause of the increased excitement at both these periods; and he states that the stimulus of light frightens some lunatics, pleases others, but agitates all.

Equally unfounded is the notion of solar influence on the same class of unfortunates, at the summer solstice especially. The whole of the excitant effect is owing to the length of the days, and the oppressive heat that usually prevails at this period. Heat is a well known irritant to the insane; and light, as we have seen, acts in the same manner: when the two, therefore, are conjoined, the effect must be still greater. On these accounts, consequently, the summer solstice may be connected with maniacal exacerbations; but the cause rests, in no respect, on direct solar influence of the kind that has been imagined.

The belief in lunar influence has not been restricted to the case of the maniac. Even the simple operation of cutting corns could not be ventured upon formerly without attending to the condition of that luminary. The satirist Butler has not failed to touch upon this superstition, in describing the qualifications of Sidrophel.

> " He with the moon was more familiar
> Than e're was almanac well-willer;
> Her secrets understood so clear,
> That some believ'd he had been there;
> Knew when she was in fittest mood
> For cutting corns or letting blood."

Strange to say, this notion still exists in many parts of Great Britain, and elsewhere,—the common people consulting the almanac to find when the moon is in the wane, in order that the operation may be performed with full advantage.

The superstitions, connected with the increase, full, and wane of the moon, were common among the ancient Kelts, and Goths. These periods were with them emblematic of a rising, flourishing, and declining fortune. In the wane, consequently, they carefully avoided entering upon any business of importance. In the Orkneys they do not marry except in the increase of the moon, and they would consider the meat worthless, were they to kill cattle during the wane. In Angusshire, in Scotland, it is believed, that if a child be put from the breast during the waning of the moon, it will fall off whilst the moon continues to wane. The superstition with respect to the fatal influence of a waning moon seems, indeed, to have been general in Scotland, where it was probably derived from the ancient Scandinavians, and hence we account for its prevalence amongst the Germans, and other nations of kindred origin. In the Swedish portion of Scandinavia, great influence is, even at the present day, ascribed to the moon, not only as a regulator of the weather, but as influencing the affairs of life in general. A number of the popular superstitions, regarding the moon, still prevalent amongst the Germans, and Dutch of this continent, acknowledge a Scandinavian origin. For example, both here and in Sweden, the farmer will decline felling a tree, for agricultural purposes, in the wane of the moon, under the fear that it may shrink, and not be durable. Opinions, however, differ on this point, as they do regarding the proper time for putting seed into the ground. Some prefer felling the trees in the wane, and period of darkness of the moon. A good housewife, too, will not kill, for the use of her family, during the wane, under the dread that the meat may shrivel and melt away in the pot.

All these superstitions, with regard to the " orb of night," seem to be equally based on a want of accurate observation, and on the fondness of the human mind for the mysterious. The *direct* influence of the moon on the human body we have said to be, in our opinion, mythical. On atmospheric changes it *may* exert some agency. The aqueous tides *may* produce corresponding impressions on the aerial medium; but these impressions are so modified by innumerable circumstances of a meteorological character, as to preclude the possibility of attaining any accurate prognostications.

There are, doubtless, physical circumstances—as we have elsewhere remarked— which occasion the shape of to day's clouds to differ from those that have passed away; but these circumstances are inappreciable by us. In all these cases the *onus probandi* must rest with the party asserting that such effects are produced by the causes assigned, and the proof must repose, not on one or two detached observations, but on a considerable number, carefully watched by those whose minds are devoid of all prepossessions on the subject. If investigations, thus conducted, should prove, that the human body is indirectly influenced by the moon,—or if even they should render it probable, that that luminary exerts any *direct* power over us,—we should have to bow to the evidence, although the testimony ought to be strong indeed before we admit such mysterious agency. (See *Manuel d'Hygiène Publique et Privée*, par L. Deslandes, pp. 4 to 12, for some sensible remarks on this subject.)

## SECTION V.

Effect of the seasons—comparative mortality amongst Adults and Children—winter residence for the consumptive—France and Italy—Madeira—Canaries—the Azores—Bahamas—Bermudas—West Indies—Havanna—Vera Cruz—Cumana—Peru—Chili, &c.—Effects of a Sea voyage—climate of Florida, &c.—Saint-Augustine, &c.—comparative merits of seaside and inland situations—due succession of seasons necessary for full mental and corporeal development—effects of unseasonable weather.

The effect of the seasons of the year upon human health resolves itself greatly into that of temperature, of which we have already treated. The succession of the seasons is necessary for vegetable existence; and if the vegetable kingdom were to fail, many of the higher classes of organized bodies would soon cease to exist also. It is favourable, likewise, to mental, and corporeal development; and the countries, which have a marked spring, summer, autumn, and winter, are those that have exhibited such development to the greatest extent. In the torrid regions, the distinction between the seasons is but slight; and the heat throughout is excessive. The enervation, and listlessness, thus induced, are well known. In the more frigid regions, again, the year is divided between winter, and summer; the former attended with benumbing cold,—the latter even hotter than in the temperate regions; both being consequently unfavourable, by their continuance, to mental and corporeal energy; whilst in the temperate regions, the winter, if severe, and the summer if hot, are of comparatively short duration; and are separated from each other by the pleasant seasons of spring and autumn, in which the excessive heat of the summer, and the rigorous cold of the winter are amalgamated and tempered, so as to form an agreeable vicissitude; and one adapted for developing the most active powers of man.

The tables of Dr. Emerson, to which we have had occasion to refer, strikingly exhibit the influence of the seasons on the mortality of both adults and children in civic life. From a series of observations, embracing a period of twenty years, the relative mortality of the different months, in Philadelphia, when arranged according to the order of their decreasing mortality stood, as follows: —the months being all equalized or presumed to be made eqnal to thirty-one days. Dr. Emerson's first essay was published in the *American Journal of the Medical Sciences* for November, 1827, and the second in the number for November, 1831.

| | | | | | | |
|---|---|---|---|---|---|---|
| 1. | August | . 6632 | 7. | April | . | 4370 |
| 2. | July . | . 5887 | 8. | November | . | 4361 |
| 3. | September . | . 5309 | 9. | February . | . | 4283 |
| 4. | June . | . 4699 | 10. | January . | . | 4112 |
| 5. | October | . 4554 | 11. | December | . | 4072 |
| 6. | March | . 4371 | 12. | May | . | 3892 |

When arranged according to the mortality of adults alone, and supposing the months to consist of thirty-one days each, placed in the order of their decreasing mortality, they would stand as follows:—

| | | | | | | |
|---|---|---|---|---|---|---|
| 1. | August | . 2845 | 7. | November. | . | 2432 |
| 2. | September | . 2716 | 8. | July | . | 2429 |
| 3. | April | . 2609 | 9. | June | . | 2409 |
| 4. | October | . 2560 | 10. | January | . | 2390 |
| 5. | February . | . 2501 | 11. | December . | . | 2252 |
| 6. | March | . 2480 | 12. | May . | . | 2224 |

The relative mortality of those under twenty years of age, in the respective months, would stand thus:—

| | | | | | | |
|---|---|---|---|---|---|---|
| 1. | August | . 3787 | 7. | March | . | 1891 |
| 2. | July . | . 3458 | 8. | December | . | 1820 |
| 3. | September . | . 2591 | 9. | February . | . | 1782 |
| 4. | June . | . 2290 | 10. | April | . | 1761 |
| 5. | October | . 1994 | 11. | January . | . | 1722 |
| 6. | November . | . 1929 | 12. | May | . | 1668 |

The bills of mortality show how much more the infant is affected by season than the adult. Dr. Emerson found, that the difference between the months exhibiting the maximum, and the minimum, —or greatest, and least proportion of deaths,—was in adults about 21 per cent., whilst in children it was no less than 55 per cent. For the purpose of investigating this interesting topic in detail, he constructed a table, showing the infantile mortality per month, at different ages. A period of five years, embracing the years 1826, 1827, 1828, 1829, and 1830, was taken, and the proportion of stillborn was deducted from the mortality under the first year. The months of the five years equalized, and given in the order of their decreasing mortality, with their respective proportions, stood as follows:—

|  | Under 1 year. | Between 1 & 2. | Between 2 & 5. | Between 5 & 20. | Totals |
|---|---|---|---|---|---|
| 1. July | 836 | 249 | 117 | 120 | 1322 |
| 2. August | 546 | 317 | 120 | 165 | 1148 |
| 3. September | 377 | 221 | 140 | 185 | 923 |
| 4. June | 510 | 148 | 84 | 105 | 847 |
| 5. February | 382 | 109 | 123 | 131 | 745 |
| 6. October | 324 | 127 | 117 | 153 | 721 |
| 7. March | 322 | 119 | 122 | 138 | 701 |
| 8. April | 342 | 107 | 125 | 122 | 696 |
| 9. December | 269 | 910 | 114 | 135 | 608 |
| 10. November | 267 | 90 | 114 | 132 | 603 |
| 11. January | 281 | 81 | 102 | 109 | 573 |
| 12. May | 250 | 98 | 107 | 107 | 562 |
|  | 4706 | 1756 | 1385 | 1602 | 9449 |

From this table it appears, that much the greatest mortality, occurring in early infancy, takes place in July, June, and August, —months distinguished from all others by their high temperature, and that heat is one of the most fatal enemies to early life in Philadelphia, and in most of our cities.

In Saint Louis,—where, according to a recent writer, (Dr. V. J. Fourgeaud, *St. Louis Medical and Surgical Journal,* for March 15, 1844) the number of deaths under 7 years of age is more than half the whole number,—the influence of seasons on the mortality of children is stated to be as follows:—

| Years. | Jan. | Feb. | March. | April. | May. | June. | July. | Aug. | Sept. | Oct. | Nov. | Dec. | Total. |
|---|---|---|---|---|---|---|---|---|---|---|---|---|---|
| 1841 | 8 | 7 | 10 | 12 | 31 | 36 | 133 | 87 | 58 | 47 | 32 | 27 | 488 |
| 1842 | 16 | 21 | 19 | 9 | 14 | 32 | 39 | 26 | 29 | 27 | 22 | 16 | 270 |
| 1843 | 16 | 12 | 16 | 4 | 17 | 24 | 141 | 209 | 67 | 60 | 40 | 39 | 645 |
|  | 40 | 40 | 45 | 25 | 62 | 92 | 313 | 322 | 154 | 134 | 94 | 82 | 1403 |

"It is interesting to observe," says Dr. Emerson, "that the destructive influence of this agent (heat) has lost much of its power after the first year of life, and that after the second year it is scarcely perceptible, there being but little variation in the columns representing the monthly mortality after this period. If we take the mortality for the months of June, July, and August, we find that the proportion, occurring under the second year of infancy, is about four times greater than that which occurred during the same months for the whole eighteen succeeding years of life; whereas, for the three months of November, December, and January, the amount of mortality,—under the two first years of life, is but little above that of the eighteen succeeding years. It will be observed, that the month of September stands among the highest months in the scale of infantile mortality,—differing, however, from those with which it is associated, by having a larger proportion of deaths distributed under the latter periods designated."

We have already said, that the cholera infantum is the great scourge of our cities during the summer months; and this affection is doubtless, in part, occasioned by excessive heat, but that this alone does not induce it is shown by the fact, that in country situations, where the heat may be as great, it is comparatively rare. It is necessary, that there should be a union of great atmospheric heat, with atmospheric deterioration, in order that the disease should exist fatally, and extensively: and this combination is met with in the confined, and deteriorated air of our towns. Although, however, infants are chiefly carried off during the summer and autumnal heats by bowel affections, these complaints prove fatal, likewise, to many of those who are greatly advanced in life. A sub-inflammatory condition occurs in the lining membrane of the intestines, which often resists every remedy, and proves too much for a system, whose elasticity has been gradually diminished by the play of the organs beyond the ordinary duration of human existence.

In another table, Dr. Emerson has classed the deaths in Philadelphia, amongst adults and children—for the different seasons during a period of twenty years—as follows:

|  | Adults. | Children |
|---|---|---|
| In March, April, and May | 7,229 | 5,264 |
| June, July, and August, | 7,606 | 9,462 |
| September, October, and November, | 7,545 | 6,369 |
| December, January, and February, | 6,900 | 5,153 |

By this it is shown, that the deaths among children, during the summer months, greatly predominate. These different tables can, however, only be regarded as affording positive results applicable to Philadelphia; although the general deductions may be extended to New York, Baltimore, Charleston, and other towns, where the temperature is elevated during the summer months.

In England it has been remarked, that the proportion of aged individuals, who die during cold weather, to those who die during summer, is as high as seven to four; and that the number of deaths of all ages is greatest in the months of January, February, and March; and least in June, July, and August.

According to Mr. Farr (*Report of the Registrar-General*, p. 102, London, 1842) the degree to which the mean monthly temperature falls in December, January or February, determines, to a great extent, the mortality of winter. In the following table, the deaths registered in the seasons of the three years are compared with the temperature;—the number of deaths having been corrected on the assumption that each period embraced 275 days.

|  | 3 Winters. | 3 Springs. | 3 Summers. | 3 Autumns. |
|---|---|---|---|---|
|  | Jan. Feb. March. | April. May. June. | July. Aug. Sept. | Oct. Nov. Dec. |
| Deaths— | 39.764 | 35.128 | 33.677 | 36.684 |
| Temp. (Fahrenheit) | 39°.8 | 53°.8 | 61°.0 | 44°.6 |

The causes of death that proved most fatal in the cold months belong principally to the pulmonary class, and the cerebral diseases of the aged; and those that proved most fatal in summer to diseases of the bowels; but in almost every class, it was found, that there were one or two diseases over the fatality of which temperature exerted a marked influence.

| Causes of death. | Winter. | Spring. | Summer. | Autumn. |
|---|---|---|---|---|
| Diseases of the Respiratory Organs | 12140* | 9890 | 8433 | 11.008 |
| Diseases of the Digestive Organs | 1.982 | 2139 | 2978 | 2.263 |

Persons affected by the following diseases were found to die in greatest numbers when the temperature was low; and Mr. Farr sug-

* The three winters contain the deaths registered in 271 days: the summer those registered in 275; and the same applies to the following tables.

gests, that many cases, arranged under apoplexy and sudden death, are the effects of congestion of the lungs—" a sort of spontaneous asphyxia," the development of which appears to be favoured by a temperature below the freezing point of water. (*Op. cit.* p. 108.)

| Causes of Death. | Winter. | Spring. | Summer. | Autumn. | Causes of Death. | Winter. | Spring. | Summer. | Autumn. |
|---|---|---|---|---|---|---|---|---|---|
| Apoplexy | 801 | 627 | 626 | 695 | Nephritis | 19 | 17 | 14 | 19 |
| Sudden Death | 618 | 524 | 381 | 547 | Diabetes | 19 | 12 | 7 | 15 |
| Paralysis | 647 | 520 | 485 | 602 | Dropsy | 1403 | 1286 | 1135 | 1457 |
| Insanity | 73 | 45 | 35 | 42 | | | | | |
| Tetanus | 23 | 11 | 15 | 19 | Diseases of child-bed | 310 | 261 | 217 | 309 |
| Asthma | 1733 | 642 | 344 | 1080 | Phlegmon | 9 | 2 | 3 | 1 |
| Bronchitis | 495 | 307 | 191 | 347 | Ulcer | 23 | 16 | 9 | 13 |
| Pneumonia | 3326 | 2454 | 1827 | 3600 | | | | | |
| Pleurisy | 70 | 62 | 39 | 51 | Mortification | 217 | 177 | 153 | 171 |
| Hydrothorax | 124 | 113 | 99 | 117 | Old age | 3437 | 2609 | 2150 | 2814 |
| Disease of Heart | 739 | 556 | 571 | 698 | | | | | |
| Rheumatism | 124 | 113 | 99 | 117 | | | | | |

On some of the fatal diseases of infants and adults the range of temperature appeared to have little effect.

| Causes of Death. | Winter. | Spring. | Summer. | Autumn. |
|---|---|---|---|---|
| Hydrocephalus | 1370 | 1330 | 1348 | 1231 |
| Convulsions | 2414 | 2298 | 2532 | 2119 |
| Consumption | 5600 | 5778 | 5501 | 5148 |
| Scrofula | 72 | 64 | 72 | 54 |
| Cancer | 276 | 230 | 264 | 262 |

It was an interesting point to determine at what degree of cold the mortality began to rise. It has been observed by meteorologists, that the mean temperature of October represents pretty nearly the mean temperature of the year and place; and the facts observed by Mr. Farr show, that the mortality rises progressively as the mean temperature falls below the mean temperature of London —50°.5 —the deaths in the week rising to 1000 and upwards when the temperature of night falls below the freezing point of water, and to 1200 when the mean temperature of day and night descends a degree or two lower than 32°. The rise in the mortality is immediate; but the effects of the low temperature go on accumulating, and continue to be felt thirty or forty days after the extremes of cold have passed away. A certain number of persons are destroyed rapidly by it: in others it occasions diseases, which prove fatal in a month or six weeks.

The relation between depressed temperature and mortality is well shown in the following table.

Temperature and mean weakly deaths in the Metropolis for periods of four weeks from Nov. 7, 1840 to April 17, 1841.

|  | Nov. 7th–28th | Nov. 29 to Dec. 26 | Dec. 27 to Jan. 23 | Jan. 24 to Feb. 20 | Feb. 21 to Mar. 20 | Mar. 21 to April 17 |
|---|---|---|---|---|---|---|
| Temperature { mean | 46°.3 | 35°.8 | 34°.3 | 37°.0 | 46°.0 | 48°.5 |
| { lowest | 33 .0 | 21 .0 | 15 .0 | 22 .0 | 34 .0 | 37 .0 |
| Weekly deaths | 905 | 1086 | 1.239 | 1.056 | 1.039 | 844 |
| Age 0—15 | 438 | 512 | 513 | 451 | 443 | 366 |
| 15—60 | 292 | 336 | 393 | 355 | 341 | 292 |
| 60 and upwards | 171 | 235 | 336 | 250 | 253 | 185 |
| From Bronchitis | 6 | 18 | 34 | 24 | 19 | 15 |
| Pneumonia | 100 | 138 | 140 | 97 | 89 | 62 |
| Asthma | 20 | 55 | 92 | 56 | 43 | 23 |

This table proves the importance of protecting the infant and the aged against the influence of cold, as inculcated in an early part of this work. " A great number of the aged," says Mr. Farr, " and those afflicted with difficulty of breathing, whether it arises from emphysema, chronic bronchitis, diseased heart, or impairment of the function of respiration, cannot resist cold sunk so low as 32°. The temperature of the atmosphere in which they sleep can never safely descend lower than 40°; for, if the cold that freezes water in their chamber do not freeze their blood, it impedes respiration, and life ceases when the blood-heat has sunk a few degrees below the standard."

It has been already shown, that not only is the general mortality of London greater than that of Philadelphia, but the deaths at the ages most liable to cholera infantum are more numerous also; a fact which confirms the remark just made,—that something more than excessive heat is, in such cases, the lethiferous agent. The same observation is applicable to the malarious diseases, which prevail to so destructive an extent in certain localities, during the heats of summer and autumn. Elevated temperature is required for the exhalation of the miasms, and these miasms are the grand exciting cause of such diseases, although many of their complications may be directly produced through the influence of heat.

It has been elsewhere remarked, that a certain degree of equability and elevation of temperature is important to the preservation of the health of such as are predisposed to consumptive affections, and that these, as indeginous affections, are almost unknown in the torrid zone. It has, consequently, been a matter of anxious inquiry, how best to escape the rigours of the winter season in temperate climes, and the great vicissitudes,—infinitely more dangerous than depressed temperature,—which are incessantly happening in spring and autumn, but especially in the former. For this purpose, the invalid has been advised to seek a milder climate during those seasons, and, where this has been impracticable, to keep his room, and have its temperature properly regulated. This can be readily effected; but the steps, which are necessary for the purpose, interfere so much with due ventilation, that the vitiation of the air of the apartment counterbalances, to a great extent, the advantages that would otherwise be derived from the elevation, and equability of temperature; and thus we may, in some measure, account for the good effects, that have accrued from allowing the consumptive, or those threatened with consumption, to take exercise in the open air, whenever it has been dry, and the temperature, although cool, equable. (Parrish, in *North American Medical and Surgical Journal*, for 1829, and 1830: and Morton's *Illustrations of Pulmonary Consumption*, p. 142, Philadelphia, 1834.) Still, when the person is unfit to bear exposure to the air without doors, a regulated temperature in his apartments becomes indispensable. The recent inventor of the *Respirator* by Mr. Jeffreys enables the patient to bear a cold atmosphere with comparative impunity. It consists of various strata of thin silver plates, perforated with numerous holes; and, although entirely effectual in tempering the cold air before it reaches the air passages, causes no difficulty in respiration. It is especially useful for such as are affected with chronic bronchitis.

We have before shown,—and shall have to recur to the subject,—that no removal to a warmer climate, and no artificial temperature can be of much service, when the lungs are ulcerated, or in other words, when the individual is in a state of confirmed consumption; but that, on the contrary, the disease seems generally, under such circumstances, to be hurried onwards in its progress to a fatal termination. Although, however, removal to another clime may be most injudicious and cruel, under the circumstances mentioned, it becomes a matter of momentous inquiry to select those situations, that are best adapted during the cooler months for such as have a tendency to, or are labouring under, pulmonary affections, which may lead to abscesses in the lungs, and to phthisis. In the summer months, the climate of most parts of the United States is sufficiently mild, provided ordinary precautions be taken, but the intense, and sudden vicissitudes of the autumnal, winter, and spring seasons render it advisable, that the invalid should, at those times, seek a more genial residence.

At one time, it was a common course with physicians—in their ignorance of the climate, and misled by the partial observations of travellers—to send, not only those threatened with consumption, but such even as were suffering under the disease in its confirmed stage, to Southern France and Italy. The tours of medical and other travellers, and residents have shown, that such a course is most unadvisable,—the climate of these parts being one of great vicissitudes, and therefore but little adapted for the valetudinarian. " The more I see of Italy," says the intelligent Matthews, in his ' *Diary of an Invalid*,' " the more I doubt, whether it be worth while for an invalid to encounter the fatigues of so long a journey, for the sake of any advantages to be found in it in respect of climate during the winter. To come to Italy, with the hope of *escaping* the winter, is a grievous mistake. This might be done by getting into the southern hemisphere, but in Europe it is impossible; and I believe that Devonshire, after all, may be the best place for an invalid during that season. If the thermometer be not so low here, the temperature is more variable, and the winds are more bitter, and cutting. In Devonshire, too, all the comforts of the country are directed against cold;—here, all the precautions are in the other way. The streets are built to exclude, as much as possible, the rays of the sun, and are now (Rome, December 20th,) as damp, and cold as rain or frost can make them. And then, what a difference between the warm carpet, the snug elbowed chair, and the blazing coal fire of an English winter evening, and the stone staircases, marble floors, and starving casements of an Italian house! where every thing is designed to guard against the heat of summer, which occupies as large a portion of the Italian year as the winter season does of our own. The only advantage of Italy, then, is, that your penance is shorter than it would be in England, for I repeat that, during the time it lasts, winter is more severely felt here than at Sidmouth, where I would even recommend an Italian invalid to repair, from November till February, if he could possess himself of Fortunatus's cap, to remove the difficulties of the journey. Having provided myself with a warm cloak, which is absolutely necessary, for the temperature varies twenty degrees between one street and another, I have been proceeding leisurely through the wonders of Rome."

Such is the testimony afforded—from personal experience of the climate of Rome—by a well informed invalid; and his statement is confirmed by the observation of Sir James Clark, who resided long in Italy, and of Dr. James Johnson, who visited that region; both of whom have published their conviction of the unsuitable nature of the climate for such as are desirous of escaping the harshness and instability of a British winter; and their remarks are equally appropriate when transferred to this country.

Yet Italy is the sanitarium to which so many hundred invalids have been, and are, annually sent,—doomed, too often, as Sir James Clark has observed, to add other names to the long and melancholy list of their countrymen, who have sought, with pain and suffering, a distant country only to find in it an untimely grave. The traveller, who bends over the lowly tombs in the burial ground at Leghorn, has melancholy testimony of the fatal character of phthisis, the too often injudicious recommendation of the physician, and the excessive and sudden vicissitudes to which Southern France and Italy are so signally liable. In all these situations, too, to which invalids are sent, pulmonary affections—especially inflammation of the chest—are very prevalent, and in many of them the deaths from consumption are as numerous as in Great Britain, and other countries, from which the consumptive are hurried for the purpose of enjoying a more favourable climate. Sir James Clark affirms, (*The Sanative Influence of Climate*, p. 232) that in the whole of Italy, inflammation of the lungs appeared to be more violent, and more rapid in its course, than in England; and Dr. Kreysig, of Dresden, informed him, that he had never witnessed such violent cases of pneumonic inflammation in Germany, as he saw during his stay at Pavia. The testimony of every medical traveller is hostile to the expectation of relief in pulmonary disorders, when at all advanced, from a residence under the beautiful skies, but uncertain climate, of Southern France and Italy. Dr. Morton remarks, that if we were to make exceptions to every place, where phthisis exists as a common disease, there would be scarcely a locality left in Europe in which the invalid could shelter himself. (*Op. citat.* p. 157.) It is too true, that no such locality does exist there, and to this the most honest and discriminating observers have borne ample testimony. It is obvious, that where phthisis is a " common disease," the locality must favour its existence, and it cannot, consequently, be as eminently salubrious for such strangers as are strongly predisposed to that affection, as if the disease were rare.

Recent observations have shown, that the climate of Algeria is exceedingly favourable to the phthisical valetudinarian. (See the Author's *Practice of Medicine*, 2nd edit., ii. 379, Philad. 1844.)

The climate, which Sir James Clark esteems best suited to consumptive patients generally, is that of Madeira; and this is the opinion of most of the British physicians; although some prefer certain situations in Southern France and Italy. Sir George Lefare (*Thermal Comfort*, Amer. edit., p. 39, New York,) recommends Valentia in Spain for its equable mildness, its moderate temperature, its calmness, and a certain degree of moisture from daily sunny showers.

In England, Penzance, Torquay, Undercliff in the Isle of Wight, Clifton, Hastings, St. Leonards and Brighton, have been recommended; and, of late, Cove, in Ireland, has attained great celebrity. In equability of temperature, the Cove of Cork would indeed seem to be surpassed by but few places. Observations, according to Dr. Stokes (*On the Diseases of the Chest*, Dublin, 1837, or Amer. edit. Philad. 1844,) have shown that the mean difference of days and nights rarely exceeds four or five degrees; and often, in the winter months, does not exceed one degree. The town is completely sheltered from the north wind, and, owing to its southern exposure, receives the full influence of the sun, and the southern breeze.

The Author, in conjunction with Professor Smith of the University of Maryland, recommended a young medical friend, who had been attacked with hæmoptysis—consequent on the existence of tubercles in the lungs, as indicated by the rational and physical signs—to take a voyage across the Atlantic, and to occupy some time in travel, so as to return to this country before the setting in of the cold weather,—in order that he might again have the advantages of a sea-voyage and milder climate during the winter, should this course be necessary. Whilst in London he consulted some distinguished members of the profession, by one of whom he was advised to go to Madeira, and remain there until May, "that no other place would do;" and by another to winter in Hyères, a small town, about two miles from the shores of the Mediterranean, and twelve from Toulon, and which is described by Sir James Clark (*Op. citat.* p. 200) as " the *least exceptionable* residence for the pulmonary invalid in Provence."

From the meteorological tables it appears, that the winter temperature of Madeira is considerably higher and more equable, and the summer heat more moderate, than at any of the European places mentioned. To individuals, consequently—threatened with, or in a state of incipient, phthisis—who can derive any benefit from climate, Madeira would seem to be an excellent residence, and the correctness of this opinion appears to have been amply confirmed by experience. Dr. Renton,—who resided there for a considerable period, and who has made some touching and appropriate remarks on the inhumanity of advising those in confirmed phthisis to undertake a voyage that can be productive of nothing but mischief and disappointment,—has published a table drawn up from the cases of which he had kept notes, during the eight years preceding, which places the subject in a striking point of view. (*Edinburgh Medical and Surgical Journal,* vol. 27; quoted by Sir James Clark, *Op. citat.* p. 268.)

| | |
|---|---:|
| Cases of *confirmed* phthisis, | 47 |
| Of these there died, within six months after their arrival at Madeira, | 32 |
| Went home in summer, returned and died, | 6 |
| Left the island, of whose death we have heard, | 6 |
| Not since heard of, probably dead, | 3 |
| | 47 |

Cases of *incipient* phthisis, - - - - - - - 35
Of these there left the island much improved, and of whom we have
   had good accounts, - - - - - - - - - - 26
Also improved but not since heard of, - - - - - - - 5
Have since died, - - - - - - - - - - - 4
                                                                                    35

What a black picture is afforded by the first of these lists, and how fearful is the responsibility, incurred by the medical adviser, who hurries his patient far from his comforts and his friends, on such a forlorn hope; and, again, how cheering are the prospects, afforded by the second table, to those, who are sent to a proper climate before the disease has made serious inroads! Yet so little is this all important difference attended to in England, that the annual importation of invalids from that country into Madeira, according to Dr. Renton, is thought a fit subject for ridicule among the boatmen, on landing these unfortunates on the island;—'*La vai mais hum Ingles a Laranjeira:* ' there goes another Englishman to the orange tree'—(the burying ground of the Protestants.)

The mean annual range of temperature is only 14°, being less than half the range at Rome, Pisa, Naples, and Nice. The heat is also distributed with great equality throughout the year, so that the mean difference of the temperature of successive months is only 2°.41; whilst at Rome, it is 4°.39, at Nice, 4°.74, at Pisa, 5°.75, and at Naples 5°.08. " But," observes Dr. Morton (*Op. cit.* p. 157.) " Notwithstanding this uniformity of temperature, no malady is more prevalent in Madeira than pulmonary consumption. Persons of all ages, and of both sexes, says Dr. Gourlay, (*Observations on the climate and diseases of Madeira*, London, 1811,) fall victims to it; nay, whole families have at times been suddenly swept away by it. And yet, as before mentioned, this climate is extremely congenial to consumptives from other shores, and probably would permanently restore the health of many, in the incipient state even of tubercular disease, was not the removal protracted to its last and irremediable stage." It is proper, however, to state, that much difference of sentiment exists amongst those, who have had the best opportunities for observation, as to the prevalence of consumption amongst the natives of Madeira. The experience of Dr. Heineken —long a resident on the island—led him to a conclusion directly opposed to that of Dr. Gourlay; and Sir James Clark states (*Op. citat.* p. 269,) that he is satisfied, from the information he has received, that tubercular consumption is a rare disease, compared with what it is in more northern climates; and infinitely more rare than it would be in those climates, were the causes, which commonly induce tubercular disease among the lower classes, applied as powerfully and generally as they are in Madeira. " The lower classes in Madeira are hard worked and miserably nourished; their food consists chiefly of crude vegetables, and hard salted fish; they are badly clothed, and worse lodged; their habitations are low, miserable huts, and their beds consist of pallets of straw, raised a foot or two only from the ground, damp during nine months of the year. That inflammatory diseases of the lungs should be frequent, under such circumstances, is not surprising; and as these are generally neglected, or badly treated, they often prove fatal in a chronic form of simulating phthisis. But even if tubercular consumption were a frequent occurrence, under the circumstances which we have stated, it would afford no reasonable ground of objection to the climate of Madeira, for persons exempted from such palpable causes of disease."

Sir James Clark farther asserts, that there is no place on the continent of Europe—with which he is acquainted—where the pulmonary invalid could reside with so much advantage, during the whole year, as at Madeira; and in support of this opinion he cites Dr. Heineken, who lived for many years in Madeira in consequence of a pulmonary affection. That gentleman found, from his own experience, that he rather retrograded during the winter, but always gained ground during the summer.

The climate of the Canaries approaches most closely, in its character, to that of Madeira, but the temperature is more equable throughout the year at the latter place; the difference between the mean temperature of the summer and winter being $9°.8$, and at Santa Cruz, $12°.3$. The heat, during the summer, is considerably higher in the Canaries, and in the months of November, and December, much rain falls. The superiority of the climate of the Canaries is therefore limited to the three winter months, but this appears to be more than counterbalanced by the greater equability of the climate of Madeira, and the much superior accommodation for invalids.

The Azores or Western Islands, which are surrounded on all sides by a vast extent of ocean are considered to afford one of the best examples of a mild, humid, equable climate to be met with in the northern hemisphere. It is slightly colder, according to Dr. Bullar, and more humid than Madeira, but probably even more equable.

A change from the Azores to Madeira, and from thence to Teneriffe, would—it is conceived by Sir James Clark (*Op. cit.* p. 281) in many cases, prove more beneficial than a residence during the whole winter on any one of the islands. Nor does this appear to be difficult. The West India steamers regularly touch at Madeira, whence a fine vessel sails with the mails and passengers to Fayal and St. Michaels, and returns to Madeira. Madeira in summer is oppressively hot, whilst the temperature of the Azores is delightful: hence, some consumptive individuals pass the winter with benefit in Madeira, and the summer in the Azores.

With respect to the islands on this side the Atlantic, and which may, with propriety, as regards their geographical position, be called *American*, their climate is somewhat modified by that of the continent near which they are situate. This is greatly the case with the Bahamas, which are subject to considerable vicissitudes of temperature, but to what extent cannot be accurately determined in the absence of careful thermometric observations, registered for a considerable period. Still, as a winter residence, they must, *cæteris paribus*, be superior to most parts of the United States.

Consumptive patients have often been sent from this country to the Bermudas, but these islands do not afford by any means the best locality for such as are disposed to incur the evils of expatriation. The northerly winds blow with considerable asperity, and are most obnoxious to the valetudinarian; but the climate is greatly better than that of many parts of the Union, and they who are predisposed to consumption might pass the winter there safely, and perhaps with benefit. When the disease is established, it is found to run its course more rapidly than in England. "There are many beautiful spots in these islands, where, protected from the northerly gales by the cedar-clothed hills, the invalid might find sufficient space to enjoy exercise in the open air, almost every day during the winter. The neighbourhood of the little town of Hamilton, situate nearly in the centre of the island, affords the most favourable situations for such a residence." (Sir James Clark, *Op. cit.* p. 293.)

Sir James has, we think, somewhat too hastily laid down the position, that the climate of the West Indies is unsuitable for the generality of consumptive patients. (*Ibid.* p. 303.) That the heat of torrid climes hurries on confirmed phthisis is a fact admitted by all, but these are not the cases that ought to be subjects for expatriation any where. Speaking of Jamaica, in his "*Observations on Diseases of the Army in Jamaica,*" Dr. John Hunter observes, that pulmonary consumption rarely originates in the island ; and a medical friend of Dr. Morton, whom he characterizes as " highly intelligent, " informed him, that he never knew a case of consumption to originate there, not even among the blacks, although among the latter class scrofula is of common occurrence. On the other hand, however, it appears from the British Army Reports, that nearly twice as many cases of consumption originate among the British Troops in the West Indies as at home:—twelve per thousand of the aggregate strength of the troops serving in the West Indies being attacked annually, whilst, of the Dragoon guards serving in Great Britain, the ratio is only six and a half per thousand. The disease, according to the same reports, is even of more frequent occurrence among the black than the white troops.

Sir James Clark thinks, that to invalids of whatever class—resorting to the West Indies—Barbadoes, St. Vincent, Antigua, and St. Kitts afford all the advantages of the country and climate, and fewer of the disadvantages than most of the other islands. Santa Cruz has been frequently selected for the phthisical valetudinarian from the United States, but it does not seem entitled to any preference, in such cases, over the other West India islands, whilst its general salubrity is said to be less than that of many. The Reverend Dr. Tuckerman, of Boston (*Boston Med. and Surg. Journal,* xvi. 363) who spent there the winter of 1836-7, has given an accurate meteorological table from December to May inclusive. It exhibits great equability of climate. He observes, however, that very small changes, as indicated by the thermometer,—3, 4 or 5 degrees for example—are scarcely less felt, and occasion a scarcely less uncomfortable state of feeling than changes of 8, 10 or 15 degrees in our own climate. Dr. Tuckerman advises an invalid from New-England not to leave Santa Cruz before the 10th of May,—after which the temperature is considered too enfeebling for the inhabitants of a colder region—and upon his arrival at New York, or any point north of it, to proceed at once to Philadelphia, or Baltimore, or farther south, and to make the last week in June or the first in July the time of return to his home. "In the healthy," he observes, "the last change to be sought for gratification is a residence in the West Indies. It will be at no small cost of physical as well as of intellectual and moral enjoyment, that one who has health, and who knows how to use it, will unnecessarily pass even five or six months there. The temperature of Santa Cruz is indeed generally a very grateful one to an invalid. It is often delicious. But the heat is sometimes very debilitating; and it is always too great either for much intellectual or physical effort."

The mean annual temperature of the West India islands near the sea, is about 79° or 80°. The mean daily range is only about 6°, and the extreme annual range not more than 20°. The mean temperature of some of the habitable spots of the mountain ranges is not more than 65° or 70°; so that various climates exist according to the elevation above the surface. In Barbadoes, the mean temperature of the seasons is as follows:—winter, 76°. 7; spring, 79°; summer, 81°, and autumn, 80°.

At the Havannah, the mean temperature is 78°, and the difference between the mean temperature of the warmest, and the coldest month, 23°.86,—twice as great as in Madeira. The mean temperature of winter is 71°. 24; of spring, 78°. 98; of summer, 83°. 30, and of autumn, 78°. 98.—The venerable and estimable Dr. Jackson, of Boston, sends his patients chiefly to Cuba. (Sir James Clark, *Op. cit.* p. 306.)

The above estimates exhibit, that the West Indies, so far as regards elevation, and comparative equability of temperature, must be favourable to those of weak lungs; but at the same time many of these places are liable to weighty objections, owing to their general insalubrity; to their being infested with musquetoes, sand flies, &c. and to the difficulties of obtaining such accommodations as are indispensable to the comfort, and welfare of the valetudinarian.

In the southern portion of our own continent,—that is, to the south of the United States,—there are many situations, which, as regards elevation, and equability of temperature, would appear to be signally adapted for the residence of those predisposed to consumption. At Vera Cruz, the mean temperature throughout the year is 77°. 72; and the difference between the mean temperature of the warmest, and the coldest month, 10°. 80; whilst at Cumaná, the annual mean is 81°. 86; and the difference between the mean temperature of the warmest and the coldest month only 5°. 22; but even greater objections, on the score of general insalubrity, apply to these situations than to any of the West India islands. Such insalubrity, it is true, prevails most at particular seasons, but it exists more or less in all.

Peru, it is said, is unusually exempt from consumption. " My friend, Dr. M. Burrough," says Dr. Morton, (*Op. citat.* p. 159,) " who resided upwards of four years in Lima, informs me, that he did not meet with a single unequivocal case, that originated there during that period; although scrofula was not unfrequent. The same intelligent gentleman mentions, that he knew many foreigners in consumption to be much benefited by a residence in Lima; but that in every instance where they had been tempted to go farther south into Chili, the effect on their constitutions was fatal."

There is another variety of atmospheric change, respecting which some difference of opinion has existed, as regards its adaptation to the cases we have been considering,—that which is afforded by a sea-voyage. At a distance from land, the temperature of the air is equable, owing to the elevation of temperature that naturally results, when the wind passes over the ocean from a cold quarter; and the depression that occurs when it blows from the torrid climes. In the equatorial seas, the difference between the maximum and minimum of the day is, at the most, one or two degrees of the centigrade scale; whilst on the continents it is five or six; and in the temperate regions—between 25° and 50° of latitude—the difference between the maximum and minimum of the day is extremely small compared with that of the continents. (*Elémens de Physique*, &c. par Pouillet, tom. iv. p. 684, 2de édit. Paris, 1832.)

When the temperature of the sea, at its surface, is compared with that of the air, we attain the following results. Between the tropics, the air, at its highest temperature, is generally a little warmer than the surface of the water, taken likewise at its highest temperature,—as will be seen by an examination of the following tables, compiled by M. Arago, and contained in the *Annuaire du Bureau des Longitudes,* for 1825.

MAXIMA OF ATMOSPHERIC TEMPERATURE OBSERVED AT SEA, FAR FROM ANY CONTINENT.

| | *Dates.* | | *Latitude.* | | *Temperature.* | *Observers.* |
|---|---|---|---|---|---|---|
| Atlantic Ocean, | Aug. | 14, 1772. | 14°·54′ | N. | 81.°5 | Bayley. |
| South Sea, . . | Aug. | 16, 1774. | 17.46, | S. | 84. | do. |
| Atlantic Ocean,. | May, | 23, 1774. | 4.5, | N. | 83. | do. |
| do. | Aug. | 13, 1772. | 14.50, | N. | 83.5 | Wales. |
| do. | June, | 22, 1775. | 11.12, | N. | 84.6 | do. |
| do. | Sept. | 29, 1785. | 0.0 | | 79.5 | Lamanon. |
| do. | Nov. | 1788. | 0.58. | S. | 81. | Churruca. |
| do. | Nov. | 6, 1791. | 9.16, | N. | 83. | Dentrecast. |
| Sea of the Moluccas, | Oct'r, | 27, 1792. | 10.42, | S. | 87. | do. |
| do. | Aug. | 2, 1793. | 0.3, | S. | 85.5 | do. |
| Atlantic Ocean, | March, | 1800. | 0.33, | S. | 82. | Perrins. |
| South Sea, . . | Feb'y, | 1803. | 0.11, | N. | 82.5 | Humboldt. |
| Atlantic Ocean, | Mar. | 16, 1816. | 4.21, | N. | 82. | John Davy. |
| do. | May, | 11, 1816. | 4.43, | N. | 81.5 | La Marche. |
| Sea of Sunda, . | June, | 20, 1816. | 5.38, | N. | 85. | Basil Hall. |
| China Sea, . . | July, | 3, 1816. | 13.29, | N. | 84.5 | do. |
| Great Ocean, . | Aug. | 7, 1816. | 2.10, | N. | 83. | John Davy. |
| Atlantic Ocean,. | Oct. | 13, 1816. | 5.38, | S. | 84.5 | Lamarche. |
| Mediterranean, . | Aug. | 3, 1818. | 39.12, | N. | 84.5. | Gautier. |
| do. | June, | 24, 1819. | 38.46, | N. | 84.5 | do. |
| Black Sea, . . | June, | 23, 1820. | 44.42, | N. | 85. | do. |

MAXIMA OF TEMPERATURE OF THE SEA AT ITS SURFACE.

| | *Latitude.* | | *Long. from Paris.* | | *Temperature.* | *Dates.* | | *Names of Observers.* |
|---|---|---|---|---|---|---|---|---|
| Atlantic Ocean, | 7°. | N. | $20\frac{3}{4}$°. | W. | 80.5 | Aug. | 23, 1772. | W. Bayley. |
| South Sea, . | $17\frac{3}{4}$ | S. | 208. | E. | 84. | Aug. | 18, 1773. | do. |
| Atlantic Ocean, | 4. | N. | 24. | E. | 83. | May, | 23, 1774. | do. |
| do. | $6\frac{1}{4}$. | N. | $22\frac{4}{5}$. | W. | 84. | October, | 1788. | Churruca. |
| do. | 2. | S. | $29\frac{1}{4}$. | W. | 83.5 | April, | 1803. | Quevedo. |
| do. | 7. | N | $25\frac{1}{2}$. | W. | 84. | Nov. | 1803. | Rodman. |
| do. | $0\frac{2}{3}$. | N. | $22\frac{1}{3}$. | W. | 83. | March, | 1804 | Perrins. |
| do. | 4. | N. | 21. | W. | 83.5 | Mar. | 16, 1816. | John Davy. |
| do. | 5. | N. | 26. | W. | 81.5 | May, | 10, 1816. | La Marche. |
| China Sea, . | $13\frac{1}{2}$. | N. | $110\frac{1}{2}$. | E. | 84.5. | July, | 3, 1816. | Basil Hall. |
| Atlantic Ocean, | $7\frac{1}{3}$. | N | $24\frac{1}{2}$. | W. | 81. | July, | 14, 1816. | Ch. Baudin. |
| Sea of Ceylon, | $2\frac{1}{2}$. | N. | $75\frac{1}{2}$. | E. | 84. | Aug. | 9, 1816. | John Davy. |
| Atlantic Ocean, | 10. | N. | $20\frac{1}{2}$. | W. | 84.5 | Oct. | 18, 1816. | La Marche. |
| Indian Ocean, | 1. | N. | 91. | E. | 85. | Nov. | 15, 1816. | Ch. Baudin. |
| To the north of Sumatra. | $5\frac{1}{2}$. | N. | 98. | E. | 84. | Mar. | 8, 1817. | Basil Hall. |

When, however, the temperature of the air, and of the water, is taken every four hours—as was done by Captain Duperrey—and the different temperatures are compared, the water is generally found warmer than the air—even between the tropics. Of 1850 observations—made by that officer, in his voyage round the world, and between 0 and 20° of northern and southern latitude—the sea was found, in 1371, warmer than the air; whilst the air was only in 479 cases warmer than the sea. In higher latitudes—between 25° and 50°—the air is but rarely warmer than the surface of the water, and in polar regions, it is always colder, and commonly much colder.

The tables, it will be observed, exhibit but a slight range between the maxima of the various places, where the observations were made; although the latitudes of some were so different.

The good effects of a sea-voyage in phthisical cases are probably more dependent upon this equability of temperature, and upon the impression made upon the nervous system, than upon any saline impregnation of the air,—on which much stress has been laid by some writers; or than upon the sea-sickness, which has occurred in some cases, and not in others, where equal benefit has notwithstanding been experienced from the voyage. Still, in many cases, full vomiting, produced in this way, has apparently been highly salutary. At one time, indeed, ordinary emetics were regarded as specifics in phthisis, and Dr. Thomas Young, (*Treatise on Consumptive Diseases*, p. 65,) observes;—" It is remarkable, that a very great majority of the cures of consumption, which are related by different authors, have either been performed by emetics, or by decidedly nauseating remedies."

Perhaps no plan, that could be devised in incipient phthisis, is more judicious than a sea-voyage; and where hæmoptysis has existed, it has not seemed to be augmented whilst at sea, even during the violent retching that accompanies sea-sickness; indeed, Sir James Clark is of opinion, that more benefit is derived from the voyage when the incipient phthisis is accompanied with hæmoptysis; and he refers to numerous cases of decided amelioration where this complication existed. Nor is it only in incipient phthisis that relief is afforded by this agency. Although a permanent cure may rarely or never be accomplished, life is occasionally protracted, and fresh, though transient, vigour acquired, long before the invalid, who leaves this country on a European pilgrimage, has reached the shores of that continent. Many an individual quits the United States, labouring perhaps under hæmoptysis, with two evident indications of serious pulmonary mischief, yet how rare is it for us to hear, that his health has not been somewhat improved, and still more rare, that death has overtaken him during his voyage.

The good effects of a sea-voyage in invigorating the lungs is farther evidenced by the great exemption of sailors from phthisical affections.

We have yet to inquire into those situations, within our own country, which seem to be pre-eminently adapted for the consumptive, or rather for those of weak lungs. From the published meteorological tables, it would seem, that St. Augustine and Tampa Bay, and certain situations deeper in the peninsula of Florida, are among the best situations for this purpose.

Accurate meteorological registers afford the most unquestionable single evidence of climate; but there may be other circumstances connected with localities, that may render them an inconvenient or insalubrious retreat. The seasons, too, differ somewhat in different years; and this fact, with the successful or unsuccessful issue of cases, defective accommodations, and the presence or absence of hypochondriasis in the valetudinarian, may somewhat explain the conflicting statements occasionally met with respecting the climate of different situations, of which it would appear to be so easy to obtain exact accounts.

This seems to be the case with St. Augustine. In the number of the *American Journal of the Medical Sciences*, for May, 1833, the Author, on the strength of meteorological registers kept by the surgeons of the United States' Army, as well as on other grounds, inferred the superior fitness of St. Augustine and of Tampa Bay, as winter retreats; but in regard to the former of these localities there has been a wide difference of sentiment.

In a northern periodical, (*Medical Magazine*, No. 12, cited in *American Journal of the Medical Sciences*, for Nov. 1833,) Dr. L. V. Bell,—now the able superintendent of the Charlestown Insane Asylum,—who resided in St. Augustine during one season, gave a most unfavourable picture not only of the climate but of almost every thing connected with the place directly or indirectly. According to this gentleman, a bar exists at the entrance of the harbour, which renders the entrance or exit of vessels, drawing more than nine, or nine and a half feet of water, impracticable. The attempt is rarely made to enter the harbour without a pilot; and, from the natural obstructions, "as well as the want of capacity, indolence, or absence of competition among the pilots, the harbour is justly esteemed one of great difficulty." Again; "the surf, breaking on the outside of Anastasia Island in certain winds, is tremendous. When heard in the city, it resembles very much the roar of Niagara Falls, a circumstance not a little annoying to the sick, before the ear becomes accustomed to the sound." The appearance of the town, and the materials of which it is built, are described as miserable in the extreme, not more than about half a dozen of the residences being "tolerably convenient and comfortable." Nor does the supply of food draw forth any commendation. "The agricultural productions of the vicinity are almost nothing. A little market place is furnished with one beef, *uniformly of miserable quality*, which is adequate to the consumption of the whole place, with fish of some variety, including a small and indifferent species of oysters, and rarely with pork and poultry. Mutton is never seen: sheep, it is said, being immediately destroyed, when turned to pasture, by a small sharp pointed bur, called the *cockspur*, which grows every where. Garden vegetables of all kinds, as well as hay, butter, apples, &c. must be brought from the north, and are generally of indifferent quality, and high prices. The market is so limited, and the number of vessels arriving so small, that there are frequently long periods in which some of the most necessary and essential articles cannot be obtained at all, or only at the most exorbitant rates; butter, for example, at seventy-five cents per pound. With a soil and climate capable of producing almost every article of vegetable use or luxury, such is the indolence and want of enterprise of the great bulk of the population, that they prefer subsisting, day after day, on fish, oysters, and the sweet potato, to the trouble and labour of raising bread stuffs, garden vegetables, poultry, &c."

The population, it farther appears, is much below the statement of any gazetteer or account, which Dr. Bell has seen; a great proportion of the whites are Minorcans, "retaining all their original ignorance, indolence and superstition." All the essentials for invalids are obtained with difficulty; even the facilities of taking exercise are almost null; there is not one pleasant landscape, or agreeable view; and the means of gestation are few, and very expensive. " In short," he observes, " (excepting the climate,—whose claims to attention we shall shortly examine,) St. Augustine possesses, in a most eminent degree, the deficiency of every thing which can amuse, improve, or restore the invalid, and the presence of every thing, which can serve to irritate his feelings, impoverish his estate, and disappoint his hopes."

After such an exposition of collateral circumstances, it could scarcely be expected, that Dr. Bell should afford any strong testimony in favour of the climate; and if we admit, as we readily do, that he had every disposition to record accurately; still, with impressions so unpropitious, this could scarcely be accomplished. He objects to the thermometrical registers kept by the medical officers of the army; and asserts, that there was an " unfair, injudicious exposure of the instruments from which the observations were made." It is impossible, however, to divine the object, which the officers could have in view by any false reports, and it must be admitted, that their official statements are more to be relied upon than the results of individual, and irresponsible observations.

Climate, is doubtless, the most important of all considerations to the invalid; but the fatigue of the voyage, the extent of accommodations when at the place of destination, and other collateral circumstances, cannot be disregarded. It matters not what may be the advantages of climate, provided they cannot be properly enjoyed. We have seen, however, that a sea-voyage is beneficial; and the fatigue in this way, when there is no after land journey, must be infinitely less than in the laborious and uncomfortable pilgrimage, which invalids have been, and are, accustomed to undergo for the purpose of wintering in Southern France or Italy, and it is difficult to suppose, that the accommodations in Florida can be much inferior to those in certain places of any of the situations we have mentioned, or to such as could be afforded in any of the foreign localities, which we have indicated as adapted for the winter residence of the consumptive. Accounts, indeed, from invalids in Florida, have spoken in the highest terms of the kindness and hospitality of the inhabitants, and of the advantages of the climate. During the prevalence of certain winds the air is cold and damp, but at such times the invalid can keep his apartment. The great questions are—whether the locality be not more favourable, for a winter retreat, than the more northern portions of the United States; and whether the invalid, by resorting thither, may not escape in a great measure the depressed temperature, and the numerous vicissitudes, for which most parts of the United States are so proverbial. In corroboration of the affirmative view of these questions, the Author is glad to be able to adduce the following interesting letter from his friend Dr. Peter Porcher—an intelligent physician at that time practising in St. Augustine, now of Charleston, S. C. For it the Author was indebted to the politeness of the late Colonel Joseph M. White—delegate from Florida—to whom he applied for information on the subject.

*St. Augustine*, March 24, 1834.

My Dear Sir—

Numerous engagements have prevented me from paying earlier attention to the letter of Dr. Dunglison, forwarded by you some time since, requesting some information on the subject of the climate, &c. of St. Augustine. The Doctor has been prompted to this inquiry by the great discrepancy, which he has noticed between the statements made by Dr. Bell, and those contained in circulars, letters, &c., which have had very general circulation, but which are characterized by any thing but a freedom from exaggeration. They are all calculated to produce too favourable an impression, and to disappoint those who may place reliance on them. Dr. Bell, however, is not free from the imputation of having gone into the other extreme. His sojourn was during a short period of a season, which he acknowledges to have been "one of rather unusual severity;" and this circumstance, together with the disappointment of high wrought expectations, has caused him to underrate the advantages to be derived from a resort to this climate. Having myself resided here five years, I shall endeavour to satisfy the inquiries of Dr. Dunglison, by giving such a statement as my own observations for that period enables me. I shall commence by confirming the remark of Dr. Bell, that the meteorological tables, which have been published, are little to be depended on,—the observations having been made under circumstances calculated to exhibit too favourable a result, owing to the unfair, and injudicious exposure of the instruments. My own tables have been made with *self-registering thermometers*, in a northern exposure, without doors, and under circumstances favourable to a correct report, but it is only for the last fifteen months that I have kept them regularly.

The " extent of vicissitudes," which is the subject of the first inquiry, is greater than has been generally reported. My record does not extend beyond December, 1832. In that time there has occurred one change of 37° in 24 hours. It may be considered a rare instance, and perhaps such a one has not taken place before for many years. Changes of 20° or 25° occur frequently every winter; in some instances even in a few hours. But they take place generally within a range, which seems to produce no serious influence on the system. They are usually between 65° and 45° or 40°. Sometimes they may extend even to 35°. To the latter point, however, the thermometer falls not more than five or six times in the course of a winter, nor does it remain so low, more than a few hours. There is an assertion in Dr. Bell's paper, as published in the Philadelphia Journal, which I am sure the Author never intended to make. " It is no uncommon circumstance," says the paper, " for a fall of 70° to 10° to be produced in about as many minutes." Such a statement would be contradicted by his own table. The meaning of the Author, I take to be that a fall of 10° in as many minutes is no uncommon occurrence. The lowest degree to which the mercury has fallen, that has been noticed, has been 20°, and on one occasion I knew ice to remain in the shade during the greater part of a day. But such an occurrence is so exceedingly rare that it may only be noted as an exception to the general mildness of the climate. I have never known the mercury to remain for twenty-four hours as low as 32°. On the contrary, frequently, when my thermometer has indicated a minimum of 32° during the night, it would be found above that point in the morning; so that the occurrence of such a degree of cold for a short period, and that too when the invalid is sheltered from its influence, may be considered of little consequence. The lowest point, to which the thermometer fell during the two last winters, was 26°— once in each winter.

The climate is, if I may use the expression of a most *relenting* character. When we do experience what may be considered cold weather for our latitude, it is seldom of more than two days' duration, and is generally followed by a long succession of days with an atmosphere the most bland and delightful. Its peculiar softness is a subject of common observation. We are liable, it is true, to north-east storms, often of long continuance, during the early part of winter, from which, by the by, no climate is altogether exempt at that season; but which are a great source of complaint to the invalid, who may be prevented from taking his accustomed exercise. But, for this inconvenience he never fails to be compensated by the prevalence of such weather, as would satisfy the most fastidious in as large an amount as in any climate of which I have any information.

Although St. Augustine has been long known, and its climate appreciated, it is only within the last four or five years, that public attention has been more particularly directed to it, by circumstances which it is unnecessary to mention. The consequence was, that the keepers of hotels and boarding-houses, who had hitherto received but a very limited patronage, and whose means did not enable them to prepare themselves but for the reception of a few visiters, found themselves suddenly called on to accommodate two or three times the number they had expected. Of course, the majority of those, who came at that time, found no provision made for their reception, and were very uncomfortably situated. This inconvenience is, however, less sensibly felt every season. In consequence of the increasing number of visiters, (more than two hundred during the past winter) there has been an immense alteration within the last two years; and there are now three or four houses capable of accommodating from twenty-five to thirty-five each, besides a number of private families, who are in the habit of receiving six or eight. It is not difficult to obtain houses at a moderate rent,—in some instances furnished. The price of board varies from six to eight dollars per week. The fare to be obtained at the boarding-houses may not be found to be equal to what it is in places having greater facilities in obtaining supplies,—almost every article of consumption being brought from Charleston and New York, except the ordinary productions of the garden, to which more attention is now paid than formerly. With the encouragement, which they are now receiving, however, there is an obvious improvement each successive season. The communication with New York is kept up by one, and with Charleston by two, regular packets, besides the frequent arrival, during the winter season, of other vessels from those ports, as well as from Philadelphia and Baltimore. They are usually laden with produce, which is bartered for oranges—the principal staple of the place. The product of the groves in the city and vicinity, the past season, was about two millions, which was a large crop; the ordinary yield being from a million, to a million and a half.

I have never visited the middle district, and can therefore say nothing of the climate; but from the inquiries I have made, I presume it does not differ materially from this. There are several situations on the river St. Johns, which runs parallel with the sea for two hundred miles, to which the invalid can retreat. Being on an average about twenty-five miles from the sea, and the intervening country a dry pine barren, its banks are sheltered from the northeast winds, which are apt to prevail on the coast during the winter season. The number that could at present be accommodated is, however, limited, as the country is thinly settled, and few persons are as yet prepared for the reception of visiters.

I am not disposed to deny the existence of objections to St. Augustine, yet I am inclined to believe it is the best resort for an invalid within the limit of our own country. The fact of its being the most southern settlement would of itself lead us to expect a milder climate, and the vicissitudes of the weather, although not unfrequent, make no serious impression on the system. As to the curative effect, which may have been absurdly claimed for the climate, and which is disputed by Dr. Bell, I would only observe, that such a character can hardly be predicated of any climate; but if air and exercise be important to the invalid, and contribute in any degree to his recovery, which they confessedly do, he cannot enjoy those advantages in any part of our country in so great a degree as here.

Of the number, that annually visit us, there is a fair proportion of cases that experience relief, and many of permanent restoration to health. Among our own citizens, there are several to be found, who have been compelled to make this their permanent abode; and in other instances it is only after a succession of seasons spent in this climate, that they have ventured to face the rigours of a northern winter. Among my own acquaintance there are several, who have had occasion to visit the different climates of the south of Europe, and who, after a knowledge of this resort, have given it the preference.

I have very briefly, and I fear unsatisfactorily, replied to the inquiries of Dr. Dunglison; and I am sorry I have not been able to comply sooner with his request. If any information it is in my power to give can be of any service to him, he may at all times command,

My dear sir, yours most truly,

PETER PORCHER.

Hon. Joseph M. White, *Washington City.*

The late Dr. H. Perrine was of opinion, that the most salubrious retreat for the valetudinarian is farther to the south than St. Augustine. In a letter to the editor of the *American Journal of the Medical Sciences,* occasioned by the remarks of the Author of this work—he challenges his professional brethren in general to name any place in the world, which, in climate and position, can combine as many natural, and social advantages, for a dry winter retreat to our invalids, as Cape Florida: and in a subsequent number of the same journal, he recurs to the subject, and suggests, that an association might be formed, with a capitol of 100,000 dollars, "which would furnish the buildings, gardens, and other conveniences requisite for the most squeamish visiter, and keep a packet running every month with passengers and effects, to and from the north." It is obvious, however, that until such conveniences exist much cannot be said of the *social* advantages, which Cape Florida possesses; and, that these are important adjuvants to the advantages bestowed by nature, and not to be overlooked in questions of this kind, is manifest. At the present time, according to a recent writer (Dr. Forry, *The Climate of the United States,* p. 259, New York, 1842) St. Augustine and Key West are the only places that afford the conveniences required by the wants of an invalid: but assuming that proper accommodations can be equally obtained at all points, Key Biscayno on the south-eastern coast, or Tampa Bay, on the Gulf of Mexico, claims a decided preference especially, over St. Augustine; and he adds—"when the period of the red man's departure shall have passed, the climate of this land of flowers will, it may be safely predicted, acquire a celebrity as a winter residence not inferior to that of Italy, Madeira, or Southern France."

The candour, which pervades the above letter of Dr. Porcher, and the standing of its author stamp it as authority on which the utmost reliance may be placed; and if we regard the advanced stages of phthisis, in which individuals are occasionally sent to those retreats, the disappointment in the minds of the attendants at the unfavourable result,—which ought still to have been anticipated,—and the hypochondriasis of many invalids, rendering them disposed to be dissatisfied with every situation, we can, in some measure, account for the unfavourable representations, that have been made of the climate.

Of the advanced condition of pulmonary mischief, under which patients proceed, at times, to Florida, we have a striking example in the work of Dr. Morton, (*Op. cit.* p. 147) who, by the way, is by no means favourably disposed towards it as a winter retreat. "The winter at this place," he observes, " is occasionally mild, and equable throughout, and, under such circumstances, has afforded a decidedly beneficial retreat. But for one such winter, I am informed, that there are three, which present a reversed picture. The late Dr. C. of this city was induced by his friends to pass the winter of 1829—1830 in St. Augustine. He had, when he left here, *purulent expectoration, hæmoptysis, and hectic fever.* The winter proved of the most favourable character, and he returned home in the spring surprisingly improved in his general health. This fact induced not only himself, but many other invalids, similarly affected, to pass the following winter (1830—1831) at the same place. But, in lieu of the mild climate of the previous year, there was an almost constant prevalence of a damp, chilly, north-east wind, so deleterious in its effects as to destroy many of the invalids collected there, and irreparably to shatter the feeble frames of others. Among the latter was my friend, who survived his return but a few months."

But, surely, such are not fair cases to be adduced against any winter retreat whatever;—cases of " purulent expectoration, hæmoptysis, and hectic fever"!—in other words, of confirmed consumption—of what Dr. Morton himself had elsewhere called " the last and irremediable stage." The great aim of all recent writers on climate has been to show, that such are precisely the cases, that ought not to be subjected to the inconveniences of expatriation under the slender hopes, that change of residence, of any kind, may be followed by any important amelioration ; and it is, consequently, no more remarkable, that they should terminate fatally in St. Augustine, than in southern France and Italy, or in any other situation to which they might be sent.

"When consumption is fully established," says Sir James Clark—an individual, who has had, perhaps, more opportunities for observing the effects of expatriation, in such cases, than any professional gentleman in England, having resided, for many years, since the peace of 1815, in southern France and Italy—"that is, when the character of the cough and expectoration, the hectic fever and emaciation give every reason to believe the existence of tuberculous cavities in the lungs; and still more, when the presence of these is ascertained by auscultation, benefit is not to be expected from change of climate; and a long journey will almost certainly increase the sufferings of the patient, and hurry on the fatal termination. Under such circumstances, the patient and his advisers will, therefore, act more judiciously by contenting themselves with the most favourable residence which their own country affords, or even by awaiting the result amid the comforts of home, and the watchful care of friends. And this will be the more necessary, as the degree of sympathetic fever, and the disposition to inflammation of the lungs, or hæmoptysis, is more considerable. It is natural for the relations of such a patient to cling to that which seems to afford even a ray of hope. But did they know the discomforts, the fatigue, the exposure, and irritation, necessarily attendant on a long journey in the advanced period of consumption, they would shrink from such a measure. The medical adviser, also, when he reflects upon the accidents to which such a patient is liable, will surely hesitate ere he condemns him to the additional evil of expatriation. And his motives for hesitation will be increased when he considers how often the unfortunate patient sinks a prey to his disease long before he reaches the place of destination, or, at best, arrives there in a worse condition than when he left England, doomed shortly to add another name to the long and melancholy list of his countrymen, who have sought, with pain and suffering a distant country, only to find in it an untimely grave. When the patient is a female, the reasons against such a journey may be urged with increased force." "There are, however," he adds,—and this is the only consideration that can justify us in having recourse to so doubtful a measure, where the disease is so far advanced—" chronic cases of consumption, in which the disease of the lungs, even though arrived at its last stage, may derive benefit by a removal to a mild climate. The cases, to which I allude, are those in which the disease has been induced in persons little disposed to it constitutionally, and in whom it usually occurs later in life than when hereditary. The tuberculous affection in such persons is occasionally confined to a small portion of the lungs, and the system sympathizes little with the local disease. In instances of this kind, a residence for some time in a mild climate, especially when aided by a proper regimen, and such remedies as the state of the general health, or any complication requires, may be the means of saving the patient. Likewise in those fortunate, but unhappily too rare, examples of consumption, where the progress of the disease in the lungs has been arrested by nature, but in which a long period must elapse before the work of reparation is completed, a mild climate may be of considerable service in improving the general health and in removing the patient from many causes, which are likely to renew irritation in the lungs. Such a climate, indeed, offers great advantages to consumptive invalids of this description. During my residence abroad, I met with several such, who passed their winters in Italy with much more comfort, and enjoyment of life than they did in England. I believe, that in nicely balanced cases life may be preserved for many years by a constant residence in a mild climate, and by sedulously avoiding, at the same time, whatever could, by disturbing the balance of the circulation, produce congestion, or light up inflammatory disease in the lungs." (The *Sanative influence of Climate*, p. 52.)

The testimony of Dr. James Johnson is less encouraging than that of Sir James Clark. In *delicate health*, without any proof of organic changes in the lungs—in what is called a " tendency to pulmonary affection," a journey to Italy—and the remark is equally applicable to the winter retreats of our own continent—and a winter's residence there, he thinks, under strict caution, offer probabilities of an amelioration of health ; and, again, in cases where there is a suspicion, or certainty of tubercles in the lungs, not softened down, or attended with purulent expectoration, an Italian climate *may* do some good, and *may* do much harm—the chances being pretty nearly balanced; but where tuberculous matter appears in the expectoration, and where the stethoscope indicates, that a considerable portion of the lungs is unfitted for respiration, a southern climate is more likely to accelerate than retard the fatal event, and takes away the few chances, that remain of final recovery. " But," he adds, " there is a large class of complaints, which *resemble* consumption, and which, I have no doubt, contribute much to the reputation of southern climates for the cure of that terrible scourge. These are bronchial affections, viz :—chronic inflammation, or irritation of the mucous membrane of the lungs. The journey to Rome, or to Pisa, and the mild air of the winter in those places, with care to avoid sudden transitions, often cure or greatly relieve these complaints, and the individuals are said to be saved from tubercular consumption. The greatest care—sometimes considerable power of diagnosis—is required to discriminate the *bronchial*, from the *tubercular* affection, and yet upon this discrimination often hangs the fate of the patient, or, at all events, the propriety of migrating to a southern clime. The science of auscultation, now so ardently cultivated, will prevent much injudicious advice being given by the profession, and much serious injury being sustained by invalids. It is also probable, that in some cases, where there is a very partial or circumscribed tuberculation of the lungs (the rest of the apparatus being unaffected,) a winter's residence in Rome, Pisa, or Nice, might be beneficial. This is the opinion, at least of Dr. [Sir James Clark;] but here the greatest care is to be taken, in examination with the stethoscope, to ascertain that the expectoration comes from a very small excavation, the lungs being elsewhere in a sound state." (*Change of air*, p. 307.)

It is not logical, consequently, to infer the insalubrity of any situation from its apparent effects on these unfortunate cases. The climate, the vicissitudes of which are within trifling limits, and the medium temperature of which is somewhat elevated, is decidedly the best adapted, *cæteris paribus*. Information on these points is afforded mathematically by accurate meteorological registers; and they exhibit, that the climate of St. Augustine, and of Florida in general, possesses these requisites pre-eminently over other parts of the United States. " Whatever situations," says Dr. Morton, " may be chosen, those will be found most congenial, which possess the nearest approach to an equable temperature." In a previous page, however, he observes :—" with respect to the bay of St. Louis, and the Passa Christiana, both on the gulf of Mexico, Dr. Hunt informs us, that the climate is not more salutary than at Sullivan's Island, or St. Augustine;"—yet he remarks, that " Passa Christiana is liable to no variety of temperature—its atmosphere is warmed by the gulf stream, and is exempt by distance, and the intervening forest from the cold air of the mountains:"—possessing in other words, we should conceive, every requisite for a salubrious retreat for the consumptive; and if St. Augustine enjoy equal advantages, it ought to be considered highly favoured by nature for the valetudinarian.

Besides, if objections apply to St. Augustine on the score of the north-east storms, they are not equally applicable to Pensacola or to Mobile. To the latter place the Author recommended a young medical friend to proceed to pass the winter, which he did with evident advantage; but the benefit was temporary only, and he ultimately sank under his intractable malady. The following extract from a letter to the Author conveys his views of the climate, and of the advantages and inconveniences to the invalid who may proceed thither.

*Philadelphia*, Sept. 1st, 1842.

DEAR SIR—It affords me much pleasure, to give you any information in my power, respecting Mobile as a place of resort for invalids.

Mobile is situate on the west side of Mobile bay—about 30 miles from the Atlantic, in a position elevated several feet above the overflow of the river. The Spanish part of the town consists principally of ancient frame, and log, and plastered buildings: the more recently improved parts, however, are handsomely built of brick.— The public buildings are not very numerous, but some of them would be an ornament to any city. The population during the winter is 15,000—and in summer 10,000:—the streets are pleasant: many of them have been paved with shells:—the roads are generally very good, and there are some beautiful rides, 5 or 10 miles from the city. Although the population consists largely of eastern and northern men, yet their manners and habits are similar to those met with so universally in the southern states. They are exceedingly kind to strangers, and it is a place in which a stranger soon feels himself at home, and surrounded by a kind and most hospitable people, by whom, morals and religion have lately received a good share of attention. For these and other reasons mentioned, it is, in my opinion, a pleasant place of resort for an invalid, so far as the place and the people are concerned.

The climate is very changeable, and damp ; but it never was so cold, during the time I was there (from 1st Nov. 1841 to April 7th 42,) as to make it an objection to my being out of doors. I was not kept in doors more than five whole days all the winter, and then it was in consequence of the heavy rains that fell occasionally.— The month of November was, indeed, delightful during the day ; but cool at night. The coldest weather we had was in the last of December, when there was a thin scum of ice formed, which was the only ice I saw all the time I was there. In January, the weather was cool and changeable. February was much warmer and more pleasant than December or January; and in March it was quite warm during the day ; and at night mild and pleasant. I could remain out of doors in the night air until 10 o'clock, in most of the nights of the month; and experienced no inconvenience from so doing. When I left, I weighed 14 pounds more than when I started from home. I noted the state of the thermometer part of the time while there, and the following table will give you a more particular idea of the climate : the observations were taken in the shade, on the north side of the house.

|  | Average temp. at 10 o'clock. | Extremes min. | max. | Rain in inches. |
|---|---|---|---|---|
| 1841 December | 56° | 47° | 76° | 4 |
| 1842 January | 63 | 50 | 77 | 5 |
| February | 64 | 50 | 78 | 8 |
| March | 79 | 60 | 88 | 3 |

There is a large number of boarding houses, and in the most respectable the accommodations are very good. Green peas, potatoes, &c. &c. are ripe by the first of April, or earlier. The water used is rain water purified by charcoal, &c. It is the best water I ever tasted. In consequence of the dampness of the atmosphere, and the frequent changes that occur, an inland situation would in my opinion be more advantageous; but of the correctness of this opinion you are well qualified to judge.

Professor R. Dunglison.

In regard to St. Augustine and Pensacola, Dr. Chapman (*Lectures on the more important Diseases of the Thoracic and Abdominal Viscera*, p. 85, Philad. 1844) states, that no comfortable accommodations are to be had in either, and that " they are less suited from their proximity to the sea-board."—He thinks, that there is the least objection to a short distance within South Carolina or Georgia; and he is inclined to believe, from what he has heard, that the town of Athens in the latter state offers great advantages. Savannah, he adds, has hitherto been his choice when called on to decide peremptorily;—yet Savannah must be more strongly liable to the objections which he brings against Pensacola, inasmuch as it has, in addition, the N. E. storms which have been considered to render St. Augustine an unsuitable winter residence for the pulmonary invalid.

In every situation within the limits of the United States, the range of the thermometer is great, and so far as this goes the climate would appear unfavourable for those of weak lungs. The medium heat is, however, higher in the southern situations we have mentioned, and this, along with other atmospheric advantages, may counterbalance the evil. Certain it is, that although the climate of the United States is proverbially one of extreme vicissitudes, the number of deaths by consumption is not as great as in England, or in many of the situations of southern France and Italy, which have been selected as the winter resort for the phthisical invalid.

It has been affirmed, that all the towns on the sea-board of the United States, and indeed of every country, are less suited for the valetudinarian than the more inland situations; or, in other words, that a mixture of sea and land air is unfavourable to those of delicate lungs, and especially where phthisis, or a predisposition to it, exists; and Dr. Morton judiciously suggests, that this is probably, in a great measure, owing to the sudden and extreme changes in the atmosphere in such situations; " for it has been observed," he adds, " that several sea-bathing places in the south of England, which are protected from the north and east winds, are congenial to pulmonary invalids; while other places, but a short distance off, and which are exposed to the winds in question, exert a decidedly noxious influence." There must, however, be an admixture of sea and land air in all these situations, and the truth seems to be, that although it has appeared to Dr. Rush, Dr. Morton, Dr. Chapman, and others, that this admixture of sea and land air is of deleterious tendency in the cases in question, the experience of others is not in accordance with theirs, and it is by no means uncommon for invalids, from the interior of some of the States, to resort to seaports in the same parallel, with the view of enjoying a milder atmosphere during the winter,—a change, however, too insignificant in extent to be likely to be productive of any marked advantage. Moreover, the greater part of the situations in southern France, and Italy, which are the resort of invalids, are on, or near, the sea; and the different seaports on the southern coast of England, and the Cove of Cork, are, as we have seen, the chosen retreats of the consumptive during the winter season. The evidence, too, adduced by Dr. Porcher in favour of the climate of St. Augustine for the consumptive, is certainly highly favourable, notwithstanding all the objections that have been brought against it; and Dr. Hulse of the Navy, (*Army and Navy Chronicle*, April 16, 1835) asserts, that he has never known or heard of a case of consumption that originated in Pensacola. There is, indeed, a great difference of sentiment amongst the profession as regards the preference to be given to a sea-side, or an inland situation; and a good deal of the difficulty, as Sir James Clark has correctly remarked, arises from the circumstance, that we have no very satisfactory comparisons on the subject, in which the nature of the climate, occupations and habits of life, &c. of the inhabitants, have been fairly and fully taken into account, so as to enable us to judge, how far the frequency of consumption, in any particular place, may be connected with the nature of the climate; and how much may depend upon the mode of living, &c.

The following table by Dr. Gouverneur Emerson, of the average mortality from consumption, and acute diseases of the lungs, in the four largest cities in the United States,—New York, Boston, Philadelphia, and Baltimore,—is strikingly elucidative of the difficulties that surround us, in accounting for either the general or particular mortality of any place, as compared with that of others.

| | New York. | Boston. | Philad. | Balt. |
|---|---|---|---|---|
| Average annual proportion of the general mortality to the population, one in | 39.36 | 44.93 | 47.86 | 39.17 |
| Average of the mortality from consumption alone to the general mortality, one in | 5.23 | 5.54 | 6.38 | 6.21 |
| Average of consumption and acute diseases of the lungs, one in | 4.07 | 4·47 | 4.90 | 5.33 |

It is proper to add, however, that this point of statistics has been recently investigated by Dr. Hayward, of Boston (*New England Quarterly Journal of Med. and Surg.*, Jan. 1843) who has found, that whilst Philadelphia has suffered less from consumption than New York or Boston during the last thirty years—the average proportion of deaths from that disease being 1 in 7.003; in Boston 1 in 6.185; and in New York, 1 in 5.547—during the last ten years, Boston has enjoyed the greatest exemption. From 1831 to 1840 inclusive, the deaths in Boston from consumption were 1 in 7.587; in Philadelphia, 1 in 7.482; and in New York, 1 in 5.952. These observations are far from according with the views of a recent writer, which certainly require the aid of statistical evidence. "It is on the lateral boundaries of our north-eastern territories, that it (consumption) extensively prevails, and greatly in New York, Newport and Boston. As we advance southerly, and particularly receding from the ocean, it sensibly diminishes. The native population of this city (Philadelphia) is nearly exempt from the disease, and the fact is important as showing the influence of locality. Equally remote from the sea and the mountains, it comparatively escapes from the austere winds of the one, and the cold blasts of the other, maintaining a more regular and moderate temperature than the latitude of its position would seem to warrant." (Dr. Chapman, *Op. cit.*, p. 28.)

The admixture of sea and land air, which must exist in some of these cities to a greater extent than in others, obviously cannot be invoked to explain the entire discrepancy. It would seem, however, that situations in cold and highly variable climates, in which the hygrometric state of the atmosphere is liable to be considerable, and which are open to cold winds from the ocean, are less fitted than others for those of weak lungs,—and yet the observations of our Army Surgeons would seem to show, that the posts on the seacoast and the lakes are less subject to catarrhal affections "than the dry and cold atmosphere of opposite localities." (Surgeon General Lawson, *Statistical Report*, p. 337. Washington, 1840.)

After all, as the Author has stated elsewhere, (*Practice of Medicine*, 2nd edit., i. 379, Philadelphia 1844,) the good effects of change of climate are mainly, if not wholly, dependent upon the revulsion produced in the *physique* as well as the *moral*; so that instead of selecting a situation for the brumal retreat of the invalid, which has equability of temperature as its sole recommendation, one ought rather to be chosen the temperature of which may be less equable, provided it be not too elevated, as in the torrid regions, or the air be not too damp. The great object is to select a situation in which the invalid can take exercise with safety in the open air every day during the winter; and the nearer the climate approaches this desideratum the better it is for the consumptive. In such a climate the patient ought to be as much as possible in the open air, and take exercise, both by walking and riding, short of inducing much fatigue.

Invalids who have passed the winter in the West Indies or in the southern part of the United States, should be especially careful not to return too early to their homes. The spring months are markedly those of great vicissitudes and trying to the delicate. Dr. Jackson, of Boston, who, as already remarked, sends his patients chiefly to Cuba, directs them to remain there until the last of April; then to go to Georgia or South Carolina, and to return end to Boston very slowly, so as not to reach New England until the of June:—and the course is precautionary and judicious. Should the invalid be unable to pursue it he should remain in his winter retreat until the end of May if possible.

Thus much, respecting the choice of a climate for escaping the severity of our winters, as well as the vicissitudes to which our autumnal, and spring months are so proverbially liable. It is often, however, an important subject of inquiry to decide as to the course to be pursued by the phthisical invalid during the summer season. When the mischief is incipient, there is nothing perhaps comparable to the revulsion, which the change of physical and moral influences, during a sea-voyage, is capable of effecting; and even in the more advanced stages, life has appeared to be prolonged by it. The facilities are so great for crossing the Atlantic, that a sea-voyage to Europe is easily undertaken, with every comfort provided that is practicable; and from the commencement of May no countries, perhaps, could afford greater advantages for a summer journey, and a temporary residence, than Great Britain or France. The invalid can remain some weeks in either, and return to his own country before the autumnal vicissitudes are experienced to any extent, so that he may be ready to make such arrangements as may be advisable for the winter. So salutary has been the influence of sea-voyages in consumptive affections, that it has not been deemed an idle or foolish proposal to have a ship fitted out for the express purpose of taking phthisical invalids to sea, and keeping them there for months and even years.

Next to a sea-voyage during the summer, travelling by land through different parts of this country may be recommended; and now, that the distance between different places has been so much reduced by rail-roads and steam navigation, a thorough change of atmospheric influences can be speedily obtained, with all the other advantages of change of society and scenery attendant upon travelling exercise. The physician must, however, use his best judgment in adapting his advice to particular cases. Pamphlets have appeared strongly recommending the Red Sulphur Springs of Virginia to the invalid during the summer season; and in many pulmonary affections, in which change of air, society, scenery, and appropriate mineral waters are indicated, few situations appear to offer more advantages. Possessing a delightful climate, and with accommodations well adapted for the comfort of the valetudinarian, it is an excellent retreat for all those for whom travelling exercise is deemed advisable,—no matter whether or not its waters possess the power of diminishing the frequency of pulse, as is affirmed by some, but denied by other observers. Were they, indeed, endowed with this virtue, they would not be applicable to all cases of phthisis; but where the waters failed, the admirable climate, with all the attendant advantages, might not the less exert its beneficial agency.

Attention has been recently directed by Professor Drake, of Louisville, to the northern lakes of this country as a summer residence for invalids of the south. (The *Northern Lakes, a Summer Residence for Invalids*, Louisville 1842.) A tour to these is said to offer advantages of novelty, great variety, magnificent scenery, a pure cool air, and many historical associations.

The due succession of the seasons and atmospheric vicissitudes, when within certain limits, are requisite for full mental and corporeal development. This we have already asserted. It is against the great vicissitudes, that occasionally take place, and for which this continent is celebrated, that we have to guard, by appropriate clothing, and by avoiding all unnecessary exposure.

It is a common feeling amongst mankind, that unseasonable weather,—as the occurrence of unusual warmth during the winter months,—must necessarily be unhealthy; and although this happens year after year, and every year, without confirming the impression, it remains as unshaken as the various superstitions regarding atmospheric prognostics, or the influence of the moon on organized bodies, which neither philosophy nor experience can recognise. There is no exact sequence of atmospheric changes, and although we may have them supervening in the most capricious manner, they do not aid us in solving the difficult problem of the causation of epidemics, which are doubtless, however, produced by peculiar atmospheric modifications, aided by a favourable concurrence of local influences.

The fallacy of our wonted deductions, with regard to unseasonable weather, is well illustrated in the remarks of one, who bestowed much time and attention on the investigation of the effects of the climate of London on the health of its inhabitants.

"The extraordinary mildness of last January," says Dr. Wm. Heberden, Jr., "compared with the unusual severity of the January preceding, affords a peculiarly favourable opportunity of observing the effect of each of these seasons, contrasted with each other. For of these two successive winters, one has been the coldest and the other the warmest of which any regular account has ever been kept in this country. Nor is this by any means an idle speculation or matter of mere curiosity; for one of the first steps towards preserving our fellow creatures is to point out the sources from which diseases are to be apprehended. And what may make the present inquiry more particularly useful is, that the result, as I hope clearly to make appear by the following statements, is entirely contrary to the prejudices usually entertained upon this subject.

"During last January, nothing was more common than to hear expressions of the unseasonableness of the weather, and fears lest the want of the usual degree of cold should be productive of putrid diseases, and I know not what other causes of mortality. On the other hand, 'a bracing cold,' and 'a clear frost,' are familiar in the mouth of every Englishman, and what he is taught to wish for as among the greatest promoters of health and vigour.

"Whatever deference be due to received opinions, it appears to me, however, from the strongest evidence, that the prejudices of the world are, upon this point at least, unfounded. The average degrees of heat upon Fahrenheit's thermometer, kept in London during the month of January, 1795, were 23° in the morning, and 29°.4 in the afternoon. The average in January, 1796, was 43°.5 in the morning, and 50°.1 in the afternoon;—a difference of above twenty degrees! And if we turn our attention from the comparative coldness of these months to the corresponding healthiness of each, collected from the weekly bills of mortality, we shall find the result no less remarkable. For in five weeks, between the 31st of December, 1794, and the 3d of February, 1795, the whole number of burials amounted to 2,823; and in an equal period of five weeks, between the 30th of December, 1795, and the 2d of February, 1796, to 1,471. So that the excess of the mortality in January, 1795, above that of January, 1796, was not less than 1,352 persons; a number sufficient surely to awaken the attention of the most prejudiced admirers of a frosty winter. And though I have only stated the evidence of two years, the same conclusion may universally be drawn, as I have learned from a careful examination of the weekly bills of mortality for many years. These two seasons were chosen as being each of them very remarkable, and in immediate succession one to the other, and in every body's recollection;"—And he concludes with the following observations on the effects of severe cold upon health.—"The poor, as they are worse protected from the weather, so are they of course the greatest sufferers from its inclemency. But every physician in London, and every apothecary can add his testimony, that their business, among all ranks of people, never fails to increase and to decrease with the frost. For if there be any whose lungs be tender, any whose constitution has been impaired either by age, or by intemperance, or by disease, he will be very liable to have all his complaints increased, and all his infirmities aggravated by such a season. Nor must the young and active think themselves quite secure, or fancy their health will be confirmed by imprudently exposing themselves. The stoutest man may meet with impediments to his recovery, from accidents otherwise inconsiderable; or may contract inflammations, or coughs, and lay the foundation of the severest ills. In a country where the prevailing complaints among all orders of people are colds, coughs, consumptions, and rheumatisms, no prudent man can surely suppose, that unnecessary exposure to an inclement sky,—that priding one's self upon going without any additional clothing in the severest winter,—that inuring one's self to be hardy at a time, that demands our cherishing the firmest constitution lest it suffer,—that braving the winds, and challenging the rudest efforts of the season, can ever be useful to Englishmen. But if generally, and upon the whole, it be inexpedient, then ought every one for himself to take care that he be not the sufferer. For many doctrines very importantly erroneous, —many remedies either vain, or even noxious, are daily imposed upon the world for want of attention to this great truth,—that it is from general effects only, and those founded upon extensive experience, that any maxim, to which each individual may with confidence defer, can possibly be established."

The animal body is necessarily exposed to so many diurnal vicissitudes, that it acquires the power of resisting many of those atmospheric conditions which might otherwise be morbific; and hence it is, that our speculations, regarding the healthy or unhealthy character of particular days, or seasons, are so often fallacious.

# CHAPTER II.

## FOOD.

### SECTION I.

Difference between the elements of animal and vegetable bodies, not great—definition of aliments—digestive apparatus of an animal indicates its food—natural food of man—sketch of the physiology of digestion—singular case of fistulous opening into the stomach, with experiments—classification of aliments—fibrin—albumen—gelatin—osmazome—fat and oil—fecula—mucilage—sugar—terms nutritious and digestible not convertible—proper digestive texture of food.

THE matters that enter into the composition of the human body are various, and some of them so difficult to be met with elsewhere, as to have caused a doubt, whether there may not exist in the powers of life a capability of forming new simple substances.— Vauquelin found, by feeding a hen for ten days on oats, that 137.796 grains of phosphate of lime, and 511.911 grains of carbonate of lime, more than could be accounted for by the food taken, were contained in the eggs, and excretions; and that of the silica— contained in the oats, on which it had been fed—34.282 grains had disappeared. The inferences from these singular facts were;— that lime, and perhaps phosphorus, is not a simple substance, but a compound, formed of ingredients existing in oats, water, or air, the only substances to which the fowl had access,—and that silica must have entered into its composition, seeing that a part had disappeared.

Since the time at which these experiments were instituted, lime has been proved to be a compound, but phosphorus still continues in the list of elementary bodies. If, however, the accuracy of Vauquelin's results be admitted, which, however, as he himself gives them, are arithmetically incorrect,—we must be compelled to regard it either as a compound formed in the plant under the vital influence, or to infer, that the same influence is capable of forming elementary or simple bodies, which seems incomprehensible.

Animals and vegetables, when examined as regards their chemical composition, afford strikingly analogous results. In both we find at least the following elements:—oxygen, hydrogen, carbon, azote or nitrogen, phosphorus, sulphur, iodine, bromine, chlorine, potassium, sodium, calcium, magnesium, silicium, manganese and iron: aluminium and copper, and, according to some, gold have been found only in plants; fluorin, and, it is said by some, lead and arsenic only in the animal kingdom. There is not, consequently, any essential difference in the elements that enter into the composition of animal and vegetable bodies. It is the particular combination and arrangement, that give rise to the diversities we observe in the two kingdoms of living nature, and in the individuals composing those kingdoms. Of these elements, nitrogen enters most commonly and in greater quantity in animal combinations; carbon most frequently, and abundantly in the constitution of the vegetable.

Thus far, we have employed the term *element* in its application to inorganic, as well as organic chemistry,—that is to designate a substance, which, in the present state of chemical science, does not admit of decomposition. We meet, however, in organized bodies, with substances that are also termed *elements*, but with the epithet *organic*, because they are found only in organized or living bodies. These are also called *proximate principles* or *compounds of organization*. They arise from the primary combination of two or more of the elementary substances in definite proportions, and go to the constitution of the different organs. They are, in the animal, protein, and its compounds albumen, fibrin, and casein, gelatin, osmazome, chondrin, globulin, pepsin, mucus, urea, uric or lithic acid, red colouring principle of the blood, yellow colouring principle of the bile—all of which contain azote: and olein and stearin, fatty matter of the brain and nerves, acetic acid, oxalic acid, benzoic acid, lactic acid, sugar of milk, sugar of diabetes, picromel, &c. which are devoid of azote. (See the Author's *Human Physiology*, 5th edition, i. 33, Philad. 1844.)

These immediate principles are more numerous in the vegetable, than in the animal kingdom; and every day is bringing to light some new substance of the kind. The organic salifiable bases are peculiar to the vegetable kingdom; and almost all the immediate principles of this kingdom, it was until recently believed, are ternary combinations of carbon, hydrogen, and oxygen; whilst those of animals are quaternary, from the union of azote with the three other elements. Modern researches, have, however, shown, that many of the principles formerly esteemed ternary in the vegetable are really quaternary.

In all cases, whatever may be the nature of the organic compound, the elements must be received from without; and, under the action of the living forces must be so combined as to constitute the different corporeal constituents; which, although themselves consisting of so many ingredients, are always identical in composition, whatever may be the nature of the food on which the organized being is nourished; or, if the organization varies, it is only within slender limits, and never to such an extent as to prevent the texture, peculiar to the animal, from being easily discoverable on intimate analysis. Thus, we can always detect—whatever may be the extraneous circumstances that influence them—the wood of the oak from that of the maple, and the flesh of the sheep from that of the ox.

Some of the secreted fluids afford us striking evidence of complexity of constitution. Messrs. Tiedemann and Gmelin detected the following articles in human saliva;—salivary matter; osmazome; mucus; perhaps albumen; a little fat, containing phosphorus; phosphate, and carbonate of lime; acetate, carbonate, phosphate, and sulphate of potassa; chloride and sulphocyanuret of potassium. Again, Dr. Henry affirms, that the following substances have been satisfactorily proved to exist in healthy urine:—water; free phosphoric acid; phosphate of lime; phosphate of magnesia; fluoric acid: uric acid; benzoic acid; lactic acid; urea; gelatin; albumen; lactate of ammonia; sulphate of potassa; sulphate of soda; chloride of calcium; chloride of sodium; phosphate of soda; phosphate of ammonia; sulphur, and silex;—all of which must have been obtained from without, and many of them combined, within the body, by ordinary chemical affinity, controlled, however, in all probability, by vital agency, but in what manner we know no more than we do of the vital processes in general. When we assert, that the operation is *vital*, we have expressed the limit of our knowledge, and the term is too often employed to protect our ignorance, when a better examination, or understanding of the subject, might have enabled us, at times, to present a more satisfactory explanation, founded on physical laws.

The physiologist is, therefore, chary in invoking this mysterious agency, and does not have recourse to *vitalism*, until other means of explanation fail him. Accordingly the tendency has been, of late years, to explain many of the phenomena of respiration, absorption, secretion, &c. on physical principles, which were, at one time, referred exclusively to vital agency, and are still so by such individuals as Lepelletier de la Sarthe, whose work on physiology has been written avowedly for the purpose of bringing back the minds of physiologists to the half deserted tenement of exclusive vitalism.

As all the substances we have enumerated—*inorganic* and *organic*—are necessary for the constitution of the secretions referred to,—and the remark is applicable to every other secretion, and to every tissue of the body,—it follows that, in strict language, they must all be regarded as *aliments*,—in other words, as substances, which, when introduced into the living body, are capable of nourishing it, and repairing its losses. Generally, however, the term *aliment* is restricted to substances, which, when received into the digestive organs, are capable of being converted into the nutritious fluid called *chyle,* and of serving to repair losses, which are constantly supervening in a living body, from the earliest period of fœtal formation to decrepitude. Accordingly, it has been affirmed, that bodies, which have possessed life, can alone be considered as affording aliment to animals. This is the opinion of Dr. Paris. (*Treatise on Diet,* fifth edition, p. 175. Lond. 1837.) "Yet," he remarks, " there exists a certain number of inorganic substances, such as water, common salt, lime, &c. which, although incapable by themselves of nourishing, appear, when administered in conjunction with the former, to contribute essentially to nutrition. The consideration, therefore, of the *Materia Alimentaria* necessarily embraces not only the SUBSTANTIVE agents above stated, but those which, from their *modus operandi,* are entitled to the distinctive appellation of alimentary ADJECTIVES." Under the head of *substantive agents* he arranges all the varieties of animal and vegetable food; under that of *alimentary adjectives,* the class of condiments.

It would seem obvious, that no substance can be regarded as adapted for full animal sustenance, which does not contain oxygen, hydrogen, carbon, and azote, combined, as we meet with them, in the animal and vegetable kingdoms; and, therefore, that inorganic bodies, which are totally devoid of these ultimate elements, or possess but a binary, or ternary combination of them, cannot be regarded as *substantive* aliments although their presence may be necessary for the due constitution of certain products of organization. Iron and silex, for example, are found in the hair, and are necessary for its perfect organization; but they can only be regarded as alimentary *adjectives*, and could afford no support against the decay of organized matter which is perpetually occurring in the living tissues, and which absolutely demands for its reparation a due supply of ultimate organic elements.

It is known, that particular tribes feed, at certain seasons, on mineral substances, or are *geophagists*. The quarriers in Thuringia eat a kind of *rock butter*, spread on bread; the inhabitants of New Scotland a kind of steatite, and the Ottomaques of South America, a fat, unctuous earth, or a species of pipe-clay; but whether these ought to be regarded as *substantive*, or *adjective* aliments—to adopt the language of Paris—has been a matter of dispute. It is probable, that they belong rather to the latter class,—serving to allay the sensation of hunger by impressing and distending the stomach, and acting as *condiments* by putting the organs into a condition for assimilating a greater quantity of the nutritious matter taken into the stomach along with them. It is true Humboldt asserts, that the quantity of clay, consumed by the Ottomaques, and the greediness with which they devour it, seemed to him to prove, that it does more than merely distend their hungry stomachs; and the organs of digestion, he thinks, may have the power of extracting from it something convertible into animal substance. We are told, however, by the same excellent authority, that the Ottomaques occasionally make an addition to this—what he terms—" unnatural fare," of small fish, lizards, and fern roots. These additions probably furnish the reparatory materials. We are in the habit of taking far more nutriment than is absolutely necessary for the repair of the wear and tear of the living machine; but the organs of assimilation appropriate no more than is requisite. The residue, consequently, is ejected from the body as excrement. But if, as in the case of the tribes in question, the sensation of hunger be postponed, by filling the stomach with inorganic matter, the activity of the assimilating organs may be augmented, and a small quantity of a substance, that has possessed life, may be sufficient, if thoroughly converted, to supply the wants of the system. This view is strengthened by the analysis, made by Vauquelin, of the greenish steatite of New Scotland; which, according to Labillardière, served to allay the sensation of hunger by filling the stomach. He was totally unable to extract any thing nutritive from it. So far as we know, there is no animal that feeds on mineral substances. The earthworm swallows considerable quantities of earth, but this is for the purpose of obtaining the organic matters that are mixed with it. The gallinaceous birds, too, require an admixture of sand, or pebbles with their organic food, but this is necessary for the due trituration, or mastification of the food in the gizzard. (See, on this subject, Truman, *On Food*, p. 66, Lond. 1842.)

The inorganic compound, respecting the nutritive properties of which there has been the greatest doubt, is water. Fordyce kept gold-fish for six months, in distilled water, and thought himself justified in concluding, that animals might live on water, and air alone; and Rondelet kept a fish for three years in a vessel containing spring water, which grew so large, that the vessel was too small for it. It has been supposed, however, that in such instances the water may contain organic matters dissolved in it; or, if not so,—as in the case of distilled water,—that the seeds of confervæ, and the ova of infusory animalcules, borne about in the atmosphere, may be received into the fluid, undergo slight development, and be swallowed by animals; but even under this explanation the facts are sufficiently singular. It is possible, that the phenomena in these cases may be otherwise explained. The human body is capable of being nourished by both animal and vegetable substances; yet, many of these contain no azote. This element must, therefore, in such cases, be obtained elsewhere, and perhaps from the air of the atmosphere. Liebig, indeed, affirms, that no nitrogen is absorbed from the atmosphere; but this is opposed to the results of all modern observation. (See the Author's *Human Physiology*, edit. cit. ii. 45, and Pereira, *Treatise on Food and Diet*, Amer. edit. p. 17, New York, 1843.) In the same way, we may conceive, that the oxygen, and hydrogen of the water may unite with azote, and carbon derived from the atmosphere, and that a product may result, which is capable of supplying the wants of nutrition. It is probable, indeed, that all organized bodies possess the power of reducing substances, taken as food, into their elements, and of recomposing them, by virtue of affinities, controlled by the vital agency. In whatever manner, the circumstance may be explained, there are cases on record in which persons have subsisted for a considerable period on water alone. Dr. McNaughton (*Transactions of the Albany Institute,* for 1836) has given the case of a man, who lived on water alone for 53 days. In the first six weeks he walked out every day, and, at times, spent a great part of the day in the woods. Until about a week before his death, he shaved himself; and was able to sit up in bed until the last day. This was a case of voluntary abstinence, and under the influence of a delusion. He asserted that when it was the will of the Almighty that he should eat, an appetite would be given him.

Much difference prevails, amongst animals, regarding the nature of their food. The inhabitants of the waters, and several land animals are *carnivorous;* many of the most useful quadrupeds and birds *phytivorous.* By inspecting the digestive apparatus of animals we can generally tell the kind of food for which they are destined by nature. The teeth of the carnivorous animal are pointed, and the chief motion of the lower jaw is in a vertical direction; those of the herbivora are broader, better adapted for grinding, and the jaws have a lateral motion; whilst the organization of the mouth of the being, that is capable of subsisting on the products of both the animal, and the vegetable kingdom, is a combination of both. The complexity, and length of the intestinal canal of the omnivorous animal hold a medium place between the simplicity of that of the carnivorous animal, and the composite character of that of the herbivorous. The arrangement of the human digestive organs is that of the omnivorous animal. Man has teeth for incising, and for grinding: he has the vertical, and lateral motions of the jaws; and his alimentary canal is not so short as that of the carnivora, whose food is nearly allied to their own organization, and therefore does not need much assimilation, nor so long as that of the herbivora, whose food requires to be detained in the alimentary tube, until it is robbed of the scanty nutriment it contains.

It has been an unprofitable discussion with some naturalists, whether the organization of man prove him to have been originally more herbivorous, or more carnivorous. Broussonet embraced the former opinion, on the ground, that of the thirty-two teeth, twenty resemble those of the herbivora, and twelve only those of the carnivora. Hence he inferred, that, in the origin of society, the diet of man must have been exclusively vegetable. Mr. Lawrence, too, concludes, that whether we consider the teeth, or jaws, or the immediate instruments of digestion, the human structure closely resembles that of the Simiæ,—the great archetypes, according to Lord Monboddo, Rousseau, and others, of the human race; all of which are, in their natural state, completely herbivorous.

These views, however, are too exclusive. If man possesses both cutting, and grinding teeth, it would seem manifest, that his organization destines him to feed on substances for which either or both are adapted; and therefore, any inference, which could be deduced from this circumstance, in favour of his being originally, or by nature, intended for one variety of food only, is not legitimate.

Yet, although man is so organized as to be adapted for living on both animal, and vegetable substances, it is not indispensable that he should be enabled to obtain both. In the frozen regions of the north, vegetable food fails him; whilst, in the torrid regions, animal food, if it can be obtained in due quantity, is not relished. Accordingly, we find nations and tribes, which subsist on animal food almost exclusively, and others by which an animal diet is rarely, if at all, employed. It is in temperate climes, that man is truly omnivorous. The products of both animal, and vegetable life are there in requisite abundance, and equally laid under contribution. But even in these climes, the young of the human family in the earliest period of their existence, are nourished on animal matters exclusively,—that is, so long as they are restricted to the breast; and there is no doubt whatever, that if from infancy, man, in the temperate regions, were confined to an animal banquet, it would be entirely in accordance with his nature, and would probably develope his mental, and corporeal energies to as great a degree as the mixed nutriment on which he usually subsists. The same may be said of an exclusively vegetable diet, which some have supposed to have been man's original food, and, as we have seen, to be most in accordance with his nature. These remarks, however, apply only to the case in which the animal, or the vegetable sustenance has been employed exclusively from birth, or until the system has become habituated to it. It is far otherwise if we lay aside our mixed nutriment, and restrict ourselves wholly to the products of the one or the other kingdom. Scurvy supervenes, whether the restriction be to the vegetable, or to the animal. Certain experiments, instituted by Magendie, show clearly, that omnivorous man—omnivorous, that is, from nature and habit—re quires variety of articles of diet. This he lays down as " an important hygienic precept;" but it is of course inapplicable to those tribes, that have been accustomed, from birth, to supply the wants of the body by a diet exclusively animal or vegetable.

At one time, from the results of these experiments,—which consisted in feeding the dog exclusively on substances, as sugar and gum, which contain no azote, and finding that they fell off in their nutrition, and died,—Magendie was disposed to infer, that they perished owing to the privation of azote. He found, however, by subsequent experiments, that if the animal was confined to a diet of white bread, the gluten of which contains an abundance of azote, the results were the same. Even when it was kept on hard boiled eggs, and on cheese, it became diseased, although casein is highly azoted, and albumen has been regarded as the peculiar source of all the animal secretions. (Paris, art. Dietetics, in *Cyclop. of Pract. Med.*, Amer. edit., Philad. 1844.) Recent experiments have shown still more forcibly, that these results were not owing to privation of azote. In the name of a committee, appointed to inquire into the nutritive properties of gelatin, M. Magendie reported that gelatin, albumen and fibrin,—all of which are highly azoted, when taken separately, —nourish animals for very limited periods only, and in an imperfect manner. They generally soon excite such insurmountable disgust, that the animal prefers death to partaking of them. These experiments led to the too hasty conclusion, that gelatinous tissues are incapable of conversion into blood. " The gelatinous substance," says Liebig (*Animal Chemistry*, Amer. edit. by Dr. Webster, p. 124, Cambridge, 1842,) " is not a compound of protein: it contains no sulphur, no phosphorus, and it contains more nitrogen or less carbon than protein. The compounds of protein, under the influence of the vital energy of the organs which form the blood, assume a new form, but are not altered in composition; whilst these organs, as far as our experience reaches, do not possess the power of producing compounds of protein, by virtue of any influence, out of substances which contain no protein. Animals, which were fed exclusively on gelatin, the most highly nitrogenized element of the food of carnivora, died with the symptoms of starvation. " In short," he adds, " the gelatinous tissues are incapable of conversion into blood."—Yet, it has been shown above, that fibrin and albumen—both compounds of protein —when exhibited alone to animals, did not nourish them more perfectly than gelatin.

Of late, great light has been shed on this subject by the researches of the organic chemist. These have shown, that the chief proximate principles of animal tissues, and those that have been regarded as highly nutritious amongst vegetables, have almost identically the same composition. (Liebig, *Op. cit.* p. 100.)

*Animal Proximate Principles, according to Mulder.*

|  | Albumen. | Fibrin. | Casein. |
|---|---|---|---|
| Carbon, | 54.84 | 54.56 | 54.96 |
| Hydrogen, | 7.09 | 6.90 | 7.15 |
| Nitrogen, | 15.83 | 15.72 | 15.80 |
| Oxygen, | 21.23 | 22.13 | 21.73 |
| Sulphur, | 0.68 | 0.33 | 0.36 |
| Phosphorus, | 0.33 | 0.36 |  |
|  | 100.00 | 100.00 | 100.00 |

*Vegetable Proximate Principles, according to Scherer and Jones.*

|  | Albumen, from wheat. | Fibrin. | Casein or Legumin. |
|---|---|---|---|
| Carbon, | 55.01 | 54.603 | 54.138 |
| Hydrogen, | 7.23 | 7.302 | 7.156 |
| Nitrogen, | 15.92 | 15.809 | 15.672 |
| Oxygen, Sulphur, Phosphorus, | 21.84 | 22.286 | 23.034 |
|  | 100.00 | 100.000 | 100.000 |

It has been maintained by Liebig, and by others, that azoted or nitrogenized food is alone capable of forming organized tissues. These, consequently, have been classed by Liebig " as plastic elements of nutrition ;" whilst the non-azoted or non-nitrogenized aliments are considered by him to be inservient only to respiration, and are, therefore, termed " elements of respiration. The following is his classification.

| Nitrogenized food or Plastic Elements of Nutrition. | Non-nitrogenized food or Elements of Respiration. | |
|---|---|---|
| Vegetable Fibrin, | Fat, | Pectin, |
| ———— Albumen, | Starch, | Bassorin, |
| ———— Casein, | Gum, | Wine, |
| Animal flesh, | Cane sugar, | Beer, |
| ———— Blood. | Grape sugar, | Spirits. |
|  | Sugar of milk, |  |

All this, however, requires proof, and is opposed by what we observe in chylification. In the small chyliferous vessels, more fat, which is non-nitrogenized, is found than can be accounted for by the fat in the food; and as the chyle proceeds along these vessels the proportion of fat becomes less and less, whilst that of the nitrogenized elements increases; hence, nitrogen must have been obtained, and a conversion has taken place of non-nitrogenized into nitrogenized matters. (*Human Physiology*, edit. cit. ii. 182.)

In the work just cited, (p. 502) reference has been made to the views, that have been entertained by different naturalists, with regard to the *natural food* of man. It was there attempted to show, that if we trace back nations to their infancy, we find that then, as in their more advanced condition, the diet has been animal or vegetable, or both, according to circumstances; and that where the influence of circumstances, which prevailed in ancient periods, has continued unmodified to modern times, the food has equally continued unchanged. We are told by Agatharchides, that along both banks of the Astaboras, which flows on one side of Meroë, in Africa, a nation dwelt, who lived on the roots of reeds growing in the neighbouring swamps. These roots they cut to pieces with stones, formed them into a tenacious mass, and dried them in the sun. Close to them were the *hylophagi*, who lived on fruits and the shoots of trees; on vegetables growing in the valleys, &c. To the west of these were the hunting nations, who fed on wild beasts, which they killed with the arrow. There were also other tribes, who lived on the flesh of the elephant, and the ostrich—the *elephantophagi* and *struthiophagi*. Besides these, he mentions another and less populous tribe, who fed on locusts, which came in swarms from the southern and unknown districts.

The mode of life, with the tribes described by Agatharchides, does not seem to have varied for the last two thousand years. Although cultivated nations are situate around them, they themselves appear to have made no progress. Hylophagi are still to be met with. The Dobenahs, the most powerful tribe amongst the Shangallas, still live on the elephant; and farther to the west dwells a tribe, the people of which subsist, in the summer, on the locust; and at other seasons, on the crocodile, hippopotamus, and fish. All history, indeed, shows, that the productions of a country are the great regulators of the food of its inhabitants. Where a country has the advantages of an extensive commerce, large supplies may be obtained from without; but these generally belong to the class of luxuries, although custom may have taught us to regard them as almost indispensable. Numerous extensive tribes of the human family possess, however, no commerce, and are consequently compelled to draw their necessaries from their own soil. In our own times we have the singular example of a people—the people of Paraguay—shutting themselves up, so as to exclude all communication from without, and, of necessity, regulating their food according to the productive capabilities of their soil and climate.

These all-controlling influences, in the absence of ready communication with other countries, have compelled the people of Æthiopia to retain their habits unmodified for so many generations; the Esquimaux, and Samoiedal Tartars, &c. to live almost wholly on animal food; and the natives of the torrid regions of many parts of the globe to subsist chiefly on the cocoa-nut, the plantain, the banana, the sago, the yam, the cassava, the maize and the millet.

Before proceeding to the classification of aliments it may be well to give a very brief view of the digestive operations, and of the nature of the gastric fluid, to the action of which the aliment is subjected.

When food is received into the mouth, it is masticated by the appropriate organs, and becomes mixed with the fluids, poured out from the salivary glands, and from the mucous membrane of the mouth. It is then passed by the efforts of deglutition into the stomach, becoming mixed in its course with the fluids of the lining membrane of the upper portion of the alimentary tube. In the stomach, it is exposed to the action of these various mucous secretions; to that of the mucous membrane itself, and of an additional secretion, which contains free chlorohydric and acetic acids, and which through the intermedium of a nitrogenized secretion would appear to be the great solvent. The identical composition of this fluid has been definitively settled by a case to which few similar have been met with; and none that has afforded a better opportunity for repeated and accurate experiments.

Through the politeness of Drs. Beaumont and Lovell, of the United States' army, under the former of whom the individual was placed, an opportunity was afforded the Author to examine the case; to analyze the gastric secretions; to test the digestibility of certain aliments, both in and out of the body, and to investigate some disputed points, connected with the physiology of digestion. (See his *Human Physiology*, 5th edit. i. 558, Philad. 1844.)

Dr. Beaumont has published the results of his various experiments and observations on this case, (*Experiments and Observations on the Gastric Juice, and the Physiology of Digestion.* Plattsburg, 1833, pp. 280,)—many of which will be referred to in the course of this chapter,—and the Author is glad to find that its reception by the profession has somewhat repaid him for the zeal and assiduity, with which he has prosecuted his researches on this interesting topic of hygiène, and physiology.

When the food is received into the stomach, it undergoes a physical change which has been termed *chymification,* or conversion into *chyme,* through the action of the various secretions to which reference has been made; and when this has been accomplished, the alimentary mass is passed into the small intestine, where a second digestion occurs, through the admixture of the fluids of the mucous membrane, of the pancreas, and liver,—but especially of the latter. The alimentary mass is now in a state to allow *chyle* or the strictly nutritive portion to be separated from it by the appropriate vessels, and the excrementitious portion is then sent on into the large intestine.

Most alimentary matters experience considerable changes in the stomach through the agency of the gastric secretions; but there are some, which undergo but little change there, and require admixture with the alkaline portion of the bile, before they are in the proper condition for having the nutritive matter separated from them.

Aliments have been variously classed by writers on Dietetics. Some have endeavoured to reduce them all to one alimentary principle, which is to aliments what the ultimate fibre is presumed to be to the different tissues, or the line to the various geometrical figures. The division, proposed by Magendie, and adopted by Dr. Paris, is according to the proximate or immediate principles that predominate in their composition. They may be separated into nine classes; according as there is a predominance of one or other of those principles:

| | |
|---|---|
| I. Fibrinous Aliments, | Flesh and blood of various animals, especially of the adult. |
| II. Albuminous Aliments, | Eggs, nerves, brain, &c. |
| III. Gelatinous Aliments, | Tendons, aponeuroses, skin, cellular tissue, flesh of very young animals, calf's foot, certain fish, &c. |
| IV. Fatty and Oily Aliments, | Animal fats, oils and butter, cocoa, olives, &c. |
| V. Caseous Aliments, | Different kinds of milk, cheese, &c. |
| VI. Amylaceous, Feculaceous or Farinaceous Aliments, | Wheat, barley, oats, rice, rye, Indian corn, potato, arrow-root, sago, salep, peas, haricots, lentils, &c. |
| VII. Mucilaginous Aliments, | Carrots, turnips, asparagus, cabbage, salsify, beet, &c. |
| VIII. Saccharine Aliments, | Sugar, figs, dates, raisins, &c. |
| IX. Acidulous Aliments, | Orange, currant, raspberry, peach, cherry, strawberry, mulberry, grapes, prunes, apples, tomatoes, &c. |

Dr. Prout (*On the Nature and treatment of Stomach and Urinary Diseases*, Amer. edit. Philad. 1843) arranges the alimentary principles in four great classes,—the *aqueous*, the *saccharine*, the *oleaginous*, and the *albuminous*. This classification is taken by Dr. Pereira as the basis of his own. (*A Treatise on Food, and Diet*, &c., Amer. edit. by Dr. C. A. Lee, p. 38, New York, 1843.) The types of the classes of Dr. Prout are found in milk, which holds, however, also saline matter. Hence, Dr. Pereira has admitted another class of *saline* elements. He has, likewise, both from "chemical and physiological considerations,"—which, however, are questionable, and becoming daily more and more so,—separated gelatin from the albuminous principles, and united the aliments in which it predominates under the *gelatinous* group. Moreover, it seemed to him to be desirable to have distinct classes for gum, sugar, starch, vegetable jelly, alcohol, and vegetable acids. Hence, he adopts the following classes of alimentary principles;—the *aqueous, mucilaginous or gummy, saccharine, amylaceous, ligneous, pectinaceous, acidulous, alcoholic, oily* or *fatty, proteinaceous,* (from protein, the organic constituent of fibrin, albumen, and casein,) the *gelatinous,* and the *saline.*

By the combination of these alimentary principles and simple aliments, our ordinary articles of food and compound aliments are formed.

Although such arrangements are the most satisfactory to the chemist, the division that would be embraced by the naturalist, is perhaps the best, inasmuch as we rarely meet with any of these proximate principles in a state of purity. They are always united, in the animal, or vegetable, with other proximate principles peculiar to those, by which the nutritive, or digestible qualities of the main ingredient are largely modified, and at times completely changed.

In the above table, the first five classes are animal, and are variously combined to form the different kinds of animal food. The last four are vegetable; and their combinations are equally multifarious. In order, however, to comprehend the properties of the various aliments, it will be well to inquire briefly into the qualities of those proximate principles, which predominate in the classification:—*fibrin, albumen, gelatin, fat* and *oil, casein, fecula, mucilage, sugar,* and *acid,*—the fibrin, albumen, and casein, whether animal or vegetable, it will be recollected, being compounds of protein, and eminently capable of being formed into new tissues. It has already been remarked, that, according to Liebig, they alone are adapted for the purpose.

*Fibrin* constitutes the great mass of the solid parts of the muscles of animals, and also of the blood. It is the base of the muscular tissue. As we meet with it, however, in muscular flesh, it is combined with gelatin, osmazome, and albumen. We have little or no knowledge of its nutritious, or digestible qualities, when it exists alone; but in combination with the substances mentioned, it is certainly eminently nutritious; and from its being so extensively diffused over the human frame, it is an important article of diet, by the facility with which it is probably assimilated. The muscular fibre contains no gelatin; but the sheaths of the separate fibres and muscles consist of cellular membrane, which has gelatin for its base.

*Albumen.* The substances, in which this proximate principle predominates, are the eggs of the gallinacea, and certain fishes; some molluscous animals,—as oysters, muscles, &c.; and the brain, liver, blood, sweetbread, &c. of certain animals. The best example is in the white of egg. Albumen is nutritious, and when raw or moderately boiled is easy of digestion.

*Gelatin.* The views of certain modern chemical physiologists, in regard to this alimentary principle, have already been canvassed. It is the predominant principle in the flesh of very young animals; in the intestines and peritoneum; in tripe; in the tendinous structures,—as in cow-heel, cow-feet, and in the skin, ligaments, aponeuroses, and cellular membrane in general. It is nutritious, but perhaps not to the same degree as either of the principles just mentioned. It has been supposed to be the most readily digestible of animal substances, but this is not precisely the case. Very young meats, and watery solutions of gelatin, are not as easily digested as the flesh of older animals. The state in which we meet with gelatin in animal jellies is not suitable to the digestive powers of many dyspeptics; and we often notice, that, with such, soups are not easily digested. Hence the origin of the French proverb:

> " Qu'après la soupe un coup d'excellent vin
> Tire un ecu de la poche du médecin."

*Osmazome*—which gives the flavour of meat to soups, is contained in too small quantity to admit of any very satisfactory experiments being made upon it. It is, however, asserted by Mr. Rostan to be the most reparative of the constituents of flesh.

*Fat* and *Oil.* All animal and vegetable oils, and fats are highly nutritious, being, perhaps, wholly assimilated or converted into chyle. They are, however, extremely difficult of digestion, undergoing little change in the stomach, and requiring the presence of the bile before their physical character is such that chyle can be separated from them.

In the case of fistulous opening in the stomach, to which reference has been made, a full opportunity was afforded for observing the comparatively feeble action of the gastric secretions on fat in that organ. Whilst other substances were chymified and passed on into the small intestine, oil was detained until the last; and even when it was finally sent through the pylorus, it appeared to have undergone but little chymification. In all the *artificial* digestions, effected by Dr. Beaumont, with gastric juice obtained from this individual, it was found, that whilst other alimentary matters underwent chymification in a reasonable time, the fatty portions were long in experiencing modification. (*Op. cit.* p. 264.) Such were, likewise, the results of some artificial digestions, made by the Author with gastric secretion, sent him by that gentleman. Yet Dr. A. T. Thomson,—professor of Materia Medica and Therapeutics, and of Medical Jurisprudence, in the University of London,—in treating of spermaceti, remarks, that " it is *readily digested* in the stomach, *in the same manner as animal fat,* and is converted into chyle with equal facility as any other animal matter!"(*Elements of Materia Medica and Therapeutics*, vol. ii. p. 629, London, 1833.)

When oleaginous matter is combined with insoluble woody fibre —as in most of the kernels—it is rendered even more rebellious, and is the cause of many attacks of disorder of the stomach and bowels, when these organs are morbidly predisposed,—as during the heats of summer and autumn. The *chincapin*—the fruit of the *castanea pumila*—is, in this way, an abundant source of gastro-intestinal irritation.

*Casein.* Opinions vary with respect to the digestibility of this substance as met with in cheese. It is usually regarded as extremely difficult of digestion, and capable of affording but little nutriment to man. In the case of the dog, the experiments of Sir Astley Cooper, related by Sir C. Scudamore, exhibit cheese as a substance of easy digestion, losing more in the same time than the common meats, as in the following table:

| Food. | Form. | Quantity. | Animal Killed. | Loss by Digestion. |
|---|---|---|---|---|
| Cheese | Square | 100 parts | 4 hours | 76 |
| Mutton, | . | . | . | 65 |
| Pork, | . | . | . | 36 |
| Veal, | . | . | . | 15 |
| Beef, | . | . | . | 11 |

These experiments were made, however, on dogs; and it need scarcely be said, that any results of experiments, regarding the comparative digestibility of substances on animals, and on such animals, ought to be applied with great caution to man. The gastric secretions of the dog are capable of overcoming the hardest bones in a short space of time; and it is not improbable but that they may act upon such matters more rapidly than upon others, which would seem to possess—in the language of Dr. Paris—a better " digestive texture," yet it would be unphilosophical to infer, that the same thing takes place in the human stomach. There is every reason, indeed, to believe, that in the case of the article in question, the experiments of Sir Astley Cooper on the dog cannot be transferred to man. In the dog, the loss of the cheese by digestion was much greater than in the case of any of the meats tested; but it is not improbable, that attention was not paid to the unmodified portion floating on the surface of the fluid contents of the stomach, which is observable when cheese is subjected, in man, either to natural or artificial digestion. The Author artificially digested 20 grains of rich old cheese in three drachms of gastric juice sent him by Dr. Beaumont; yet, although the solid cheese had disappeared, there was a supernatant substance, nearly equal in amount to the cheese placed in the fluid, whilst the fluid below it appeared but little modified. So far, therefore, as regards the changes effected in the stomach, we cannot regard cheese to be easy of digestion. It probably requires admixture with the secretions poured into the small intestine, to give it the necessary physical constitution, that chyle may be formed from it. (See the *Table of the Comparative Digestibility of Various Substances*, at the end of the volume.)

It has been supposed, that cheese ought to be highly nutritious, as casein is, of all the azoted immediate principles of aliments, the one in which azote is contained in the greatest proportion; but it is questionable, as before remarked, whether a deficiency of azote detracts materially from the nutritive properties of alimentary substances, as it can be so readily obtained.

Casein is one of Liebig's plastic elements of nutrition. " The young animal," he remarks, (*Animal Chemistry*, Amer. edit.,) " receives in the form of casein, which is distinguished from fibrin and albumen by its greater solubility, and by not coagulating when heated, the chief constituent of the mother's blood. To convert casein into blood no foreign substance is required, and in the conversion of the mother's blood into casein, no elements of the constituents of the blood have been separated. When chemically examined, casein is found to contain a much larger proportion of the earth of bones than blood does, and that in a very soluble form, capable of reaching every part of the body. Thus, even in the very earliest period of its life, the development of the organs in which vitality resides is, in the carnivorous animal, dependent on the supply of a substance, identical in organic composition with the chief constituents of its blood."

## FECULA OR STARCH.

*Fecula* or *starch*. This principle is very extensively diffused through the vegetable kingdom. It exists in considerable purity, in rice, barley, Indian corn, &c. It is combined with gluten in wheat; with saccharine matter in some grains—as in oats; and in many leguminous seeds,—as haricots, beans, peas, lentils, buckwheat, chestnuts, potatoes, &c.; with viscid mucilage,—as in the seed of the cerealia, especially rye, in the garden bean, and the potato; with fixed oil and mucilage in the emulsive seeds,—as in the almond, hazelnut, cocoa, in linseed, rapeseed, hempseed, poppyseed, the seed of the palma christi, &c.; and, lastly, with a poisonous matter,—as in the manioc (janipha manihot,) bryonia—the different species of arum, &c. This poisonous matter can generally be readily separated from the fecula.

Starch is artificially prepared in great purity from various substances. In the form of *starch*—so termed—we have it from wheat, and the potato. *Bermuda arrowroot* is the starch of *maranta arundinacea*, and of various species of arum, and is sold at a considerable price.—*Florida arrowroot* is procured from the genus Zamia. The root is called *Coonti Root* in Florida, and the farina prepared from it is also called *Coonti*. (Carson, in Amer. edit. of Pereira's *Elements of Materia Medica and Therapeutics*, ii. 160, Philad. 1843.) The fecula of the *saw palmetto, chamærops serrulata*, is also used by the Florida Indians as food. It is liable, however, to induce bowel complaints. (*Amer. Med. Intelligencer*, 1838.) The starch of the potato, when carefully prepared, is, in the Author's opinion, as agreeable as arrowroot, and probably as nutritious. It is often, indeed, substituted for it, and the difference is not easily distinguishable. In order to procure the potato starch, the root must be peeled, and rasped, until it is reduced to a pulp, which must be placed on a hair sieve, and water be poured upon it, until all the fecula is extracted. This, after its subsidence to the bottom of the water, is collected and dried. Potatoes contain about fifteen or seventeen parts of fecula in the hundred; so that every hundred weight of potatoes may be expected to yield fifteen pounds of the starch; and, consequently, an article very much cheaper than the genuine arrowroot. This substance is called, *French Sago, petit sague,* and *common arrowroot*. The starch of the *arum maculatum* or *wake-robin* is called *Portland Island sago*.

*Tous-les-mois* or *Canna Starch* is the starch of the rhizome of *Canna Coccinea* of the West Indies. *Cassada* or *cassava flour* is the powdered compressed pulp of the root of *Janipha Manihot*, the Cassava or Tapioca plant; *salep* is obtained from the *orchideæ* in general; *sago* from the pith of various species of palm, from the *Sagus Rumphii, S. Lævis*, and *Saguerus Rumphii;* and *tapioca* from the root of *Janipha Manihot. Sowans* is a starch prepared from the husks of oats.

*Mucilage* or *gum* is a great ingredient of alimentary vegetables. In Africa, and the East Indies, it is obtained abundantly from various species of mimosa, and is occasionally used in diet. The Africans of Senegal are affirmed to subsist entirely upon it during the gum harvest,—eight ounces being the daily, and sufficient allowance for each man. It is asserted, also, that the caravan, which passes from Abyssinia to Cairo, employs gum Arabic, when other food fails.

Mucilage is combined simply with green colouring matter, in the leaves of beet, and spinach; with bitter matter, which may be prevented by the process of blanching,—as in endive and lettuce; or by using the plant very young—as in asparagus. It exists, also, in every part of every individual of the mallow tribe; in many roots, —as salsify, Jerusalem artichoke, &c., and in the receptacle of the flower of the artichoke. It is combined with an acid in sorrel leaves; with saccharine matter in many fruits,—as in the fig and date; and in roots,—as the carrot, parsnip, and beet; with slight acrimony in the turnip, in cabbage-leaves, cauliflower, and broccoli; and with more acrimony in the radish, cress, and mustard. It exists in considerable abundance, combined with a peculiar, nauseous principle, in onions, garlic, leeks, &c.; and, lastly, in small quantity, with much aroma, in those vegetables, that are used only for seasoning, as parsley, thyme, &c.

Linnæus regarded gum alone to be highly nutritive. It are one of the many substances which do not contain azote, and is yet inservient to animal nutrition. It probably, however, is not possessed of powerful nutrient properties; and is not very digestible, fermenting in the stomachs of those of feeble digestive powers, who, by the way, afford the only criteria by which we can usually judge of the comparative digestibility of alimentary substances. It often, according to Dr. Chapman, passes through the bowels very little changed. This, he says, he has " a hundred times observed." (*Elements of Mat. Med. and Therap.*, 6th edit., i. 352, Philad. 1831.)

*Sugar*, chymically considered, presents several varieties. It is found in greatest quantity, combined with mucilage, in the juice of the sugar-cane, sugar-maple, manna ash tree, and beet root. It seems to be a constant attendant on the inflorescence of vegetables, and is a constituent of all the subacid, and sweet fruits, in combination with vegetable jelly. It is collected by various animals. Of these the bee is most familiar, which culls the honey from various flowers. A species of locust in Australia covers the trees and ground with a variety of sugar.

Sugar also is a non-azoted substance, yet it is highly nutritious,—the azote being obtained elsewhere, and uniting with the elements of the sugar to constitute the substance of the animal, to which it has to serve as aliment. It has been a common prejudice, that its use injures the teeth; but the idea seems to have originated in frugality, rather than in philosophy. Children are fond of sugar, and this bug-bear has been presented to prevent them from indulging in a luxury, which has been at times extravagantly expensive. During the sugar season, the negroes of the West India islands drink copiously of the juice of the cane, yet their teeth are not injured; on the contrary, they have been praised by writers for their beauty, and soundness; and the rounded form of the body, whilst they indulge in the juice, sufficiently testifies to the nutrient qualities of the saccharine beverage.

The ancients had a high opinion of the nutritive properties of the fig, which is saccharine, and formed a principal article of diet with the athletæ; and, when served up with bull beef, was esteemed a banquet fit for Hercules.

According to the statistical tables of M. César Moreau, it would seem, that France then consumed about five pounds weight avoirdupois for each person, the United States ten pounds, and England fourteen pounds. The quantity, consumed in the island of Cuba, is so enormous, that France required, for her own necessities, only three or four times as much, although the population of the island did not exceed 340,000 inhabitants.

The quantity of sugar consumed in the world is astounding. The following has been given as the amount brought into the markets of the world in the year 1838. (Ure's *Dictionary of Arts, Manufactures*, &c.)

|  | Tons. |  | Tons. |
|---|---:|---|---:|
| British West Indies | 160.000 | Bourbon | 20.000 |
| Mauritius 35.000 and British East Indies 20.000 | 55.000 | Cuba | 100.000 |
| Java | 36.000 | Brazil | 95.000 |
| Manilla and Siam | 30.000 | France and Belgium, from beet root | 65.000 |
| Dutch West Indies | 25.000 |  |  |
| St. Thomas and St. Croix | 7.000 | United States | 65.000 |
| Martinique and Guadaloupe | 80.000 | Total | 738.000 |

In a memorial presented to the Congress of the United States in December 1837, it is stated, that the sugar then produced in Louisiana averaged only about 4½ pounds per head for the population of the United States, or about 70.000.000 of pounds annually; which is but a small part of the consumption,—enormous sums being paid to foreign countries for sugar, as the following table shows—(*American Almanac* for 1840.)

| In 1832 value of sugar imported | $2.933.688 |
|---|---:|
| 1833 | 4.752.343 |
| 1834 | 5.537.829 |
| 1835 | 6.806.184 |
| 1836 | 12.514.551 |

The *acid*, in the different acidulous aliments, is probably possessed of no direct or *substantive* nutrition, but it may act as a condiment, by enabling the digestive powers to separate a larger quantity of nutritious matter from the other principles, usually contained in such aliments, than they would otherwise be able to accomplish. Almost all the acidulous aliments, when ripe, are extremely grateful, and refrigerant. Hence they are valued articles of diet in sickness, as well as in health.

Lastly, to these proximate principles may be added a vegeto-animal principle, called *gluten*, which is a vegetable compound of organization, containing a notable portion of azote in its composition. It has been called the most animalized of the vegetable principles, although fungin and asparagin are equally vegeto-animal in their nature. Gluten is very generally met with, but only in a small proportion, in the vegetable kingdom; in all the farinaceous seeds; in the leaves of the cabbage, cress, &c., in certain fruits, flowers, and roots, and in the green fecula of vegetables in general; but it is especially abundant in wheat, and imparts to wheat-flower the property of fermenting, and making bread.

Gluten is highly nutritious, and is capable, when taken alone, of the prolonged nutrition of animals, (Magendie, *Comptes Rendus*, Août, 1841,)—in this respect differing from all organic immediate principles, which in every instance, in the experiments instituted by a Committee of the Royal Academy of Sciences, excited greater or less aversion in the animals obliged to subsist on them solely.

The superior nutritious powers of wheat flour, over that of all other farinaceous substances, sufficiently attest, that, in combination with starch, it is highly reparative; and it has been conceived, that the gluten of the green fecula may supply a certain portion of azote to the herbivorous animal, which may be requisite for its support; but it is scarcely necessary to have recourse to this hypothesis to account for the presence of a gas, which exists so extensively in the atmosphere.

From what has been said, it may be altogether unnecessary to observe, that the nutritive properties of a substance bear no proportion to its digestibility. Yet the terms *nutritious*, and *digestible*, are occasionally used synonymously. Although one ounce of fat meat is estimated to afford nutriment equal to four ounces of lean, it requires far more labour on the part of the digestive organs; it undergoes no change whatever in the stomach, and remains much longer in that organ. This is a singular physiological fact. It has been generally conceived, that the pylorus or valve at the lower orifice of the stomach acts, as its name imports, the part of a *janitor*,* and that it does not permit the food to pass into the small intestine, until it has undergone the physical process of chymifaction—that is, solution in the gastric secretions. Yet castor oil proceeds onwards with rapid progress, whilst a blander oil is detained longer than any other kind of aliment; and vegetable substances pass on unchanged, or but little changed,—much sooner than animal substances that are more easy of assimilation. These circumstances have induced Broussais and others to infer, that there is an internal gastric sense, which exerts an elective agency, and detains those substances, that are eminently capable of affording a chyle for the nutrition of the animal, whilst it suffers those to pass, that yield a sparing or less appropriate nourishment.

* From πυλωρος, a 'porter.'

As the process of digestion in the stomach is one of solution, the mechanical character of the same aliment—as regards the solidity and tenacity of its texture—may influence its solubility; and the object of the culinary art is frequently more to modify these mechanical properties of aliments, than to interfere with their chemical constitution. "The healthy stomach," says Dr. Paris, (*Op. cit.* p. 185,) "disposes most readily and effectually of solid food, of a certain specific degree of density, which may be termed its *digestive texture:* if it exceeds this, it will require a greater length of time, and more active powers, to complete its chymification; and if it approaches too nearly to a gelatinous condition, the stomach will be equally impeded in its operations. It is, perhaps, not possible to appreciate, or express the exact degree of firmness, which will confer the highest order of digestibility upon food : indeed this zero may vary in different individuals; but we are taught by experience, that no meat is so digestible as tender mutton. When well conditioned, it appears to possess that degree of consistence, which is most congenial to the stomach."—"It will not be difficult," he adds, "to understand, why a certain texture and coherence of the aliment should confer upon it digestibility, or otherwise. Its conversion into chyme is effected by the solvent power of the gastric juice, aided by the *churning*, which it undergoes by the motions of the stomach; and unless the substance introduced possess a suitable degree of firmness, it will not yield to such motions: this is the case with soups and other liquid aliments; in such cases, therefore, nature removes the watery part before digestion can be carried forward. It is on this account, that oils are digested with so much difficulty; and it is probable, that jellies, and other glutinous matters, although containing the elements of nourishment in the highest state of concentration, are not digested without considerable difficulty; in the first place, on account of their evading the grappling powers of the stomach, and in the next, in consequence of their tenacity opposing the absorption of their more fluid parts. For these reasons, I maintain, that the addition of isinglass and other glutinous matter, to animal broths, with a view to render them more nutritive to invalids, is a pernicious custom."

Another epithet, which has been applied to aliments, since it has been the fashion to assign the bile an undue weight in the production of indigestion, and of diseases in general, is apt to lead to erroneous inferences, pathologically, as well as therapeutically, and therefore ought to be discarded. This is the term *bilious*, which, if employed in the sense of 'difficult of digestion,' can induce no error; but if meant to convey a notion, that the aliment produces an undue flow of bile into the stomach is objectionable.

In the case of fistulous opening into the stomach, before referred to, bile was not usually perceptible in the stomach during digestion, but occasionally, without any apparent cause of a satisfactory nature, the gastric secretions, when withdrawn, were strongly tinged with it; so that its presence in that viscus may occur, consistently with health and it is not improbable but that an indirect action may be exerted on the liver, when food, difficult of digestion, is contained in the stomach. The irritation, caused by its presence there, may be propagated to the liver, which may augment its secretion; and the natural inverted action from the small intestine to the pylorus, which takes place during healthy digestion, may be augmented so as to cause the bile to clear the pylorus, and enter the stomach. Such may be—but probably is not commonly—the case, when food, difficult of digestion, is taken; but that any aliment can possess the property of being *bilious* can hardly be presumed. " There is no error," says Dr. Beddoes, " more common or more mischievous among dyspeptics, hypochondriacal, and hysterical invalids, than to suppose themselves bilious. *The bile! the bile!* is the general watch word among them, and they think they can never sufficiently work it off with aloes, magnesia, &c." Since Dr. Beddoes's time, calomel has become a sort of universal expeller of bile, or " cholagogue," as it is technically termed; is appealed to on all occasions; and too often with the effect of inducing the very state,—undue secretion of bile,—which it is employed to remove. The bile being generally regarded, by the vulgar, as a purely excrementitious secretion, its retention, or accumulation is looked upon as the cause of most maladies. The gourmand, who has eaten largely of food, injurious by quantity no less than by quality, cannot consent to curtail his enjoyments, or to ascribe his uneasy feelings to the sources of his pleasure, but assigns them to the bile; has recourse to his bilious pills—composed of calomel, and other cathartics—which carry off the results of his surfeit, and thus remove the mischief, without perhaps materially affecting the biliary secretion.

## SECTION II.

Animal aliments—quadrupeds—character of their meats according to age, sex, food, climate and season, fatness or leanness, incipient putrefaction, mode of slaughtering, &c.—birds; white fleshed, dark fleshed, aquatic, and rapacious—effect of feeding, or killing, &c.—reptiles—fish—icthyophagi—fancied evils of a fish diet—fondness of the ancients for fish—poisonous fish—esteemed parts of fish—effects of feeding, castration, age, season, crimping, &c.—shell fish—crustacea—insects.

WITHOUT meaning to affirm, that the arrangement of the naturalist is positively the best for a treatise on dietetics, we shall adopt one of that character, inasmuch as it enables us to compare substances, which, in vulgar belief, are closely associated, and to indulge in general remarks, which are applicable to a multitude of substances. For this purpose, two great divisions may be made, namely,—*animal aliments,* and *vegetable aliments.*

### 1. ANIMAL ALIMENTS.

In the classification of alimentary substances, according to their predominant principles, animal aliments embrace the five first classes;—*fibrinous, albuminous, gelatinous, fatty* and *oily,* and *caseous,* and all the combinations of these, that give occasion to the diversity of animal products in the same animal, and in different animals.

In considering these, we shall separate them, according as they are obtained from *quadrupeds, birds, reptiles, fishes, the mollusca, crustacea,* or *insects;* all of which minister, more or less, to human sustenance.

The mammalia, and birds, when in a state of health, are universally safe articles of diet. Lower down in the scale, however, this safety does not exist. There are many kinds of fish, that are positively poisonous, at particular seasons at least; and in the very lowest tribes of animated nature, there are many species that are universally unwholesome, and several so virulently poisonous, as to prove most rapidly fatal.

There is perhaps, no part of a quadruped which has not been

employed as food, if we except certain secretions; but the *muscles* of voluntary motion—constituting the flesh—are used most frequently; and least of all, perhaps, the *uterus* and external organs, with the contents of the gravid uterus, and the secundines. The Chinese and Siamese eat many creatures during the earliest periods of their existence; and in a condition which would be loathsome to us; and Mr. Holman the blind traveller, states, that at an entertainment given him by the king of the Island of Fernando Po, the uterus of a sheep containing two lambs, each about six inches long was served up as a great treat, the dish being first presented to him as a mark of respect. (Truman, *On Food*, p. 11, Lond. 1842.) The *vulva* of the sow was regarded amongst the choice parts, by the ancient Romans; and it was not uncommon to serve up the *fœtal pigs* in the gravid uterus, when the sow had been killed in the manner to be described presently. The *placenta* is, at the present day, a *bonne bouche* with many of the Tartar tribes.

In the oldest dietetic precepts extant, we find certain parts excluded from the table, probably, however, from political motives, because the taste, if indulged, might interfere with the reproduction of the species; as *blood* was forbidden amongst the Hebrews, owing, probably, in part, to the fear entertained, that its use might render the people too familiar with that fluid, and diminish the horror felt against shedding it.

No organ of the body is perhaps positively unfit for human sustenance; yet animal substances, when healthy at the time of death, occasionally acquire deleterious properties afterwards. In the two following cases, it would seem, that the meat must have become unwholesome after the death of the animal, or else that the changes had occurred prior to dissolution, in consequence of morbid action.

In the autumn of 1826, four adults, and ten children, living on the Galloway coast, partook, at dinner, of a stew made with meat taken from a dead calf, which was found on the sea shore, and of which no history could be procured. Three hours afterwards, they were all seized with pain in the stomach, retching, purging, and lividity of the face, succeeded by a state of stupor like that caused by opium; excepting that when roused, the patient had a peculiar, and wild expression. One of the persons died comatose in the course of six hours. The rest, being freely purged and vomited, eventually did well; but for some days they required the most powerful stimulants to counteract the exhaustion and collapse, which followed the state of stupor. The meat, it was said, looked well enough at the time it was used; but the remains of the dish had a black appearance, and a nauseous smell; and some of the flesh, which had not been cooked, had a white, glistening appearance, and was so much decayed, that its odour excited vomiting and syncope. (*Lond. Med. Repository*, third series, vol. iii. p. 372.)

The second case is given by Dr. Christison, (*Treatise on Poisons*, p. 565,) and was communicated to him by Dr. Swanwick of Macclesfield. A family of five persons took, for dinner, broth made of beef, which, owing to its black colour, the master of the family had previously said to his wife he thought bad, and unfit for use. In the course of a few hours two boys were attacked with nausea and vomiting, but were soon well, owing perhaps to their having speedily got rid of the poison. Next morning, a washerwoman, who had dined with the family, was seized with violent intestinal pain; diarrhœa; intense pain and weakness in the limbs, and did not recover for ten days. On the evening of the second day, the master of the house was similarly affected, and was ill for a fortnight; and a day later his wife was also seized with a similar disorder—preceded by soreness of the throat, and tongue, with difficulty in deglutition—which ended fatally in fourteen days. She had been previously in delicate health, and subject to disorder in the stomach, and bowels. Dr. Christison thinks there is little reason to doubt, that unsound meat was the cause of the morbid phenomena; but the cases are not unequivocal, as the symptoms, in some of them, were so long in manifesting themselves; and the true source of the mischief may have been some other agency, to which the family were all equally exposed.

An account has been given recently of nearly 500 out of 600 persons having been poisoned at a fête in the Canton of Zurich in June 1839 by eating cold roast veal and ham. Of this number, four persons died. (*Edinb. Journal of Med. Sciences*, Aug. 1842; cited in Davidson, *Treatise on Diet*, p. 375, Lond. 1843.)

Highly putrid food, it has been asserted, has occasioned sickness and death; and of late years a poison appears to have been noticed in Germany, developed from sausages made of blood and liver, and to which they have given the name *Allantotoxicum*, German, *W u r s t g i f t*, but respecting the precise nature of which much difference of sentiment exists. It is said to have committed, at times, great ravages in Germany, especially in the Würtemberg territories, in which two hundred and thirty-four cases of poisoning by it occurred between the years 1793 and 1827; and of these one hundred and ten proved fatal. Recently, an account has been given of eight persons who were poisoned by sausages, prepared from the liver of a healthy pig, eight days before. The sausages had a peculiar taste, and one person did not partake of them on that account. Three out of the eight persons died. (*Edinb. Med. and Surg. Journal*, 1843.) In some experiments made on a poisonous sausage by Buchner, he found that cold alcohol removed a granular fatty matter, which, when purified by distilled water, had a yellowish colour, a peculiar nauseous smell, and a disagreeable oleaginous taste, followed by extraordinary dryness of the throat for several hours. To this fatty acid he gives the name *Botulinic* (*w ü r s t f e tt s a ü r e.*) Both the *l e b e r w u r s t*, and *b l u t w u r s t*—the liver and blood sausage—are described as of large size, the ingredients being put into the swine's stomach; and they are cured by drying and smoking in a chimney with wood smoke. Those that have been found to act as poisons possess an acid re-action; are soft in consistence; and have a nauseous, putrid taste, and an unpleasant sweetish sour smell like that of purulent matter. (Kerner, Dann, W. Horn, Buchner, and Schumann, in Christison, *On Poisons*, p. 555.)

Bacon, and other cured meats have occasionally produced symptoms like those resulting from the poisonous sausage, and probably from an analogous change in their chemical nature.— Cheese and milk have also been found possessed of deleterious properties, as described under those articles.

The tame quadrupeds, chiefly used for diet, are the *ox, sheep, hog,* and *goat,* and the wild animals of the same class,—as the *deer, hare, rabbit, opossum, wild boar, hedge-hog, &c.* The flesh of the *horse,* and that of the *dog* when fed chiefly on vegetable matter, are also eaten in some places; and it is to be feared, that the use of human flesh, as an article of diet, still exists, and that it is enjoyed by certain tribes;—the relish being chiefly, however, occasioned by associations of savage vengeance, and cruelty.

The ancient Romans, distinguished for their gastronomic habits, ate the young of the *common ass*,—probably as a luxury. It was served upon the table of Mæcenas himself, when he entertained Augustus and Horace;—the young of the *asinus*, according to Pliny, being preferred to that of the *onager* or wild ass. They were also fond of young and well fattened puppies—*catuli lactantes*—which were considered, at one time, a dainty in Corsica; but Cardan asserts, " that they made the people like to dogs, that is to say, cruel, stout, rash, bold and nimble"! To this day, they continue to be eaten by the Chinese, and Esquimaux, but without appearing to be followed by the consequences mentioned by Cardan! The *glis* or *dormouse* (*myoxus muscardinus*, L.) was also an esteemed article of diet, the use of which was, however, restricted,—and probably for some satisfactory reason,—by the consul Scaurus, A. U. 639 : B. C. 116. (Plin. viii. 82.) Varro gives a long account of the mode of fattening them in the dark, by means of acorns, walnuts, and chestnuts, in cages, called *gliraria*, of which one is described by Winckelmann, as having been discovered at Herculaneum. The *glires* are still eaten by the Carniolans, Calabrians, &c. (See an article, by the Author, on the *Gastronomy of the Romans*, in the 4th No. of the *American Quarterly Review*.)

It has already been remarked, that muscular flesh consists of fibrin, gelatin, osmazome, and albumen, the gelatin being chiefly derived from the cellular membrane surrounding the muscular fasciculi; that the tendons, and aponeuroses, the different membranes, ligaments, and skin are constituted chiefly of gelatin;—the brain and nervous substance in general; the pancreas, (sweetbread,) and the various glands, of albumen chiefly; and that the fat and suet are different forms of fixed oil. The cellular structure of the bones contains a considerable proportion of gelatin, which has been separated from them, and was attempted to be converted to useful purposes, even on a large scale, chiefly through the labours of a distinguished native of this country—Count Rumford—and of M. D'Arcet. In the Report, however, made to the Academy of Sciences in Paris by the Gelatin Commission, it was affirmed, on the faith of experiments, that we cannot by any known process extract from bones an aliment, which either alone or mixed with other substances can be substituted for meat. It would appear that the gelatin is even less nutritious than the bones that yield it. The Commission found, that dogs, fed solely on raw bones and water for three months, continued in perfect health, and lost none of their weight. The bones contain other alimentary principles as fatty and albuminous matter, which, when mixed with gelatin, are nutritious. The views of Liebig on the subject, and the value of gelatin as an alimentary matter have been considered already. It may be proper, however, to add, that the confidence of M. D'Arcet in the valuable alimentary properties of the gelatin of bones is undiminished. In a recent essay (*Amélioration du Régime Alimentaire des Hôpitaux, des Pauvres, et des Grands Réunions d'Hommes Vivant en Commun*, Paris, 1844) he thus remarks. " The Hôpital Saint Louis, one of the largest in Paris, has used gelatin for fourteen years and four months : gelatin has been employed with entire success and for many years to ameliorate the nourishment of the poor at Lille, Metz, Lyons, Strasburg, in almost all the large cities of Holland, and in more places than I am able to cite. Moreover, it is well known, that gelatin forms the basis of meat soup, and of a great number of other aliments ; that it is employed in large quantity by the makers of alimentary preserves; and that it is sold by the principal dealers of spices for the use of restaurateurs and the cooks of large houses. On the other hand, has it not been demonstrated over and over again, that with a properly arranged apparatus and skilful management, it is easy to procure gratuitously gelatin from bones, sufficient, when dissolved, to animalize all aliments of a vegetable nature?"

Besides the proximate principles, described as being present in muscular flesh, different secretions are met with in the parenchymatous and cellular substance of muscles,—some of which are concrete ; others fluid. These are—the serous fluid, which is contained in all cellular parts for their lubrication ; and the fat deposited in the cellular membrane. The former is albuminous, and when the meat is boiled, it is coagulated, and constitutes the scum that forms on the surface of the water ; and the latter constitutes the round flattened drops or disks, which swim on soups, and become congealed on the surface, as the water cools.

In the same animal species, the character of the food differs considerably, according to numerous circumstances, of which the following are some.

1. *Age.* The flesh of young animals is much softer and more

viscid,—the organs abounding more in gelatin than those of the adult, and aged;—the latter containing more fibrin and osmazome. Accordingly, the flesh of young animals is more soluble in water. It is not, however, on this account, more digestible. Very young meats are, indeed, by no means as easy of digestion as the older. This is strikingly exemplified in the cases of very young veal, and beef; and of lamb and mutton. Yet, even in the fœtal state, meat is not unwholesome; and, consequently, it is not easy to account for an enactment,—passed in the reign of the first James of England,—that no butcher should kill any calf to sell, which was under five weeks old. Calves are frequently sold by the butchers, that have been taken from the uterus at, or near, the full period; and some prefer them. By the English butchers, according to Dr. Roget, (Article *Food*, in *Encyclopædia Britannica*,) calves are killed at from six to sixteen weeks old, but they are reckoned best at ten or twelve. Lambs are usually killed at from eight weeks to half a year. In this country, the common age is perhaps somewhat earlier.

Young animals differ from the older in the distribution of the fat. In the former, it is generally collected in the cellular membrane surrounding the muscles; whilst in the latter, when they are in good condition, it is situate more in the cellular membrane between the muscular fasciculi; so that when the muscle is cut transversely, the flesh has that marbled appearance—from the alternate distribution of fat and lean—which is so much admired.

The beef of the larger breeds of oxen is considered, in the London market, to be in perfection, when the animal is about seven years old: that of the smaller breeds a year or two sooner. Cow beef, on the contrary, it is thought, can scarcely be too young. The flesh of a young heifer is highly esteemed; that of an old fattened cow is considered very bad. This last notion has perhaps been maintained in consequence of the feeling, that advanced age may render the attempt at fattening idle, in consequence of the fancied dry, and innutritious nature of the muscular fibre. Some, however, of the best beef we have eaten in certain parts of the United States has been furnished by an old cow under such circumstances. The meat has been marbled, and the fibre so mellowed by the fat, as to be tender, and digestible. Wether mutton, or the flesh of the castrated animal, is considered in England to be in perfection at five years. It is the sweetest, and most digestible. Ewe mutton is best when about two years old. Sucking pigs are killed about three weeks old. The hog is at the best age for bacon at about two years. The shote is killed under one year.

2. *Sex.* Tourtelle asserts, that the flesh of animals of both sexes is the same when they are very young, and that they differ only as they become older. It would appear, however, that every day the testes are permitted to remain, even though apparently inactive, injures the delicacy of the veal of the bull calf. Daubenton directs, that male lambs should be castrated at from eight to fifteen days after their birth, although it is not usual to perform the operation until the age of three weeks, or even five or six months. Their flesh is never so good as when they are castrated at eight days.

The flesh of the female is always finer grained and more delicate than that of the entire male. As a general rule, the females of animals after puberty participate more in the constitution of infancy, and the flesh is softer, less tenacious and more soluble; and again, the removal of the ovaries in the female, and of the testes in the male improves the meat in a remarkable manner,—the neutral animal seeming to be better adapted for the table than either the entire male or female. In the castrated animal, a greater deposition of fat takes place over the whole body, wherever cellular tissue exists; and hence the muscular fibres become supple and mellow. The difference is great between the flesh of the bull, and of the ox; of the ram and of the wether. Castration must, however, be performed some time before puberty; otherwise, much of the rankness and coarseness of the entire male will remain after the operation. The males of those animals, in which the testes are active only during certain seasons,—as the deer,—have the rankness of the entire male disagreeably predominant at these periods. Buck venison, except at such seasons, is highly esteemed; and the boar is preferred for making brawn.

3. *Food.* The different effects of food on the nature of the flesh are strikingly exhibited in the carnivora, and herbivora. The flesh of the former is rank, and repulsive; whilst that of the latter is devoid of any disagreeable qualities; and if an animal, like the dog, naturally carnivorous, but by custom omnivorous, be restricted from an early age to vegetable food, the flesh loses its objectionable points,

and becomes edible. Dog's flesh, under such circumstances, is a part of the materia alimentaria of the New Zealanders.

At one time it was the custom, in England, to feed oxen, intended for the market, on oil cake, but this practice appears to be now almost laid aside, in consequence of the beef acquiring an unpleasant rancidity. The effect of feeding is strongly exemplified in the case of the hog, and it accounts for the reputation which the bacon of certain countries has acquired over that of others. In particular parts of Virginia, the hogs are fattened chiefly on the refuse from the stills after the distillation of whisky, or they are—to use the expression of the farmers—" still-fed." The inferiority of the meat, when thus forced,—compared with the result of feeding the animal upon corn, and allowing it to roam abroad, and obtain its food from the acorns, chestnuts, &c. in the woods,—is universally admitted. The Sardinian pork probably derives its celebrity from the mode of fattening the animal resembling that generally adopted in Virginia. In antiquity, the same diversity existed in the reputation of the bacon of different places. The Romans do not seem to have acquired the art of making either good bacon, or good sausages, but imported them, according to Varro, in large quantities, from the Gauls, by whom they were prepared in great perfection. The inferiority of the Roman bacon probably arose from their mode of fattening the hog, which was kept up, and fed with milk, figs, and mulse—a combination of wine and honey.

4. *Climate* and *season*. Tourtelle asserts, that climate has a great effect upon meats. In the warmer regions they are more compact and drier, and therefore nutritious, but heavy and difficult of digestion. In the cold and moist countries of the earth, they are soft and mucous; and, therefore, he asserts, acescent, indigestible and unwholesome; whilst, in temperate climates alone, they are devoid of these objectionable qualities. It is probable, however, that climate has but little influence, except so far as it regulates the supply and character of the food; and the same may be said of the seasons. The flesh of most full grown quadrupeds is in highest season during the first months of winter, after having had the advantage of the abundance of fresh summer food; in spring they become lean in consequence of deficiency of food. Pork is considered to be out of season during the summer months, and in many countries is eaten only during the winter. In several parts of the United

States, it is rarely eaten at any time in the form of pork,—that is in the fresh condition; but bacon is extensively used at all seasons. The meat of the *shote* or young hog is eaten fresh. The males of the deer tribe are in best condition during the summer months; after which they begin to rut, when their flesh is rank; and, after the rutting season, they are thin and exhausted. In general, females advanced in pregnancy, or that are giving suck, or have lately suckled, are not in condition. The hog is killed in this country to be formed into bacon in the latter end of autumn,—in November, or the commencement of December. In the southern states it is an article of daily consumption; and the quantity salted and smoked on some farms is immense. A friend of the Author, who is by no means a large landholder, annually prepares fifteen thousand pounds of bacon, which is consumed on his own estate.

5. *Fatness* or *leanness*. In lean animals the fibres are dry and close, and the meat is accordingly hard and coriaceous; in the fat animal, the fibres, fasciculi and muscles, are separated by fat, which renders the meat more soluble; hence the lean of fat meat is infinitely preferable, on account of its greater digestibility and nutritive qualities: the fat, also, with which it is interlarded, renders the meat more nutritious, although it detracts from its digestibility. Animals that use much exercise, or that are subjected to hard labor, are lean; and the fibres of their muscles are extremely dense and hard; on the other hand, rest disposes to obesity, and the muscles not being put so often on the stretch are comparatively tender.

6. *Incipient decomposition*. Nothing tends so much to the digestibility of all kinds of meat as to keep it until evidences of decomposition are about to occur; or, in the case of some meats, until they have actually occurred. Whenever the meat is cooked soon after the death of an animal, it is tough and difficult of digestion; yet if the same meat were kept until putrefaction were about to be established, it would be tender and digestible. The more vulgar meats,—as beef, mutton, veal and pork,—are never kept, by design, until these sensible evidences exist; but game is, in England, universally preferred by the *gourmet*, when it is even repugnant to the olfactory organs. This repugnance, however, soon ceases, and the *fumet* comes to be regarded as one of the most pleasing anticipations of the future repast. Venison is never put upon the table

until the signs of its having been for some time killed are unequivocal; and the same may be said of the hare, and of various *gibiers.* In this country, food is generally dressed too soon after life has ceased; and in travelling it is by no means uncommon to see, on arriving at a house of entertainment, the fowl running about, which has soon after to be served up at table. Under such circumstances, it is, of course, scarcely eatable. The taste, however, for game in a state of incipient putrefaction, requires in man a true education; but the meat is so much more agreeable that it is soon attained. By many animals, putrid food is preferred; and amongst some nations it is eaten as a luxury. A rotten egg, especially if accompanied with the chick, is highly esteemed by the Siamese.

It might be imagined, that feeding on putrid aliments would render the breath disagreeable; but this is not the fact. The gastric secretions, which, as we have seen, contain free chlorohydric and acetic acids, are so strongly antiseptic as to rapidly deprive putrid substances of their disagreeable odour. In some experiments, which were performed by Dr. Beaumont and the Author, —in the presence of the Author's friend, Mr. Trist, ex-consul of the United States at the Havannah,—with gastric juice, obtained from the individual with the fistulous aperture in the stomach, the odour of putrid food was as speedily removed as by the solution of chlorinated soda, which was employed at the same time on other portions. It is probable, however, that unless an individual were accustomed to highly putrid aliment from an early period, he could not have recourse to it with impunity afterwards. When putrid miasmata are very concentrated, they would seem to be taken into the blood; to excite considerable indisposition, and at times, it is said, death.

It may be affirmed, then, that in order that the flesh of animals, especially of the upper classes, may be as tender as possible, it ought to be kept until its constituents are about to assume new affinities, or until the force of cohesion between its particles has been diminished. Meat cannot, in fact, be kept too long before it is dressed, provided only that its flavour has not been interfered with; and even when it has been so long kept as to attain a *fumet*, or the smell of putrefaction—in particular articles of food, included under the head of game—the epicure soon learns to disregard the offensive odour, owing to the extreme tenderness of the meat.

7. *Mode of slaughtering.* The mode of killing quadrupeds for

the table has differed in different countries, in all ages. The Greeks strangled their swine, and ate them with their blood. The Romans thrust a red hot spit through the body, and suffered them to die without bleeding ; but if a sow were about to farrow, they trampled, at the same time, upon her belly, bruising the fœtal pigs and the mammary glands, with the milk and blood, and serving all up as a delicate dish. This mode of slaughtering was replete with objections, if regarded in an alimentary point of view only. The flesh of animals, thus killed, is dark coloured, owing to the retention of blood in the vessels, and hence it becomes speedily putrid. Within the last few years, however, it has been proposed by Dr. Carson, of Liverpool, to slaughter animals in such a manner that the blood may be still retained in the tissues without these objections accruing. The Author has not been able to lay his hand upon Dr. Carson's paper, but as far as he recollects it, it consists in making an aperture into each pleura, so as to occasion the collapse of the lungs. The blood cannot, consequently, be distributed to these viscera, and remains, to a certain extent, diffused through the tissues, so that the meat is said to be increased in weight, and to be more tender, and digestible. The Author is not aware, however, whether the plan has been adopted by others. In many places, it is the custom to knock down the large cattle by striking them on the head with a pole-axe, or to shoot them, and then divide the vessels of the neck by cutting the throat. When the animal is gentle, it is bled to death in this fashion, without the previous striking, or shooting. In some European countries, the operation of *pithing* is performed, which consists in passing a sharp pointed knife into the spinal marrow; and, as soon as the animal falls, dividing the vessels. Death is, in this way, immediate, and therefore it is the most humane plan that could be devised, but it has not been generally employed in Great Britain, although great encouragement was given by certain *zoophilists*—if they may be so termed—for its adoption; and Dr. Roget (*Loc. citat.*) says, he has been told, that the flesh of cattle—killed in this way, in Portugal—is very dark, and becomes soon putrid;—probably, as he suggests, from the animal not bleeding well, in consequence of the action of the heart being interrupted before the vessels of the neck are divided.

The smaller animals are all bled to death by cutting the vessels of the neck.

When an animal is killed accidentally, without bleeding, its flesh is not unwholesome, although it may not be palatable in consequence of the blood remaining in the vessels. The wild animals that are cought by snares, and those that are killed by hounds, are exactly in these conditions; yet many of them are cherished articles of diet. The blood is the most putrescible of all fluids, and consequently, animals, under such circumstances, do not keep sound so long as when they are bled to death.

Caution should always be observed in eating animals that have died from, or been killed during, disease. Although the meat may often be innoxious, at other times it would seem to be capable of producing disease, and even death. All writers on hygiène agree in this. Fortunately, this can rarely be put to the test with us. The prejudice is so strong against frauds of the kind, that a butcher would scarcely run the risk of inevitable ruin, by attempting to sell the meat of diseased animals. Fodéré refers to several instances, in which families were morbidly affected, after having eaten of animals, that had laboured under disease, especially under epizootic disease,—and although it is possible that many of these cases may not have been fairly referrible to the cause assigned; and that cookery may, in such instances, be capable of correcting the morbific qualities, which may be supposed to exist in the raw meat, it is well to be cautious in the use of such aliment.

Animals are often subjected to some preparation before they are slaughtered. They are commonly kept for a time without food; as, if killed with full stomachs, their flesh is considered not to keep so well. Yet they must not be made to fast too long, or they may fall off, and become feverish.

Dr. Lister affirms, that nothing contributes so much to the whiteness, and tenderness of veal, as bleeding the calf often, by which the colouring matter of the blood is diminished; but according to Dr. Roget this is not a common practice. It is denied, at least, by the feeders, and not confessed by the butchers.

A cruel method of preparation for slaughter prevailed, at one time, with regard to the bull, but it is now, happily, obsolescent. It is to be feared, indeed, that the original object of its adoption was too frequently lost sight of, and that it was followed, in too many instances, as an inhuman sport. Bull beef has always been esteemed difficult of digestion, requiring the most vigorous powers for its assimilation; hence, the mythical legend of Hercules feeding on bull's flesh and green figs. To remove these objectionable qualities of the flesh, bulls have been, from the earliest times, either baited by dogs, hunted by men, or torn by lions. By some ancient municipal laws of England, no butcher was permitted to expose bull beef for sale, unless the bull had been previously baited,—a regulation adopted for the reason already assigned; for whenever animals have undergone great fatigue immediately before death, or have suffered from a lingering death, although their flesh may sooner become rigid, it also sooner becomes tender, than when they have been suddenly deprived of life, when in a state of health. The flesh of hunted animals is soon tender, and speedily spoils, and upon this principle, the flesh of the pig is rendered more digestible by the revolting cruelty—recommended in our older works on the culinary art, and said to be still practised in some countries—of whipping the animal to death. In the *Booke of Cookrye*, by A. W. 1591, there is a receipt "*to make a pig taste like a wild boar.*" —" Take a living pig and make him swallow the following drink, viz:—boil together, in vinegar and water, some rosemary, thyme, sweet basil, bay leaves, and sage: when you have let him swallow this, immediately whip him to death, and roast him forthwith." And another: "*How to still a cocke for a weake bodie that is consumed:*"—" take a red cocke, that is not too olde, and beate him to death."

It has long been a custom to cause old cocks to fight before they are killed; and the Moors of West Barbary, according to Mr. Jones, before they kill a hedgehog, which is esteemed a princely dish with them, as it was of old with the Greeks, " rub his back against the ground, by holding his feet betwixt two, as men do a saw that saws stones, till it has done squeaking, and then they cut its throat." (*American Quarterly Review*, loc. citat.)

It is not improbable, but that the vinegar was administered to the pig in the above receipt, for the purpose of rendering the flesh more tender. At least, it is a common opinion in many parts of England, that a spoonful or two of vinegar, given to poultry some time before they are killed, renders the fibre so mellow, that they may be dressed almost immediately. The Author has adopted this plan in his own establishment, and he has conceived with decided advantage. The acetic acid may act upon the fibrin of the muscles in the living or recently dead frame in a mode analogous to what we witness out of the body. Berzelius found, that when fibrin is digested in concentrated acetic acid, it swells, and becomes a bulky, tremulous jelly, which dissolves completely, with the disengagement of a little azote, in a considerable quantity of hot water.

All BIRDS, and every part of them, as well as their eggs, are capable of serving for human sustenance, although, as in quadrupeds, much diversity exists in the character of the meats they furnish.

There is considerable difference in the different muscles even of the same bird. In the common fowl, the meat of the breast and wings is much lighter coloured, and somewhat more tender than that of the legs: and the muscles, that lie on the side bones, seem to be even more tender than those of the breast, and are also much darker coloured. Many epicures prefer this part of the fowl. It is certainly more juicy, and flavorous. The same may be said, but to a more limited degree, of the flesh of the legs, when the bird is young—has been long kept—and when justice has been rendered it in cooking.

As continued exercise produces rigidity of the muscular fibre, it happens, that those parts of birds, which are most exercised, are, as a general rule, by no means equal to the others; and this is one cause why the legs of the common fowl are more rigid, and tenacious than the wings. In the duck, however, whose motions are leisurely, and never long continued, there is not much difference between the flesh of the legs and that of the wings, and some prefer the former. The *woodcock*, and *partridge* afford us examples of the principle laid down. The former flies more than the latter; the latter walks more than the former. The wing of the woodcock is always comparatively tough,—that of the partridge tender; and hence the old saying,—

"If the partridge had but the woodcock's thigh,
He'd be the best bird that e'er doth fly."

It is difficult to make any classification of the different varieties of the flesh of birds; as they run into each other by insensible gradations. They have been divided into,—1. The *white-fleshed*, as the common fowl and turkey. 2. The *dark-fleshed*, as game,

—grouse, &c. 3. The *aquatic*, as the goose, and duck ; and 4thly, the *rapacious*, as the hawk, the owl, &c. and this is perhaps as good a division as can be adopted. As a general rule, the meat of the first class is less digestible, and less nutritious, than that of the second, the solubility of which is amazingly increased, as well as the luxury of the repast, by keeping it until it has attained the requisite *fumet*; which indicates, that incipient putrefaction is diminishing its cohesion.

Aquatic birds are extensively eaten, and some of them are highly delicate. Our canvass-back duck—*anas Vallisneria*—is one of the greatest luxuries furnished to the table by the animal kingdom. Aquatic birds are not, however, as easy of digestion,—taken as a class,—as the two first divisions. They are disposed to become fat, and the adipous secretion, in many aquatic birds, has a rancid and fishy taste, which may be somewhat obviated by skinning the bird, and removing the inside fat before cooking. The *common goose, duck*, and *aquatic birds* in general, are highly nutritious. Stark, in his experiments on diet, found, that when he fed upon roasted goose, he was more vigorous, both in body and mind, than upon any other food. Aquatic birds are not, however, very easy of digestion. Gesner quaintly asserted, that " the best part of a duck is its feathers;" and feasting on goose is considered a sufficient apology for a small quantity of raw brandy, whisky, or kirschwasser, taken as a digester or " peptic persuader"—as the eccentric Kitchner would have called it.

Lastly, of the rapacious birds, or birds of prey, none are eaten ; chiefly because all the objections, that lie against the flesh of the carnivorous mammalia, on account of its rankness and coarseness, apply to them.

*Age* has the same effect upon the flesh of birds as upon that of quadrupeds; the young grown bird being more tender, and digestible, than the more aged. The same may be said of the *sex*. By removing the sexual organs at an early age, as is a common custom in Great Britain, both sexes are much improved for the use of the table, becoming larger, fatter, and more tender. The male of the common fowl, when castrated, is the *capon*; the spayed female is the *poulard*, both of which are large, tender, finely flavoured and much esteemed.

As in quadrupeds, the manner in which birds are fed affects both their fatness and flavour. In the various older writers, "*de re rustica*," we find, that great attention was paid to the fattening of edible animals in general, and many of their plans are pursued at the present day. Birds seldom get very fat in their wild state,—or when domesticated, if they be allowed to go at large. We have some examples, however, of wild fowl, that are extremely fat,—the canvass-back, for example,—but its food is so abundant in our rivers, that much exercise is unnecessary.

It has been asserted, that the flesh of the grouse, and of the partridge, becomes poisonous, by feeding on the buds of the *kalmia latifolia, mountain laurel,* or *ivy,* but this is denied by Wilson—the ornithologist.

At the present day, the fattening of fowls for the markets of large towns—and especially for that of London—forms a considerable branch of rural economy. The mode, pursued, is to put them into a dark place, and cram them with a paste, made of barley meal, mutton suet, and some molasses, or coarse sugar, mixed with milk: at the expiration of a fortnight, they are found to be completely ripe; but if kept longer, the fever, induced by the continued state of repletion, renders them red, not vendible, and frequently kills them.

This plan of keeping them in dark places, with the occasional, and barbarous substitution of *stitching up the eyes*, and of cramming them, was well known to the Romans, and largely practised. (Aves quæ conviviis comparantur, ut immotæ facilè pinguescant, in obscuro continentur.—Senecæ *Epist.* 123.) It was considered to make the flesh more tender, sweeter, whiter, and also, as was supposed, more wholesome. It has long been imagined, however, and seems now to be very generally admitted, that animals, brought to this state of artificial, and forced obesity, are never so well flavoured in the flesh, and probably not so salubrious as those of the same species, fattened in a more natural way; but there are some, that refuse their assent to this conclusion. Fowls, which are fattened artificially, are preferred by them to those called *barn-door fowls;* and Kitchener asserts, that he has known such persons say, that " they would as soon think of ordering a barn-door for dinner, as a barn-door fowl."

By the way, Dr. Paris has commented upon the folly, as he terms it, into which many popular writers have fallen, of stating such and such an article to be wholesome or otherwise. "The wholesomeness of an aliment," he affirms, "must depend upon its fitness to produce the particular effect, which the case in question may require." This is very true; but the writers, alluded to, meant no more, than that the article would be wholesome to the generality of mankind. Its unwholesomeness in particular cases must be regarded as an exception to the rule. Van Swieten has a similar idea to that of Dr. Paris. "To assert a thing to be wholesome," he says, "without a knowledge of the condition of the person for whom it is intended, is like a sailor pronouncing the wind to be fair, without knowing to what port the vessel is bound." Perhaps the best opinion as regards the wholesomeness of an aliment, in the case of any particular individual, is comprised in the answer of the facetious Mandeville, who, when asked by the ladies of the court, whether this or that article of diet were wholeseme; asked whether they liked it and it agreed with them? If so, it was *wholesome*.

There are particular parts of birds, which have been selected as *bonnes bouches* by the epicures,—frequently, perhaps, more on account of their rarity, and costliness, than of any superiority of flavour. In ancient Rome, the *brains of the ostrich and peacock*, and the *tongues of the flamingo and nightingale* were largely prized. The Emperor Heliogabalus, according to Lampridius, had the brains of six hundred ostriches served up at one repast. Apicius is said to have first discovered in the tongue of the flamingo the exquisite flavour, which was afterwards so much *recherché*. Lampridius reckons amongst the excesses of Heliogabalus, that he had dishes on his table, filled with the tongues of the phœnicopterus or flamingo, and it was a common dish at the table of Vitellius. Some comparatively late voyagers, whether from their own impressions, or guided by the prejudice of the ancients, have spoken highly of the tongue of the flamingo. Dampier describes it as—"*un mets digne de la table des Rois.*" At the present day, the *trail of the woodcock* is highly esteemed, and every drop that falls from it in roasting is carefully received on bread. "This bird," says the *Almanach des Gourmands*, "has so insinuated itself into the favour of refined gourmands, that they pay it the same honours as the grand Lama, making a ragout of its excrements, and devouring them with ecstacy." The *enlarged liver of the goose*, of which we have had occasion to speak under another head, (see page 27) is likewise in high favour, especially with the people of continental Europe. When subjected to heat, and crammed, in a confined space, the liver, morbidly enlarged by this artificial process, has been known to weigh one or two pounds!

The time of the year, at which birds are in season, is dependent on their time of breeding, on the greater or less abundance of food, and on their migrations. Whilst breeding, they are less delicate. The migrating birds can, of course, only be obtained in any region for a time; and, if valued at all, it must be during that time. Accordingly the canvass-back, and the various kinds of ducks are in season in winter.

The mode of killing birds is much the same every where. Game is universally shot. Domestic birds, on the contrary, are killed by dislocating the neck, by decapitation, or by dividing the cervical vessels. In the two first modes, the blood is retained in the vessels; in the latter, not. The former processes are, consequently, less adapted than the latter, where it is desirable to keep the meat some time after death, but they are perhaps the best in a gastronomic point of view,—the flesh being more tender, and no disagreeable taste being communicated, owing to the greater delicacy of the blood in them than in the quadruped.

It is considered advisable to keep domestic birds without food for a day before they are killed, that their crops may be empty,— as food left in them, is apt to taint the flesh. We have already alluded to the practice of giving them vinegar as a preparation for death.

Not many individuals of the class of REPTILES are employed as food. It includes, however, some of the greatest luxuries of the table,—as the *green turtle, terrapin,* and many other species of the *testudo;* which are nutritious, and generally easy of digestion, when cooked in a simple manner. Several of the *lizard kind* are also eaten—by the Asiatics especially—and the *eggs* of many, both of the *testudo* and *lacerta* kind, are used, although the flesh may be reputed bad. The *flesh of the viper,*—and especially its broth,—was at one time constantly advised as an analeptic or restorative diet to invalids; and that of the *Rana esculenta* or esculent frog is employed by the French. It, as well as the *Rana taurina* or bull-frog, is occasionally eaten here. The flesh is delicate, and greatly resembles that of the chicken.

The flesh of animals, belonging to this division, is doubtless affected by the general circumstances, that influence that of other animals, as regards age, sex, &c. but we know little on this matter. The best size for a turtle, according to Kitchener—as respects taste—is from sixty to eighty pounds—scarcely a tenth part of the weight they at times attain; so that it would seem they are best before they reach the adult age.

FISH in the abstract is not so safe an aliment as any of the kinds of flesh we have considered. Essentially it consists of fibrin, gelatin, and albumen, in more equal proportions than are met with in quadrupeds or birds, but there is no osmazome. It is regarded to hold a middle place—as respects its nutritive properties—between the flesh of warm blooded animals, and vegetables; but the particular degree of its nutritive powers, and of its digestibility, is greatly dependent upon the portion of oleaginous matter it contains; which, in certain fishes—as the eel—is considerable.

There are many nations of the globe, that are almost wholly piscivorous; and many tribes in antiquity were designated from their food—*Ichthyophagi*. Such tribes are generally in a state of great moral and physical abjection. Content to subsist on fish left behind after inundations, or with the slender efforts required in catching them, they are usually indolent and debased; but multiplying—like the poor inhabitants of Ireland, who are equally contented with a miserable supply of food and clothing—to an extent not witnessed where the customs of society require more exertion for the maintenance of a family. It is remarked by Mr. Gallatin, (*A Synopsis of the Indian tribes within the United States, east of the Rocky Mountains, and in the British and Russian Possessions in North America,*) that a greater and more uniform supply of food is afforded by fisheries than by hunting; and we find accordingly, that the Narragansetts of Rhode Island were, in proportion to their territory, the most populous tribe of New England. A limited view of anthropology has caused this great multiplication of the species in ichthyophagous tribes to be ascribed to the diet. (Muffett, *Health's Improvement*, p. 54, Lond. 1655.) Tourtelle (*Elémens d' Hygiène*, tom. ii. p. 178,) asserts, that fish seems to furnish prolific matter abundantly. "We see more children," he observes, "in sea ports than any where else. The population is immensely great in Japan and China, where scarcely any other kind of food is ever met with; so that the founders of religious orders, as Montesquieu has judiciously remarked, who were desirous of subjecting their unhappy victims to the impracticable law of chastity, totally failed in their object by prescribing the constant use of fish."

The ancients had numerous prejudices with regard to the salubrity or insalubrity of certain fish employed as food, yet the taste for fish appears to have been as great then as, or even greater than, it is at the present day. The fishmonger of Athens was an important personage, and we have many instances recorded of his insolence, pride and rapacity. (Athen. *Deipnosoph.* lib. vi. p. 224-5.—Edit. Schweighäuser.) With the Greeks οψον probably signified fish, originally; but in the course of time, it was applied to every dainty; and οψοφαγια, and φιλοψια attained the same signification as the French words *gourmandise*, and *friandise:* οψον became applied, subsequently, to every kind of food, and from it originated the Latin word *opsonium* or *obsonium*, of similar acceptation among the Romans.

The Egyptian priests were forbidden to eat fish of any sort: and particular kinds were prohibited to the Hebrews by the law of Moses. In the 11th chapter of Leviticus it is said:—"These shall ye eat of all that are in the waters; *whatsoever hath fins and scales* in the waters, in the seas, and in the rivers, them shall ye eat."—*Whatsoever hath no fins nor scales* in the waters, that shall be an abomination unto you." These dietetic regulations were probably founded upon the fancied general unwholesomeness of the articles prohibited,—that is, of those inhabitants of the waters that have neither fins nor scales: the precise grounds of their rejection, however, we know not. It has been supposed, that the idea prevailed, that they increased lust, or were the cause of leprosy. We have referred to the inaccuracy of the former supposition; and the latter is probably equally untenable. Dr. Paris, (*Op. cit.* p. 210,) seems, however, disposed to support the idea that the cutaneous system may be morbidly affected by a fish diet. "It has been usual," he says, "to attribute all the cutaneous affections which follow the liberal use of fish, as depending upon the sympathy of the skin with the stomach. This, I believe is, in general, the true explanation, since the effect is merely temporary; and when the process of digestion is finished it departs. Its departure may even be hastened by the operation of an emetic removing the noxious aliment. At the same time, the fact must not be everlooked that the oily principle, upon which depends the odour of certain fish, is absorbed from the alimentary canal and carried into the blood; this is evident from the peculiar flavour of the flesh of certain birds, who live upon fish: from the ready access, which the hogs in Cornwall have to pilchards, the pork of that county is very commonly deteriorated by a fishy savour. It is also well known that persons confined for any length of time to a diet of fish secrete a sweat of a rancid smell. It is not, therefore, improbable, that certain cutaneous diseases may be produced, or at least aggravated, by such diet; and, in hot climates, this effect may be less questionable. The priests of Egypt may, therefore, have been prohibited from eating fish upon just principles, in order that the leprosy might be averted; and the great legislator of the Jews was no doubt influenced by some such belief, when he framed his celebrated prohibition." This is plausible, but not the less hypothetical.

Numa Pompilius made a law for the Romans greatly resembling that of Moses, whether owing to the influence of authority or to the experience of his people, does not appear. The law, however, could not have continued long in force, or have been rigidly observed, for we find several such fish reckoned amongst the greatest luxuries of the emperors. The *murœna*, for example—probably the *murœna Helena* of Linnæus, or Roman eel or lamprey—was held in the highest estimation. Pliny remarks, that it engenders with the land snake; and this notion existed also amongst the Greeks, and may have, in part, given rise to the prejudice entertained at one time against it! Even at the present day, their resemblance to snakes, and the unpleasing essociations connected therewith, occasionally excite a prejudice, which excludes them from the table.

Of the fondness of the Romans for this fish we have some ludicrous stories. Hortensius—the orator—is said to have wept when one died. The Licinii family assumed the cognomen *Murœna* because the head of the family delighted in that fish. At the banquet of Nasidienus, the muræna was served up in a gravid state and swimming in shrimp sauce.

> "Affertur squillas inter *murœna* natantes
> In patina porrecta. Sub hoc herus. "Hæc gravida, inquit,
> Capta est, deterior post partum carne futura." —Horat. *Sat.*

> "In a large dish an outstretch'd lamprey lies,
> With shrimps all floating round: the master cries,
> 'This fish, Mæcenas, big with spawn was caught,
> For after spawning time its flesh is naught.'"

The common eel—*anguilla, (murœna anguilla* of Linnæus,)—was also held in high account by the ancients; and in Greece, it was regarded as one of the most annoying wishes, that could be directed towards any one,—that there might be Copaic eels in the market, and the obnoxious person's arrival be retarded until they had all been sold.

In tropical climates, especially at particular seasons, different species of fish become absolutely poisonous, and hence considerable care is required in selecting the innocent and nutritious. No fish appears to partake of a poisonous property, unless it has undergone some morbid change; so that the poison is probably *sui generis,* and always most active, after the vital powers of the fish have ceased. The following is a list of poisonous fish, on the authority of Dr. Burrows, who bestowed much attention on this subject. *Balistes monoceros* (old wife :) *tetrodon sceleratus* (tunny ;) *ostracion globellum* (smooth bottle-fish ;) *tetrodon ocellatus* (blower or blazer ;) *murœna major* (conger eel ;) *coryphœna splendens* (dolphin ;) *sparus chrysops* (porgee ;) *coracinus fuscus major* (gray snapper ;) *coracinus minor* (hyne ;) *perca major* of Browne (esox barracuda, barracuda ;) *perca venenata* (rock fish ;) *perca venenosa* of Catesby (grooper ;) *scomber maximus* (king fish ;) *scomber thynnus* (bonetta ;) *another species of scomber* (cavalloe, horse eye ;) *scomber cœruleo argenteus nudus* of Browne (Spanish mackerel ;) *mormyra* of Browne (blue parrot fish ;) *clupea thryssa* (yellow billed sprat :) *cancer astacus* (sea lobster ;) *cancer ruricolus* (land crab ;) and *mytilus edulis* (mussel.)

The *clupea thryssa*, or yellow billed sprat, is said to be the most dangerous of these;—producing itching over the whole body; violent colic; contraction, and pungent heat of the œsophagus; nausea; heat of skin, and great acceleration of the pulse; giddiness; loss of sight; cold sweats; insensibility and death. At times, the fatal result occurs speedily;—convulsions ending in death ensuing immediately after swallowing the fish. Chisholm, indeed, asserts, that persons have been known to expire with the sprats in their mouths unswallowed; but the clupea is the only fish—that produces immediate death—within the tropics. The symptoms, occasioned by the other species in the catalogue, resemble the above in all essential particulars.

The cause of this poisonous property has given rise to much speculation. It has been supposed to be owing to the fish feeding on poisonous substances, as on copper-banks, medusæ, and holothuriæ, or on the manchineel apple; but these are mere speculations. Dr. Chisholm was inclined to believe in the first of these hypotheses; but on examining the argillaceous stone of the banks, near Antigua, it was not found to contain any copper. The fact, that it is only at certain seasons, that any poisonous fish are found in the Caribbean sea—as in May, June, and July, after they have spawned—is in favour of the view, that ascribes the production of the poison to a morbid process. The poison has by some been supposed to exist in the gall, and it is said, that if the peritoneum, and all the entrails be speedily, and dexterously removed, the flesh may always be eaten without danger. Dr. Burrows, however, concludes after a sedulous examination, that the poison does not exist in the skin, or stomach and intestinal canal, or in the liver and gall-bladder, exclusively, although there is no doubt, that persons have been poisoned from eating these parts; but that it pervades the whole substance of the fish, being formed probably in climates of highly elevated temperature at the moment vitality ceases, and, possibly before; although decomposition, which can occur but imperfectly in the living state, but which supervenes so readily in tropical regions, and under favouring circumstances in the fish itself, is probably the cause of its formation. What the character of the poison is we know not.

In the temperate and frigid regions of the globe there is no fish, which is positively poisonous,—to the extent at least of destroying. Perhaps we ought to except the *Bogmarus Islandicus*, which is reputed poisonous by the Icelanders, because the crows refuse to eat it. (Art. *Food*, in supplement to *Encyclopædia Britannica*.) There are many, which, in particular habits, are productive of much gastric disorder, and sympathetic cutaneous efflorescence, of the kind produced by mussels, crabs, &c. to which allusion will be made hereafter. It may, indeed, be laid down, as a general rule, that all kinds of fish, in a state of incipient decomposition, are positively unwholesome, and may be regarded as septic poisons.

Almost every soft part of fish is nutritious, and is eaten. Of old, it was imagined, that they afforded but little nutritive matter, and we have a foolish story, told by St. Jerome in his "Epistles," that Seneca, upon some conceit, abstained so long from flesh, feeding only upon fish and fruit, that when, by Nero's command, he was bled to death, no blood could be made to flow from his veins. The story exhibits the notions, entertained at the time, of the want of nutritive properties in fish; and, at the present day, when a trainer at Newmarket wishes to *waste a jockey*, he is not allowed pudding, if fish can be obtained.

Some of the smaller and more delicate fishes as the white bait, *Clupea alba*, are eaten whole. In most fishes, the skin is removed, but in some, the soft gelatinous skin is admired. *Cod-sounds*, which consist almost wholly of gelatin, are the swimming-bladders of the larger cod, and are prized by many epicures. The swimming-bladder of the *Acipenser huso* furnishes isinglass, which is much used in various culinary processes, especially in the preparation of jelly; isinglass consisting entirely of gelatin. The roe of most fishes is eaten; yet that of the barbel has been esteemed unwholesome. Muffett (*Op. cit.* p. 175.) asserts, that "assuredly the eggs or spawne of barbels is very sharp, griping, and corrosive, driving many into bloody fluxes that have eaten them fasting." Much difference of opinion, however, exists, whether it be really possessed of any unwholesome properties. Some have denied this altogether; but according to Dr. Roget, Dr. Crevelt, of Bonn, has published cases, which leave little doubt, that in some instances, the roe was actually injurious, although the flesh of the fish, whence it was obtained, was eaten with impunity. The preserved roe of the sturgeon and of some other fishes is the *caviare, caviale,* or *ickari,* which is an article of national food. The roe is separated from the skin which incloses it; is salted; and after eight days pepper and finely minced onions are added. It is then dried, and serves as a relish with toasted bread, and bread and butter. The best caviare is that from the Crimea. It is said, that from Kerch and Jenikale, in that province, 1500 barrels are annually exported to Moldavia, and the countries on the Danube. If we credit an old Italian saying, it would seem, that formerly no great care was taken in its preparation.

> "Chi mangia di caviale
> Mangia moschi morti ed sale."

The roe of the sturgeon of our rivers is very acrid and indigestible, and often produces violent gastric and intestinal disorders, and Dr. Christison, (*Op. citat.* p. 566,) asserts, that he has several times known severe cholera induced by the oily matter about the fins of *kipper* or cured salmon.

With regard to the *age* of fishes that best adapts them for food, it is difficult to lay down any thing precise. As a general rule, we may say, that a moderate sized fish is to be preferred. When they attain the full size of which they are capable, they are often coarse, and unsavory.

*Food* and *locality*, also, materially influence the flavour of fishes; and hence, the essential difference between the same fish according as it inhabits different coasts, and rivers, or different parts of the same river. The flesh of the trout, in a river, far from the source, is often delicious, whilst the same species inhabiting the small tributary streams is dark-coloured, loosely cohering, and by no means flavorous. Nay, we have often observed the trout of one side of a small lake differing essentially in aspect, and alimentary character, from those of the opposite shore, where the bottom of the lake has been different. The diversity, produced, in this way, was well known to the ancients. Thus, Horace, in the second Satire of his second book.

> "Unde datum sentis, lupus hic Tiberinus, an alto
> Captus hiet: pontesne inter jactatus, an amnis
> Ostia sub Tusci."  HORAT.

> But say, by what discernment are you taught
> To know that this voracious pike was caught,
> Where the full river's lenient waters glide,
> Or where the bridges break the rapid tide;

> In the mild ocean, or where Tiber pays,
> With broader course, his tribute to the seas?"  FRANCIS.

Juvenal, also, speaking of the portly epicure, Montanus, observes:—

> ——" Nulli major fuit usus edendi
> Tempestate mea. Circeis nata forent, an
> Lucrinum ad saxum, Rutupinove edita fundo
> Ostrea, callebat primo deprendere morsû."

> " And in my time none understood so well
> The science of good eating : he could tell,
> At the first relish, if his oysters fed
> On the Rutupian or the Lucrine bed."  GIFFORD.

and he asserts, that the epicure could say—even by the appearance of the *Echinus,* or sea urchin—the shore where it had been taken:—

> " Et semel adspectû litus dicebat echini."

Modern gastronomers rival the ancient. The Thames salmon is preferred, in the London market, to any other, and some epicures pretend to be able to distinguish, by the taste, in which reach of the river it was caught.

The fish of lakes and streams, the water of which is clear, and the bottom gravelly, are generally superior to those bred in foul water, and on muddy bottoms.

With respect to the *sex* of fishes, the rule, applicable to the quadruped, does not seem to prevail;—the male or *melter* or *soft-roed* being generally preferred. Whilst the fish is in season, the sex is but little attended to: when out of season the male is decidedly preferable, but the discrimination of the sexual characters is less easy than in the animals already considered. As on them, castration, and spaying were at one period practised to some extent; but the operations seem to be now entirely abandoned. A Mr. Tull, of Edmonton, was the first operator, and his method is given in the "*Philosophical Transactions,*" for 1754. His object was to prevent the excessive increase of fish in some of his ponds, where, owing to their numbers, none of them could attain an advantageous size. By castration, however, the increase was not only prevented, but the castrated fish grew much larger than usual; were fatter, and—what was an important consideration—were always in season. The operation consisted in dividing the vas deferens, and then stitching the wound up. It was performed in May, when the spermatic vessels, and ovaries are full;—and few died of the operation. In France, the Baron De la Tour operated so successfully, that out of two hunded carps he did not lose four.

The *season of the year* has a decided influence on the quality of fish, as connected with their spawning. In general, they are best some time before they begin to spawn; and they are unfit for some time afterwards. Fishes, that have not attained the age of spawning, are in season all the year.

To improve the quality of fish they are occasionally subjected to the process of *crimping*. Sir Anthony Carlisle has examined this operation physiologically, and the effects produced by it on the flesh of the animal. Whenever the rigid contractions of death have not taken place, the process may be successfully practised. The sea-fish, destined for crimping, are usually struck on the head when caught; which is said to protract the term of this capability, and the muscles, that retain the property longest, are those about the head. Several transverse sections of the muscles having been made, and the fish immersed in cold water, the contractions, called *crimping*, take place in about five minutes; but if the mass be large, it often requires thirty minutes to complete the process. Sir Anthony found, that by being crimped, the muscles had both their absolute weight, and their specific gravity augmented; water would therefore seem to be absorbed, and condensation to take place. It was also observed, that the effect was greater in proportion to the vivacity of the fish, so that the object of crimping is first to retard the natural rigidity of the muscles, and then, by the sudden application of cold water, to excite it in the greatest possible degree, by which means it acquires the desired firmness, and keeps longer.

Fish are not improved by keeping. The sooner they are dressed after death the better. The eel, which is tenacious of life, is sometimes put in the vessel before it is dead, but this is an unnecessary piece of cruelty. The Roman epicures, according to Pliny, were so fastidious as not to tolerate the mullet, unless it died whilst on the table. This spectacle, during which the fish changed its colour in a singular manner until entirely lifeless, was so pleasing that the dying fish was exhibited in a glass vessel to the guests before dinner;—" oculos antequam gulam pavit." By the way, the prices paid for the *mullus* or mullet, are characteristic of the luxury and gastronomy of the times. It was obtained from Sicily or Corsica; was highly prized, and therefore immensely expensive. Octavius is said to have purchased one for five thousand sestertii, upwards of one hundred and eighty dollars. Seneca, Juvenal and Tertullian mention others sold at six thousand sestertii—about two hundred and fifteen dollars. Asinius Celer, according to Macrobius, bought one for seven thousand H. S.—about two hundred and fifty dollars; others were sold for eight thousand H. S.,—upwards of two hundred and eighty dollars: and Suetonius remarks that the emperor Tiberius complained bitterly, that three mullets had been sold for more than thirty thousand sestertii,—one thousand and seventy dollars. The following anecdote is told of this emperor. A mullet, of an extraordinary size—weighing fifty pounds—having been given to him, he sent it to the market, observing, that, if he was not deceived, either Apicius, or Octavius would purchase it, nor was he mistaken. The two gourmands bade against each other, and it was ultimately knocked down to Octavius, for five thousand sestertii—about one hundred and eighty dollars.

The Italians have a proverb,—"*La triglia non mangia chi la piglia,*"—implying, that " he who catches a mullet is a fool if he eats it," and does not sell it. It does not appear, from Athenæus, that the mullet was as much esteemed by the Greeks as by the Romans.

As a general rule, the white kinds of fish—the *turbot, sole, whiting, cod, rock, flounder,* &c. are less nutritious, but more digestible than the oily—as *eels, herrings, sprats,* &c., which by no means agree with those of weak digestive powers, and require the use of condiments. If fresh, they appear to be more manageable; but where they have been caught some time,—as they must necessarily have been when carried inland to a distance from the place where they have been taken,—they are by no means wholesome.

SHELL FISH—comprising the molluscous, and crustaceous animals, —have been extolled by some physicians as nutritive, and easily digestible. Some of them are, however, assimilated with great difficulty. The *oyster* has obtained all the encomiums, that have been passed upon shell-fish in general. When raw, although this is perhaps the most digestible form—(see the table at the end of the volume)—it does not agree with every dyspeptic, and requires the addition of cayenne, or of some stimulant: when scolloped, it is digested with still more difficulty,—the albuminous part being coagulated, and heated butter added, which is itself as indigestible, perhaps, as any article of food that is ordinarily taken. In a raw state, they are eaten at times in considerable quantity, and with impunity. It is said, that one of the most distinguished French physiologists of the present day was in the habit of declaring, that he did not care about eating oysters, unless he could be supplied with at least twelve or fourteen dozen for his own share;—a number he was continually in the habit of taking, without experiencing any symptoms of indigestion. (Truman, *Food and its Influence on Health and Disease*, p. 7, Lond. 1842.) It is a common remark, that oysters are never good except in a month, in the name of which the letter R occurs. The reason of this is, that they spawn in the month of May, after which they are sick, and unfit for food; but in June and July they begin to recover, and in August are perfectly well.

Oysters have been regarded as aphrodisiac, and Tourtelle agrees with the popular opinion; but it is probably altogether without foundation. The liquor surrounding them has also been esteemed a useful excitant to feeble, or sluggish stomachs: and M. Mérat has prescribed it in several diseases, "believing," says Bricheteau, " that this animal and mineral water is not inferior, as regards its medicinal virtues, to the most accredited mineral waters;" but whatever efficacy it possesses is ascribable, perhaps, to the saline impregnation. Instances are on record, where oysters would appear to have acquired poisonous properties, and to have induced considerable gastric and intestinal irritation. Many of these cases were probably, however, dependent upon other causes. Dr. Clarke was of opinion, that even wholesome oysters have a tendency to act prejudicially on women soon after delivery. He affirms, that he has repeatedly found them induce apoplexy, or convulsions; that the symptoms generally came on the day after the oysters were taken, and that two cases of the kind proved fatal. (*Transactions of the London College of Physicians*, vol. v. p. 109, and Christison, *On Poisons*.) This would be a singular circumstance, if correct. It may be well to bear the remark in mind, although we are disposed to refer the morbid phenomena to other agency.

The *loligo*—ink-fish—and *sepia*—cuttle-fish—were eaten of old, according to Apicius, as sausages, made up with lard, and other ingredients.

The *limpet, periwinkle, whelk,* &c. are eaten at the present day, and are moderately digestible. The *snail,* too,—*cochlea, helix pomatia,*—is said to be reared, and fattened with great care, in some cantons of Switzerland, and is exported pickled. It was an article of luxury amongst the Romans. Fulvius Hirpinus—not long before the civil war between Cæsar and Pompey—made several snail parks in his garden, keeping every variety distinct. He had the white snails of Reate, the gray, and large snails of Illyricum, the fruitful snails of Africa, and the Solitan snails, regarded as the most famous and excellent of all. They were fed upon a pap, made of sweet wine, honey, and flour, and under this diet, they became so wholesome and delicate, and were so much esteemed, that they were sold for eighty quadrants the dishful. The white snails are eaten in many places, and are all, perhaps, wholesome. They are gelatinous, and viscid, and are frequently swallowed raw. In this way they have been recommended as a nutritious aliment to consumptive individuals. The *helix pomatia* was transported to England, from the south of Europe, by the celebrated Sir Kenelm Digby, for his lady—when in a decline—on account of its reputed analeptic or restorative virtues. Pectoral decoctions or *bouillons* are also made of it, which are administered with similar views. They consist chiefly of gelatin.

Most of the univalve shell-fish resemble, more or less, the snail in their alimentary properties.

Next to the oyster,—the *mussel, clam,* and *cockle,* amongst the bivalves, are most eaten, but they are more indigestible than the oyster. The mussel, especially, is apt to excite all those symptoms, that accompany the ingestion of fish poison, and death has occasionally been the consequence, especially where the mussels have been for some time dead, and an interval has been allowed for the development of the poison, as in the case of the poisonous fish already described. Dr. Burrows has given an interesting history, in the London Medical Repository, of two youths, who died in consequence of having eaten about a dozen small mussels, which they had picked from the side of a fishing smack, at Gravesend, in England. The mussels were in a state of decomposition. It was this melancholy circumstance, that directed the attention of Dr. Burrows to the subject of poisonous fish, which he has elucidated so ably. Vancouver relates, that in his voyage to the coast of America, several of his men were taken ill from eating some mussels, which they had collected, and roasted for breakfast. In an hour after, they complained of numbness of the face and extremities, sickness, and giddiness. Three were more affected than the rest, and one died.

The usual symptoms, produced by mussels, when they act injuriously, are,—violent oppression, and anxiety; tumefaction of the face, and, at times, of the whole body; a scarlet efflorescence over the surface, more or less resembling urticaria; great thirst; tormina, and vomiting; and—if the case eventuates in death—coldness of the extremities; feeble and rapid pulse; hiccough; delirium; and occasionally, coma.

The *crustacea* are pretty generally eaten. Most of these belong to the *cancer*, or *crab* family, comprising the different varieties of crabs,—the *lobster, shrimp,* and *prawn*.

The lobster and crab are nutritive, and delicious aliments, but they are not easy of digestion; frequently disagree with the stomach and bowels, and occasionally induce all the symptoms caused by fish poison. In this country, the effects are not fatal, so far at least as we know; although they might readily be so to the feeble and irritable. The shrimp and the prawn are somewhat more easy of digestion.

Not many INSECTS are used as food. Of old, the *cossus* or *cossis*—a sort of white, short, and thick worm, found in trees, logs of wood, &c.—was considered a great luxury. According to Pliny, it was fattened with meal, served up at feasts as a delicious article of diet, and also used as a cure for ulcers. " Cosses qui in ligno nascuntur sanant ulcera omnia." The Orientals,—and especially the Greeks,—were fond of the *nympha* of the *cicada* genus; and at the present day, the *locust* is said to be consumed in some countries, in great quantities,—both fresh and salted. *Centipedes* are eaten in South America, the *white ant* by the Indians in Brazil; and the negroes in the West Indies are said to be fond of a *caterpillar* found on the palm tree. (Truman, *On Food,* p. 26.)

## SECTION III.

Milk—various kinds—frangipane—cream—butter—cheese—buttermilk—eggs—vegetable aliments—congenerous vegetables possess similar virtues—farinaceous vegetables—bread—maccaroni—vermicelli—buckwheat—millet—cassava flour—potato—rice—Indian corn—sago—tapioca, &c.—leguminous vegetables—peas, beans, &c.—different kinds of kernels—potherbs—beet, carrot, parsnip, radish, leek, lettuce, cucumbers, cabbage, &c,—mushrooms—fruits—preserved fruits.

THERE are some animal substances, which require a special notice. These are milk, cream, butter, cheese, buttermilk, whey, and eggs.

MILK.—This is the sole food of the infant, and is, consequently, sufficiently nutrient to maintain life, and to minister to the growth during the earliest periods of existence. It is essentially an emulsion of albumen, oil, sugar, and a peculiar principle,—suspended in a large quantity of water; and although apparently homogeneous, when first obtained from the mammæ, it can be resolved into three compounds of organization,—*cream, curd,* and *whey,*—and in the stomach is turned, by admixture with the digestive secretions, into a solid curd, and a fluid; the former of which undergoes digestion, like any other solid; and the latter probably enters the blood vessels by imbibition, and goes directly to add to the mass of the circulating fluid.

From the physical constitution of milk, its nutritive properties may be understood. It is amongst the least nutritious of animal substances, but holds a higher place than any vegetable. At one time, the opinion prevailed, that it requires no digestion in the stomach; that it passes on into the small intestine, and enters the chyliferous vessels; but this is erroneous. It undergoes the separation, that has been mentioned, and the solid portion experiences true chymification. Still, as a general rule, it is easily assimilated, and, therefore, well adapted for the sick and the convalescent, especially when united with certain farinaceous substances,—as arrowroot, sago, &c.

It is scarcely necessary to say, that being prepared by animals for their young, milk is the most natural nutriment, during the first term of existence. In many countries, the infant is altogether restricted to the breast until teeth have begun to issue; but in others, the child has certain articles of liquid sustenance administered much earlier than this. Dr. Cullen thought, that hardly in any case should vegetable aliment be given till the infant is five months old. It is difficult to lay down any precise rule on the subject, nor this is necessary. We are so much the creatures of habit, that if ordinary caution be employed in their administration, any kinds of aliment, that possess the necessary fluidity, may be inservient to the nutrition of the infant. If there be no reason for modification, the most natural rule perhaps would be, to keep the infant on the mother's milk until the appearance of teeth, and then to give aliment, prepared from the milk of the cow, with additions from the vegetable kingdom of a farinaceous character.

It has been a question, also, how long the child should be kept at the breast; and the custom, here again, differs in different countries. Dr. Cullen thought, that either less than seven, or more than eleven, months is generally hurtful, and he prefers the common term in Scotland of nine months. There would seem, however, to be no good reason, connected with the infant, for weaning it at this period. Milk is an appropriate nourishment at all ages; and is more so the nearer to birth. In this country, females occasionally suckle for upwards of two years, to prevent the rapid succession of children, as well as on account of the pleasure, which most mothers feel, in affording the infant nutriment from their own bosom. In the second year, however, the supply becomes scanty, and altogether insufficient for the wants of the infant; and menstruation, which had previously been arrested, recurs, and indicates that the uterus is again adapted for conception. When this happens, it ought always to be regarded as a hint from nature in favour of weaning; and if the child be kept at the breast, the nutriment, thus obtained, is generally very inadequate.

Milk is an agreeable article of diet at all ages, and is generally readily assimilated; but, in certain habits, it does not digest so easily,—giving rise to headach, and to various other symptoms of indigestion. That this is owing to the cheesy part of the milk seems to be proved by the circumstance, that in many of the cases cream does not disagree. Under certain conditions of the stomach, or of its secretions, the milk is firmly coagulated; remains for hours in the stomach, and is rejected by vomiting; or it may pass through the intestinal canal almost unchanged.

A prejudice exists with many against the use of milk in cases of chronic inflammation of the stomach and small intestine, or in those that are often termed *bilious*. The milk is supposed to augment the flow of bile; or there is a notion that the milk itself is *bilious*; but whether by this is meant, that it augments or diminishes the secretion or flow of bile, is not clear. The experience of the Author does not accord with these notions. On the contrary, except in particular idiosyncrasies, he has generally found a milk diet to agree better than any other. Occasionally, where the raw milk disagrees, boiled milk digests readily; yet boiling does not produce much change in its character. The pellicle, that forms on the surface, consists of coagulated albumen, which is not very digestible, but it is only in small quantity. There are some persons, again, with whom raw milk ordinarily disagrees, that can take it with impunity if a little salt be added.

In certain stomachs, milk is apt to excite acescency;—whether owing to the development of an acid produced by the reaction of its own elements on each other, or to its presence in the stomach exciting an undue secretion of the gastric acids, or to both, is not settled. This tendency to acescency is said to be obviated by boiling, especially with some farinaceous substance, or by the addition of lime water; and Dr. Paris asserts, that he has occasionally seen benefit from such a practice, especially in cases of *tabes mesenterica*.

Owing to the digestible and nutritious properties of milk, it is the common diet in phthisis pulmonalis: the milk of the ass is usually preferred for this purpose; but as it is not readily attainable, it is not so much used as that of the cow.

When milk is evaporated to dryness, and is mixed with pounded almonds and sugar, the compound is termed *Frangipane*. It is emollient and nutritive.

The milk of different animals varies somewhat in composition. That of the human female contains more sugar, milk and cream, and less casein than cow's milk. *Asses' milk* resembles human milk, of which it has the consistence, smell and taste, but it contains a little less cream, and more soft caseous matter. *Ewe's milk* affords more cream than cow's milk; but the butter is softer.

The casein, on the contrary, is fatter and more viscid. It contains less serum. *Goats' milk* resembles that of the cow; but the butyraceous portion is more solid. Lastly, *mares' milk* contains only a small quantity of fluid butyraceous matter; a little casein, softer than that in cows' milk, and more serum.

The following is the composition of various kinds of milk, according to competent chemists. (MM. O. Henri and Chevallier, *Journal de Pharmacie*, xxv. 340, Paris, 1839.)

|  | Milk of the | | | | |
|---|---|---|---|---|---|
| Constituents. | Cow. | Ass. | Woman. | Goat. | Ewe. |
| Casein | 4.48 | 1.82 | 1.52 | 4.02 | 4.50 |
| Butter | 3.13 | 0.11 | 3.55 | 3.32 | 4.20 |
| Sugar of milk | 4.77 | 6.08 | 6.50 | 5.28 | 5.00 |
| Various salts | 0.69 | 0.34 | 0.45 | 0.58 | 0.68 |
| Water | 87.02 | 91.65 | 87.98 | 86.80 | 85.62 |
|  | 100.00 | 100.00 | 100.00 | 100.00 | 100.00 |

(See, also, *Cours de Microscopic*, par Al. Donné, p. 376. Paris, 1844.)

From a considerable number of experiments, Messrs. Deyeux and Parmentier have classed the six kinds of milk they examined, according to the following table,—as regards the relative quantity of the materials they contain.

| Casein. | Butter. | Sugar of Milk. | Serum. |
|---|---|---|---|
| Goat<br>Sheep<br>Cow | Sheep<br>Cow<br>Goat | Woman<br>Ass<br>Mare | Ass<br>Woman<br>Mare |
| Ass<br>Woman<br>Mare | Woman<br>Ass<br>Mare | Cow<br>Goat<br>Sheep | Cow<br>Goat<br>Sheep |

If, then, we are desirous of substituting the milk of the cow for that of the human female, it will be necessary to add about two thirds water and some saccharine matter; as cow's milk contains much more caseous and oleaginous matter, and less sugar than human milk.

The milk of animals differs in quantity and character, according to the quantity and character of the food;—a circumstance which was one of the great causes of the belief, that the lymphatics convey the materials for the secretion directly to the mammæ. In this respect, however, milk resembles the urine, which varies in quantity and quality according to the amount and kind of solid or liquid food taken. The milk is more abundant, thicker, and less acid, if the female lives on animal food; and it possesses the opposite properties when vegetable diet is used. It is apt, too, to be mixed with heterogeneous substances taken up from the digestive canal. The milk and butter of the cow indicate clearly the character of the food, especially if the animal has fed on the turnip, wild onion, &c.; and the same thing doubtless happens in the case of the human female. Accordingly, we can understand how particular articles of diet may affect the milk, and that the infant may be disordered by irregularities in the diet of the mother. This is not so apparent if she has accustomed herself to variety from an early period after the birth of the child; but it is often strikingly so, when she has restricted herself to particular articles of diet, avoiding those of the acescent or acid character, and then indulges occasionally in the forbidden food. The disorder of the gastric and intestinal functions, occurring as often as these aberrations take place, sufficiently and constantly indicates the change. The milk, which is indirectly obtained from vegetable food, especially from the succulent vegetable, or which contains acid, appears to disagree with infants more than any other. In like manner, certain medicines administered to the mother may act on the child by imparting their properties to the fluid of nutrition. A marked instance of this kind occurred in the Author's knowledge. A dose of morphia was administered to the lady of a professional friend, which produced such powerfully narcotic effects on her babe—a few days' old—as to occasion serious apprehensions for its safety. It is not, consequently, unimportant that the nurse should be attentive to what she takes, especially where the child is delicate and subject to derangement of the stomach and bowels. The mammæ, again, like the rest of the glands, are under the influence of the nervous system, and we can understand, that if the nervous influx be modified in any manner, the secretion may be diminished or be imperfectly accomplished; but there is no reason for the belief entertained by the older writers, (Muffet, *Op. cit.* p. 123) that the intellectual and moral powers of the offspring can be influenced by the nurse's milk, except so far as they may be modified by its greater or less nutrition.

It would seem, that milk may occasionally acquire poisonous properties. Of this, an instance occurred a few years since at Aurillac, in France. Fifteen or sixteen customers of a dealer in goat's milk were attacked simultaneously with all the symptoms of cholera, and about twenty-four hours afterwards the goat was taken ill with the same affection, and died in three days. Professors Orfila and Marc, who were appointed by the Society of Medicine of Paris to report upon the case, stated it as their opinion, that in this, and similar cases, some poisonous change had taken place in the milk, which gave occasion to the formation of new principles under the vital process. (*Archiv. général. de Médecine*, vol. xv. 460; and Christison, *On Poisons*, p. 562.)

In some of the Western States, and in certain localities of them, the cattle are liable to a disease, *milk-sickness* or *trembles*, in which the milk becomes poisonous, and produces a disease of the same name in the human subject.

a. *Cream.*—Cream, when carefully skimmed from the milk beneath, contains a certain quantity of casein and whey, along with the butter, which gives it its chief alimentary character. Owing to its oleaginous nature it is not very easy of digestion, yet as it contains little casein and whey, it is not so much disposed to turn acid in the stomach as milk. On this account, many dyspeptics and valetudinarians can digest it with less inconvenience; and there are some, who, owing to idiosyncrasy, are unable to take milk, and yet can take cream with impunity, especially when diluted with water. In this diluted state, sweetened with sugar, it forms a good article of diet for infants that are strongly disposed to acescency; and, as a general rule, when diluted, and sweetened in the manner before mentioned, it agrees better with them than cow's milk.

b. *Butter.*—As this substance is the oleaginous part of the cream, separated by the process of churning, it is not liable to the objection that occasionally applies to cream,—of becoming acescent; and, consequently it may be digested where cream cannot. It possesses the digestible, and nutritious properties of the fixed oils in general, none of which are easy of digestion, but all nutritious.

If butter be kept too long it becomes rancid, in which state it is acted upon with still more difficulty by the digestive organs, and ought to be regarded as unfit for use. When it is exposed to heat, it is rendered empyreumatic, and disagrees with those of feeble stomachs, giving rise to heartburn, and other dyspeptic symptoms. Hot buttered toast, and melted butter, are hence very objectionable forms of preparation.

c. *Cheese.*—Allusion has already been made to the digestible, and nutritive qualities of cheese, which is nothing more than the curd of milk, pressed, salted, and partly dried, with a portion of the butter,—which owing to its having been enveloped in the curd, cannot afterwards be separated from it. The common opinion is, that it is one of the least digestible of aliments, and that it is adapted only for strong stomachs, and for such persons as use great, and constant exercise. It is, however, capable of affording much nutriment. By many, it is supposed to be an excellent condiment, and, accordingly, it is often systematically taken at the end of dinner, as a *digestive*, in accordance with the old proverb:—

> " Cheese is a surly elf
> Digesting all things but itself.

Dr. Kitchener considers this notion to be an absurd, vulgar error; but he himself was far from being devoid of prejudices, and this is perhaps one of them. The presence of a small portion of a stimulating cheese may not be sufficient to oppress the stomach; and the fermented, and alcalescent varieties—as those of Cheshire, Gruyère, &c.—may excite the organ, so as to expedite the physical changes that the food undergoes in it.

When cheese is toasted, it is looked upon as still more rebellious, owing to its acquiring a tenacity of texture, which interferes with the action of the gastric secretions. Yet many persons of weak stomachs find the *Welsh rabbit* wholesome; that is—in the language, ascribed to Mandeville, " they like it and it agrees with them;"—so that practice does not in this, as in many other cases, exactly accord with theory.

The Welsh rabbit is a favourite article for supper, and has long been so:—

> " Happy the man that has each fortune tried,
> To whom she much has given, and much denied;

> With abstinence all delicates he sees,
> And can regale himself on toast and cheese."
> King's Art of Cookery. (1740.)

It would seem, that cheese has been occasionally poisonous, producing—like poisonous sausages—various degrees, and combinations of inflammation of the stomach and bowels. Hünefeld and Sertürner have rendered it probable, that the poisonous property resides in two animal acids, analogous, if not identical, with the caseïc and sebacic, so that poisonous cheese would seem to belong to the same class as poisonous sausages. No precise rules are laid down for detecting it. It has hitherto been met with only in Germany, but Dr. Christison (*Op. citat.* p. 562,) affirms, that from information, communicated to him by Dr. Swanwick, of Macclesfield, there is reason to think, that an analogous poison is occasionally met with in Cheshire, on the small hill farms, where the limited extent of the dairies obliges the farmer to keep the curd for several days before a sufficient quantity is collected to form the larger cheeses.

The soft curd of milk, as in our s c h m i e r k ä s e, is much less difficult of digestion than the salted and dried.

Milk, in a coagulated state, is used in Ireland, and in this country, under the name of *bonny-clabber*. The coagulation has here taken place spontaneously; and the compound contains all the oleaginous, albuminous, serous, and saline constituents of the milk; and hence it differs from buttermilk,—the fluid remaining in the churn after the separation of the butter. Milk, in the state of bonny-clabber,—or in that of *slip*, made by turning the milk with rennet,—is much liked by those habituated to it, and is not difficult of digestion;—that is, not more so than milk in its fresh state, and probably less.

The Scotch employ milk in the coagulated state, in another shape, under the name *Corstorphin cream*. It is so denominated from a village, near Edinburgh, where it is largely prepared. A portion of skimmed milk is put into a wooden vessel, deeper than it is wide, and having a hole in the bottom, stopped up by a peg, which, on being taken out, allows of fluid being drawn from the vessel. This vessel is set in another, which is wider and deeper, so that the smaller vessel may be surrounded with boiling water. When this is done, the vessels are allowed to remain for one or two days, more or less according to the state of the weather; after which time, the milk is found to be coagulated, and the watery portion, separated from the coagulum, has subsided to the bottom of the vessel. This acid liquor is now drawn off at the aperture, and the smaller vessel being once more stopped up, it is again set in the large vessel, to be surrounded with boiling water as before. After it has remained in this state twenty-four hours longer, more acid water is found to have separated from the coagulum, and this being drawn off, the coagulum, which is now of a pretty thick consistence, is stirred briskly with a wooden stick, and in this condition it is brought to table.

"It is an aliment, says Cullen, (*Materia Medica*, vol. i. p. 353,) "tolerably nourishing; and by the quantity of acid still retained in it, it is moderately—but gratefully—acid, and cooling. I have frequently prescribed it to phthisical patients; and neither in these, nor in any other persons, have I ever known any disorders of the stomach or intestines, arising from the free use of it."

d. *Buttermilk.*—This fluid differs according as it has emanated from milk that has been but a short, or a long time kept, before the butter was separated from it. In the former case, it may be entirely sweet when fresh; in the latter, it is more or less acid. Where it is fresh, it does not differ much in its properties from milk. It has lost the greater part of its oleaginous portion, and is consequently somewhat more digestible, but much less nutritious; hence it is employed in fevers, and whenever a light refrigerant article of diet is demanded. When still more acid, its refrigerant properties are augmented, but it is more apt to disagree with the stomach and bowels.

e. *Whey.*—Serum or whey is the least nutritious part of milk. Besides its sugar, which appears to be the base of the lactic, saccho-lactic, and acetic, acids, and certain salts, which it holds in solution, it contains a portion of butter, and cheese, on which, as well as on the sugar, its nutritious properties are dependent. These are not considerable, and hence whey forms an agreeable, and nutrient beverage in acute diseases; but it is apt to become acid in the stomach, and therefore does not always agree with the dyspeptic. A whey, prepared by boiling wine with milk, and separating the curd, is a pleasant drink in cases of catarrh, where the stimulation of the wine is not contra-indicated.

Owing to the presence of saccharine matter, milk is susceptible of the vinous fermentation, and hence it is employed by the Tartars for making an intoxicating liquor, which they call *koumiss*. Mare's milk is selected for the purpose, on account of its containing a larger proportion of sugar than that of the cow.

*Sugar of milk* resembles, in its nutritive properties, saccharine substances in general (See page 199.) It is employed by the homœopathists as the vehicle for the exhibition of their remedies. It is extensively manufactured in Switzerland by evaporating whey to the consistence of syrup. (Davidson, *Treatise on Diet*, p. 256. Lond. 1843.)

Eggs, in point of nutriment and digestibility, are classed by Dr. Paris next to milk. They certainly are more nutritious, and in most, if not all, forms of preparation, less digestible. They consist of *white* and *yelk*; the former almost pure albumen; and the latter animal oil, united with albumen.

Of albumen, in different states of coagulation, mention has already been made. It was stated, that when lightly coagulated, it is more digestible than when raw or hard boiled; and the same thing applies to the whole egg,—the light boiled being more digestible than the raw or hard boiled.

Eggs contain a large quantity of nutritive matter in a small space, and, accordingly, they are not very proper where a rigid diet is required; but, when lightly boiled, and given in small quantities,—as a teaspoonful every now and then,—they are a nutriment of value where the stomach rejects other food, or wherever it is desirable, that a small quantity of aliment should be offered at a time. The yelk is less digestible, in this state of preparation than the white.

Coction alters the qualities of eggs in another way. When light boiled, they are more laxative than otherwise, but when hard boiled they induce constipation. The form of preparation has much to do with their digestibility. Perhaps the lightest mode is to boil them only as long as is necessary to coagulate slightly the greater part of the white, without depriving the yelk of its fluidity. Next, or equal to this, is the poached egg;—the "beauty of which" —to use the language of Kitchener—" is, for the yelk to be seen blushing through the white, which should only be just sufficiently hardened to form a transparent veil for the egg." The worst form of all is the fried egg,—especially if over done. In this state, the albumen is hardened, and the animal oil of the yelk is rendered empyreumatic, and extremely difficult of digestion.

In one or other of these forms, eggs are usually brought to table, but the French writers on the culinary art reckon as many as six hundred and eighty-five modes of preparation. There are many individuals, who are unable to use the slightest portion of any part of them; and when they have undergone decomposition —even if it be incipient—they are apt to be very offensive to the stomach, and are said to be even noxious; but we have not many opportunities for witnessing their effects under such circumstances in this part of the globe. In other regions, we know they are eaten with impunity when disgustingly putrid;—so completely is man the creature of custom!

The eggs of the common fowl are usually employed by us. Those of the Guinea fowl, partridge, &c., are more delicate. The egg of the duck, goose, &c. is strong, and is, consequently, rarely or never eaten. Of old, the eggs of the peahen were greatly preferred to those of the hen.

The yelk of eggs, when diluted with warm water, and with the addition of aromatics, constitutes the *lait de poule* of the French, which is a pleasant and nutritious emulsion.

In the present complex condition of the culinary art, we are constantly taking some preparation of egg without being aware of it. Eggs are, indeed, indispensable to the cook in the formation of most of the richer dishes; but they are never employed without rendering the aliment more difficult of digestion. As a general rule, indeed, all dishes, that contain a large quantity of nutriment in a small space, are more unmanageable by the stomach; and hence every preparation of eggs, and every made dish, are more or less rebellious.

## 2. Vegetable aliments.

The vegetable kingdom furnishes numerous articles of human sustenance. In certain countries of the east, it forms almost the sole diet; and, amongst the poorer classes of society, in many countries, but little animal food is used. The potato, with the addition of buttermilk, is the chief diet of the poorer orders of Irish.

## VEGETABLE ALIMENTS. 247

When we reflect upon the elements that compose the vegetable, and compare these with the elementary constituents of animal substances, we find—as before remarked—that there is generally one element more in the latter than exists in the former,—*azote;* and hence we would infer, that vegetable food must be less easy of assimilation—that is of conversion into the nature of the animal— than animal food. Such is probably the case; but an enlarged view of bromatology instructs us, that there are not only nations of mankind, who subsist almost exclusively on vegetable, but that many animals use no other. Yet the flesh of the herbivorous animal equally contains azote; but as this element cannot be obtained from the food, it must be received from some other source, and probably from the air of respiration. So that there must exist, as we have elsewhere attempted to show, a power in the chylopoietic organs of the animal, and in the vessels of nutrition of the vegetable, to decompose alimentary substances into their elements, and then to recompose them; so that they may be adapted to the nutrition of the being they are destined to nourish. Where the food of the animal is vegetable, an additional element has to be supplied; and where the food of the vegetable is of an animal nature, the same element has to be abstracted;—thus affording signal examples of the complex processes of chemistry, which must be constantly going on in organized bodies, under the influence of vitality, and the precise nature of which we shall probably never be able to comprehend.

Vegetables are by no means as generally esculent as animals. Those, that are employed by man, are very numerous; but there are many that are positively deleterious,—as the catalogue of acrid, narcotic, and acro-narcotic poisons sufficiently testifies. Great caution is, therefore, necessary in making use of any plant, or part of a plant, when we are ignorant of its properties. De Candolle has shown, that there is considerable analogy in the action, on the animal economy, of vegetables, which resemble each other in their external characters, or botanical relations; and hence, that the arrangement of vegetables into natural groups or families is calculated to aid us in estimating the edible or medicinal properties of untried vegetables,—a method of investigation, which might be turned to useful account by such as are cast away upon foreign shores, and are compelled to subsist chiefly on unknown vegetables;

and one of great value to the scientific naturalist, in his appreciation of the various new plants, which he may have occasion to examine—as respects their utility in rural economy, or in medicine. Attention was first drawn to this method of investigation by Camerarius, and since his time it has been further treated by Murray, Linnæus, De Jussieu, Cassel, Dr. B. S. Barton, and especially by De Candolle.—(*Essai sur les propriétés médicales des Plantes.*)

Many medicines, obtained from the vegetable kingdom, and some of them of the most active kind, were considered, in the infancy of the meteria medica, to belong to a single plant. Subsequent examination proved them to belong to several congenerous species. The Peruvian bark, for example, is obtained from all the species of the true *cinchona*; rhubarb from several species of *rheum;* opium from many of the *poppy* species; turpentine from most of the *pines*, &c.; and several species of the same genus afford medicines so like each other, that they were united under the same name before their history was known. This analogy is, at times, so marked, that the whole family of plants participates in the same virtues. All the *gramineæ* for instance, have farinaceous and nutritive seeds; the *Labiatæ* are stomachic and cordial; the seeds of the *umbelliferæ* are tonic, and stimulant; those of the *euphorbiaceæ* acrid, and purgative; the juice of the *coniferæ* is resinous; and the bark of the *amentaceæ* is astringent, and febrifuge. Such is the general fact, but there are some very striking exceptions to the rule; for example, the deadly cicuta is alongside the useful and innoxious carrot; the sweet potato touches the acrid jalap; the bitter colocynth may be mistaken, by the eye, for the melon; the potato is classed amongst the poisonous solana; the lolium temulentum, of deleterious agency, is amongst the cerealia; and the deadly cherry-laurel is amongst the plums and cherries. (De Candolle, *Op. cit.*)

The FARINACEOUS VEGETABLES administer most copiously to the sustenance of man. It is from them that our various kinds of bread —properly termed the " staff of life"—are made; and some of them are employed in diet, without having undergone any such preparation.

The *flour of wheat* contains a mucilaginous, saccharine matter, fecula or starch, and the vegeto-animal principle, termed gluten to the quantity of which it owes its pre-eminence for the formation of bread. Wheaten flour is often employed, united with milk, for the food of infants, and in the formation of pottages for those of larger growth; and if it be so mixed as not to constitute too tenacious a mass, it is tolerably digestible, and certainly nutritious. It is the basis, also, of the various forms of pastry, but the texture it acquires, and the many substances, difficult of digestion with which it is apt to be mixed, cause it to be very unmanageable by the powers of the stomach.

*Wheaten bread* is either leavened or unleavened; that is, the paste is either made to ferment by means of the addition of yeast or barm, or of leaven; or it is prepared without such additions. In cities, where large breweries are in constant operation, barm is employed as the ferment, and if it be added in the appropriate quantity, the bread will be light, and free from all acidity. In the country, where there are no facilities for providing yeast, old paste or leaven is constantly kept on hand, and a portion of this is added to the newly made paste, which speedily excites fermentation in it. It is not always easy, however, especially in hot weather, to accurately regulate the quantity of leaven, and, accordingly, the resulting bread is sometimes acid, and at others dense and heavy. In this process, the flour has undergone a thorough conversion, so that none of its quondam constituents can be detected in it. It is much more miscible with water than dough, and this is of course favourable to its action as a nutriment. The precise chemical changes have not, however, been appreciated; but it would seem, that a quantity of water, (or its elements) becomes consolidated, and combined with the flour; and that the gluten forms a combination with the starch and water, which gives rise to the nutritive compound.

Bread, prepared without leaven, agrees better with the stomach than the fermented, especially if the latter be at all acid. It is on this account, that plain biscuits and crackers are so advisable for the dyspeptic. Butter is often added, with the view of rendering them less hard, and more soluble, but the addition renders them more indigestible. All sweet cakes are objectionable on this account, especially as they usually contain eggs, and always sugar, neither of which is readily disposed of by the digestive organs; and the same applies to the different varieties of pastry, which were regarded by Dr. Kitchener as so objectionable that he would not admit them into the body of his "Cook's Oracle;" but he neutralized his good intentions by giving them in an appendix!

The dietetic qualities of bread differ according to the mode of preparation of the flour whence it is formed. In Great Britain, three great varieties are met with,—the *whiten, wheaten,* and the *household.* In the whiten, the whole of the bran is separated; in the wheaten, only the coarser part; and in the household, none at all. The finest bread is, consequently, made of the pure flour; wheaten bread of a mixture of finer bran with the flour; and, in the household, the whole substance of the grain is contained. The latter has been regarded as a bread peculiarly fit for the dyspeptic, and hence has acquired the name *dyspeptic.* It is certainly more laxative, and more nutrient,—not on account of its containing more nutritive matter, for it has less, but on account of the stimulant effect of the bran on the mucous membrane of the stomach and small intestines, which causes a larger quantity of nutritive matter to be separated from the starch and gluten of the bread, than could be obtained from the bread of pure flour. The bran, in this case, acts like the shell of the walnuts employed in the fattening of fowls; or, like the charcoal, which, in the rural districts of England, is mixed with the meal with a like intent. In many kinds of leavened bread, eggs, milk, and butter enter as ingredients, but although they may add to the nutrient properties of the bread, and render it more agreeable to the palate, they detract from its digestibility.

Wheaten bread is preferable to that of the other cerealia in being less viscid, and more nutritious and digestible. *Barley bread* is, however, used in some countries to a great extent by the poorer classes of society; and rye, or a mixture of wheat and rye, is frequently employed. All these breads are apt to lie heavy on the stomach, and to become acid; but the last is the least objectionable in these respects. In the north of England, and Scotland, *oaten bread,* or as it is called there *haver bread,* (German, h a f e r, *oats*) is almost exclusively eaten by the multitude. " The *bannock, clap bread, bitchiness bread,* and *riddle cakes,*" says Dr. Paris, " are the names, which such productions (oaten cakes) have received. The *jannock* is oaten bread made into loaves. It is evident from the health and vigour of the people, who use this grain as a principal article of diet, that it must be very nutritive; but the stomach will require some discipline before it can digest it. In those, unaccustomed to such food, it produces heartburn; and it is said to occasion, even in those with whom it agrees, cutaneous affections." This has always appeared to the Author a prejudice. In the northern parts of England, oatmeal is as much employed as in Scotland, yet cutaneous affections, according to his experience, are not more common, than in parts of England where other varieties of bread are eaten. It has never appeared to him to produce any morbid effects, but on the contrary to be remarkably wholesome.

Connected with the subject of oaten cake, the Author may allude to a singular idiosyncrasy in his own person. Owing to some accidental association in very early life, whenever oaten cake—which is very brittle, as usually prepared—is broken in his presence, a spasmodic contraction of the appropriate muscles takes place, so as to draw the left corner of the mouth momentarily upwards; and although this singular sympathy occurred farther back than he can trace, he cannot, at the present day, hear a thin biscuit broken, or even think of the act, without an almost invincible effort occurring in the same muscles to assume this action.

*Rice* is also eaten as bread, and occasionally the potato, mixed or unmixed with flour; and the bread from either is sufficiently palatable and wholesome. On this continent, and in some parts of Europe, the Indian corn—*zea mays*—ministers largely to human sustenance. It may, indeed, in certain climes, be regarded as one of the most valuable of the gifts of God to man. Like the farina of the wheat, it is formed into bread, alone or with various additions,—as milk, eggs, &c. It is a wholesome and nutritious aliment, but, with those that are unaccustomed to its use, it is apt to produce diarrhœa, in consequence, probably, of the presence of the husk, with which it is always more or less mixed, in the state in which it is brought to market. It is on this account, that it has been regarded as bread but little adapted for those liable to, or labouring under, bowel affections, or in times when a choleric predisposition exists.

In the Lombardo-Venetian plains, where a loathsome and peculiar disease—the *pellagra*—has sprung up within the last one hundred years, and which is said, at this time, to affect a sixth or a seventh part of the population, the maize has, strangely enough, been looked upon as a grand exciting cause. Such seems to be the view of professor Spedalieri of Pavia,—founded, however, on very insufficient data. The experience of this country proves, that the pellagra cannot be engendered by the use of corn, to whatever extent indulged. The causes are, doubtless, in the locality; but what these causes are we know no more than we do of those of any of the endemic diseases that prevail in certain districts, and are perhaps unknown in every other. It is a subject, as elsewhere remarked, on which we are profoundly ignorant, and it is well to say so, in order that our investigations may be directed into new channels, although it is probable that it may ever escape our researches.

A bread—in the form of cakes—is made from buckwheat flour —*Polygonum fagopyrum*—which is much used in the United States, but is not very easy of digestion, especially when covered with melted butter, except for those who are habituated to it. The flour is also, at times, an ingredient in pottage, pudding, and other food, especially in Germany.

In some parts of France, the grain of the millet—*milium, panicum miliaceum*—is made into bread; but like the buckwheat cake it is viscid, heavy, compact, and is not ready of digestion. It is also, at times, used for making puddings; for which purpose it is preferred to rice by some.

In South America, bread is formed from the starch of the *Jatropha manihot*, without the aid of leaven. It is termed *cassava* or *cassada bread*, and possesses the nutrient and digestible properties of the amylaceous breads in general.

Well-made bread is an important article of diet, whatever may be the alimentary substances that are taken along with it. It is especially necessary where strong soups are used, the gelatin of which is not very readily digested; but if rendered more solid by being mixed with bread, the digestive process goes on with greater facility. In cases, too, where substances are eaten that contain a large quantity of nutriment in a small space, the addition of bread diminishes the evil. On this and every account, it is a useful adjunct to the dinner table, and especially where rich dishes prevail. In this country—in many parts at least—wheaten bread is eaten new and hot; in which state, it is by no means as easy of digestion as when stale. Dr. Paris asserts, that this is owing to its swelling like a sponge in the stomach. It is not easy to account for the difference in the two cases, which, doubtless, depends greatly upon texture; but the fact is certain, although we cannot readily convert those to the belief, who have been accustomed from early life to the use of the former. In such cases, habit becomes " second nature:" but if one, accustomed to the use of stale bread, or whose digestive powers are feeble, be restricted to it, the effects are obvious.

We have already spoken of *pastry* in general, which Dr. Paris designates as " an abomination," and expresses his belief, that one half, at least, of the cases of indigestion, which occur after dinner parties, may be traced to its use. For the valetudinarian, the boiled *bread-pudding* is the most advisable; *batter-pudding* is more difficult of digestion, on account of the egg necessary for its formation; *pancake* has the same objection, and moreover the process of frying renders the butter empyreumatic, and thus adds to the indigestibility. Neither, too, possesses the best digestive texture. *Suet-pudding* is the worst of all preparations of the kind;—the suet itself, like all fats, experiencing but little change from the action of the gastric secretions.

*Macaroni* and *vermicelli* are preparations of fine flour, the former of which is eaten in various ways, but generally when boiled and mixed with cheese. It is a national and wholesome diet with the Neapolitans. The latter also is much used in Italy, added to soups, broths, &c. Both are common at our tables.

Of the different farinaceous aliments much need not be said. The *potato* is the most employed. Of the two kinds—the 'waxy' and the 'mealy'—the former is preferred by many individuals, but its tenacity renders it comparatively indigestible; and where the digestive powers are enfeebled, it is frequently noticed to pass through the intestinal canal unchanged. In this state, it is often seen in the evacuations of young children labouring under diarrhœa. The mealy potato is nutritious and digestible, and is eaten with the same view as bread,—especially where the food contains much nutriment in a small compass, or where the proximate animal principles are taken in too liquid a form. Roasting and boiling until they are ready to fall to pieces are the best modes of preparation. Overboiling deprives them of some of their nutritive properties.

The sweet potato—*convolvulus batatas*—is a nutritious root. The English name indicates that a saccharine quality is united to the fecula. It is not as easy of digestion as the common potato.

Rice is a farinaceous aliment largely used amongst the orientals, as well as in temperate climes. In the southern part of the United States, and in Southern France and Italy, it forms a considerable portion of the vegetable diet of the inhabitants. It is nutritious, and when mixed with other food is an excellent aliment. It has been supposed to be possessed of astringent, or binding properties, but no astringent principle can be detected in it. It contains but little saccharine matter, and is not disposed to acescency and fermentation. Perhaps the cause of its having had astringent properties assigned to it is its long retention in the stomach when that organ is debilitated. This is probably owing to its possessing but little stimulating power. In hot climates, where the digestive organs are relaxed and enfeebled, this deficiency of stimulation is supplied by the use of capsicum and other spices; and hence the universality of *curry*, as an aliment in India and other torrid countries. When not freed from the water in which it has been boiled, rice is mucilaginous—but not to the same extent as barley—and has been recommended in bowel affections; the mucilage shielding the interior of the stomach, and the bland influence being communicated by continuous sympathy to the part of the lining membrane of the intestinal canal labouring under irritation. Its advantageous use, in such cases—although dependent upon another principle—may perhaps have favoured the notion of its being possessed of astringency.

Formerly, the idea prevailed, that rice, when habitually eaten, is possessed of poisonous properties. Bontius, who practised in India, affirmed that it appeared to him to produce blindness; and the same assertion has been made by others; but, if such were the case, we ought to have had numerous proofs of it in this country. The cause of the blindness ought to have been looked for elsewhere. In 1786, Bernard, a physician at Béziers, in France, read a communication before the academy of that place, in which he attempted to point out, that the use of rice is not devoid of danger. In this *Mémoire*, he cites the opinion of Bontius, and refers to the case of a merchant of Béziers, who, whenever he partook of it was attacked with fits of sneezing, and puffiness of the face, which

## VEGETABLE ALIMENTS.—FARINACEOUS. 255

disappeared with the completion of digestion. Such cases are evidently dependent upon idiosyncracy, and there is perhaps not an aliment, which does not disagree, from this cause, with particular individuals. No one, however, presumes that such aliments necessarily contain any poisonous principle; yet, strange to say, Tourtelle, on no better evidence than that we have given, ascribes the possession of such a principle to rice: and Bricheteau, in the last edition of the "*Hygiène*" of Tourtelle, vaguely observes:— "I should not have much difficulty in believing—without, however, having any evidence[!]—that rice contains a poisonous principle, similar to that met with in many other alimentary vegetables. And perhaps the action of this noxious agent is not foreign to the production of the diseases experienced by the cultivators of rice, and which are commonly attributed exclusively to the influence of humidity." This is mere hypothesis, without the least evidence, as M. Bricheteau himself admits, to support it. More recently, statements have been made by Dr. Tytler—long a practitioner in India—which would seem to show, that in certain states of the grain—the result probably of disease—much gastric and intestinal disorder may be induced. Dr. Tytler, (*Lancet*, vol. i. for 1833-34,) goes so far, indeed, as to assert, that such bad rice may be the cause of cholera, which he even proposes to call *morbus oryzeus*, as if the disease were induced by rice alone!

It is well known, that rye, and maize are subject to a disease, which renders them noxious to animals; the *spurred rye*, as it is termed, giving rise to convulsions, and to dry gangrene; and the spurred maize, it is said, to the loss of the hair, and sometimes of the teeth. (Christison, *On Poisons*, p. 780.)

Next to rice, *Indian corn* or *maize* is one of the most common farinaceous aliments, but it is by no means so easy of digestion as either of the cerealia just described. The young grains, constituting the "roasting ears," make a delicious vegetable, ready for the table, too, after the season for green peas has gone by. When very young, corn, in this state, is in its most digestible condition,—the husk being comparatively tender; but when old, a considerable part of the grain withstands the digestive operation, and passes through the bowels unchanged. It need hardly, therefore, be added, that where bowel affections are rife, this vegetable ought to be used with caution.

Corn meal, mixed with cheese, and baked into a kind of pudding, forms the dish which the Italians call *polenta*. The admixture with cheese does not add to its digestibility.

Of the other aliments, in common domestic use, which owe their properties to fecula,—such as sago, tapioca, salep, arrow root, &c.—enough has been said elsewhere, (p. 197.) They are rarely employed at table, but are frequently administered—boiled in water or milk—to the sick, or the convalescent. When the digestive powers are enfeebled, so that solid food cannot be taken, or where the bowels are disordered, these solutions of starch form a bland nutriment. The simple solution in water is not, however, as digestible as might be presumed, the mucilaginous form being by no means the easiest managed by the stomach in any case. When milk is added, it is coagulated, so that a solid is formed in the stomach, which somewhat corrects the disadvantages attendant upon the mucilaginous character of the solutions of all these feculaceous preparations.

The LEGUMINOUS VEGETABLES, or pulse, are much employed for human sustenance. When the seeds are perfectly ripe and dried, they can be readily reduced to a kind of meal similar to that of the gramineæ, but more unctuous to the feel, and of a more saccharine taste. When triturated with water, they form a milky mixture, and when heated, and pressed in the entire state, an oily matter exudes. It is in these respects, principally, that they differ from the grains. They are chiefly composed of fecula, and are highly nutritious, but not as digestible as the pure farinaceous grains, on account of the oil they contain. For this reason, they are improper for those of feeble digestive powers,—occasioning, in such, flatulence and colic. In all ages, they have been celebrated for producing these effects, and there are many popular notions, which exhibit the general belief. They are eaten in one of two states,—fresh, or dried. In the former condition, their texture is tender, and they are more easy of digestion, consequently less flatulent; but they contain less nutritive matter in the same space. In the latter state, they are far more nutritive, but extremely difficult of digestion, and therefore adapted for those only, who are possessed of a vigorous digestion. These remarks are especially applicable to peas, and beans, the latter of which are not easy of digestion, in any form of preparation, or at any degree of maturity. When peas are made into a pudding, they are rendered still more indigestible, owing to the addition of other substances, as well as to tenacity of texture. Some of this class of vegetables—as the kidney bean—are eaten with the pod. In such case, they are plucked for the table in their immature state, and like all the succulent vegetables, should be well boiled. They are not as easy of digestion as the pure farinacea.

The different varieties of pulse have been made into bread, but they are not well adapted for this purpose,—the bread being somewhat heavy and indigestible.

The KERNELS are nearly allied, in their nutrient and digestible properties, to pulse, but they are still more objectionable. With us they are scarcely ever used except as an article of desert. They contain fecula united with oil, and a considerable amount of insoluble woody matter. The *almond, walnut, hazelnut, chestnut, chincapin, hickory nut,* and *shellbark,* are commonly eaten. Of these, the four last are the most objectionable, and are not unfrequently the cause of serious gastric, and intestinal disorder.

In times of scarcity, the acorn—notwithstanding its astringent property—has served for food; and the chestnut is said to form a considerable part of the aliment of the inhabitants of the Apennines, and of the Siennois,— different preparations being eaten, under the names *nicci, polenta, castagnacio,* &c. There is, perhaps, no article of diet so well calculated to disagree with the dyspeptic as the various nuts, and it would be wise, as Dr. Paris has observed, to banish them entirely from the table.

The greater part of the OLERA, or *potherbs* are sweet, and almost insipid, containing only a small quantity of mucilaginous matter, so that they are but slightly nutritive. Those that are very sapid are employed more as condiments than as aliments. As a general rule, their texture is tender, and they are soluble, but extremely acescent,—so that thay give rise to acidity, and flatulency, where the digestive function is feebly performed.

Of some of the olera, the roots alone are used, whilst of others the whole herb is eaten. Of the roots, the *beet, carrot,* and *parsnip* strongly resemble each other. They are nutritive from the quantity of saccharine matter they contain; but when old they are stringy, and consequently difficult of digestion,—the fibrous matter passing through the bowels unconverted. They should be eaten when young, and be well boiled. The same may be said of the *turnip,* and *salsify.* The *radish* may be regarded more as a condiment,—containing but little nutriment, but stimulating the stomach by reason of a peculiar acrid matter, chiefly resident in the cortical part of the root. The *onion* likewise contains a large portion of acrid matter, which is greatly dissipated by boiling; so that there is a material difference between the stimulating properties of the raw, and the boiled root. It contains a considerable quantity of mucilage, and hence is much more nutritive than the radish. It is difficult, however, to understand why this vegetable should have been one of the few, not proscribed by the board of health of one of our cities, during the prevalence of cholera, in the summer of 1832.

The *garlic, leek,* and *shallot,* are scarcely ever used in cookery, except as condiments by virtue of the acrid matter they possess.

The different esculent herbs are eaten either in the raw state, or boiled. Perhaps, as a general rule, in the former condition they are less digestible than in the latter; but the exceptions to this rule are so numerous, that it is difficult to speak positively. With many individuals, for example, the heart of the *cabbage* digests more rapidly when uncooked than when cooked; and, in the experiments of Dr. Beaumont, it was found to yield readily to the gastric powers, whilst the boiled was more than twice as long in undergoing chymification. The K o h l s a l a t ("cabbage salad") of the Germans,—generally pronounced "cold slaw,"—is a salad, prepared of sliced cabbage dressed with vinegar and oil, and the Author has found it agree with dyspeptics, when the boiled cabbage could not be taken. The same may be said of the s a u e r K r a u t, or 'sour cabbage,' which consists of cabbage, salted and permitted to undergo the first stage of the acetous fermentation, and which the Germans consider to be wholesome, easy of digestion, and antiscorbutic. This ready digestion may with them be partly explained by the fact of its forming one of their common aliments from early childhood; and it is perhaps also dependent, in part, on the addition of vinegar, which seems to facilitate the digestive changes when vegetables are taken. Acetic acid, as we have seen, is one of the natural agents of digestion,—and probably of the digestion of vegetables especially; and, perhaps, in all cases a slight addition of vinegar may favour the process. It has been a matter of dispute, whether salads should be dressed with vinegar, and oil, or not. From what has been already said, it need hardly be remarked, that the addition of vinegar is useful. There may be more doubt as respects the oil, which is itself susceptible of but little change in the stomach. We meet, however, with many, who can digest salad with the addition of these condiments, and not without. This may be owing to the property that oil possesses of checking the fermentation, which is so apt to result in the stomachs of dyspeptics when vegetable food has been taken.

All this must, however, be a matter of experience in individual cases; but, as a general rule we may fearlessly assert, that if salad is eaten at all by those of feeble digestive powers, it is less likely to disagree when the ordinary condiments—salt, mustard, oil, and vinegar—are added, than when the herb itself composes the entire dish.

*Lettuce* and *celery* are the most common vegetables employed as salad, and their texture renders them as well adapted for the purpose as any. The different kinds of *cress,* however, contain an aromatic property which cannot but favour their digestion. *Cucumbers* have been properly regarded as the most unwholesome of all raw vegetables. They are generally dressed with salt, oil, pepper, and vinegar, but notwithstanding the presence of these condiments,—during the season when they are common, and when the disposition to affections of the stomach, and bowels prevails,— they frequently occasion great mischief; and Dr. Parrish properly remarks, that they should be avoided as poison by dyspeptics.

The chief vegetables, that are eaten after having been exposed to some culinary process, are the different kinds of *Brassica* or *cabbage, spinach, asparagus, squashes, tomatoes,* &c. Of the *cabbage genus,* Pliny and Cato have described many varieties, and have assigned to one or other the virtues of a panacea. Cato considered it as a vegetable, " quæ omnibus oleribus antistat;" and Columella, as food for both kings and plebeians.

> ——" Toto quæ plurima terræ
> Orbe virens pariter plebi, regique superbo."

The Greeks and Romans, too, fancied that it had the power of preventing or removing the effects of repletion, whether produced by eating, or drinking. Julius Africanus gives a receipt, in which this property of the cabbage is mentioned. "*That a person drinking much wine may not be inebriated.*" "Having roasted the lights of a goat, eat them; or, when fasting, eat five or seven bitter almonds; or first eat *raw cabbage*, and you will not be inebriated."

The heads of the *cauliflower*, and *broccoli* are the parts decidedly most tender, and they are consequently preferred. The whole plant of the *common cabbage* is eaten, but unless well boiled, it is very prone to undergo fermentation, and give rise to acidity and flatulence; and, indeed, when well boiled, is not very easy of digestion. In this country, it is common to boil bacon with greens, so that the vegetable becomes impregnated with the fat, and a compound is formed, which, as a general rule, is extremely improper for the dyspeptic. They, who have been accustomed to the vegetable in this state, from childhood, cannot readily comprehend this, nor are such the best tests of comparative digestibility. Let one whose digestion is feeble, and who has not been habituated to its use, taste but a small portion, and the effects will be soon, and signally apparent. The same remarks are applicable to the admixture of melted butter with cabbage. There are but few stomachs, that are not incommoded by it.

The texture of *spinach*, when sufficiently boiled, is tender, and it is somewhat mucilaginous. None of these vegetables, however, contain much nutriment. *Asparagus*, when of the proper age, is sufficiently soluble, as well as the *squash* or *cimblin*, which is obtained from a species of gourd.

In Europe, the *tomato* or love apple is chiefly employed as a sauce; but in the United States it is one of the most useful vegetables, although—like the potato—belonging to a family of plants some of the individuals of which are extremely poisonous. The acid of this vegetable does not agree with every one; but, on the whole, it may be looked upon as one of the most wholesome, and valuable esculents, that belong to the vegetable kingdom.

The mushroom or *champignon*, and the truffle, (*tuber cibarium*,) have been regarded, even in antiquity, as *les ragoûts des dieux*. The *Boletus*, of which Cicero, Horace, Pliny, Suetonius, and others speak—probably the *amanita aurantiaca*—has been esteemed by gourmets as the finest, and most delicate of the fungi, and reckoned more rare than silver or gold:—

"Argentum atque aurum facile est ⸻⸻⸻
Mittere, boletos mittere difficile est."—MARTIAL. xiii. ep. 41.

## VEGETABLE ALIMENTS.—MUSHROOMS.

Juvenal speaks of the boletus as a great favourite, and placed before the rich, while their parasites were provided with an inferior variety:—

> "Vilibus ancipites fungi ponentur amicis
> Boletus domino."—JUVENAL, Sat. v.

They are delicious; nutritive; but not very digestible; and in some idiosyncrasies act like shell-fish, almonds, &c. Their nutritive properties are probably somewhat dependent upon a vegeto-animal principle which they possess, and which distinguishes them from most other vegetables. Care, however, is required in the selection of the edible varieties, as there are many that are positively and virulently poisonous. Several writers on hygiène and toxicology have attempted to lay down rules for distinguishing the deleterious. It seems, that most *fungi*, which have a warty cap, and more especially of membrane adhering to their upper surface, are poisonous. Heavy fungi, which have an unpleasant odour—especially if they emerge from a *vulva* or bag—are also generally hurtful. Of those, which grow in woods, and shady places, a few are esculent; but the greater part are unwholesome; and if they are moist on the surface, they should be avoided. All those that grow in tufts or clusters from the stumps or trunks of trees ought equally to be rejected. A sure test of a poisonous fungus is an astringent styptic taste, and perhaps also a disagreeable, but, certainly a pungent odour. Some fungi—possessing these properties—have found their way to the table of the epicure, but they are of a questionable quality. Those, whose substance becomes blue soon after being cut, are invariably poisonous. *Agarics* of an orange or rose-red colour; and *boleti*, which are coriaceous or corky in texture, or which have a membranous collar round the stem, are also unsafe.

Such are the rules for detecting deleterious fungi, which, as Dr. Christison (*Op. citat.* p. 771) has remarked, rest on fact and experience; but they will not enable the collector to recognise every poisonous species. It has even been considered advisable to distrust all fungi except the cultivated; and it is farther stated, that so strongly was the celebrated botanist, M. Richard, impressed with the prudence of this course, that he would never eat any except such as had been raised in mushroom beds, although no one was better acquainted than he with their distinctive characters.

The common mushroom—*agaricus campestris*—is the only one of the species *agaricus*, which has been selected for cultivation in gardens; and in Europe four varieties of it are employed for this purpose. Some of the varieties are brought to our markets in great abundance in autumn; and it is occasionally cultivated. A friend of the Author, in Virginia, was in the habit of supplying his table from the produce of his garden, during the proper season.

According to the Author's friend, Professor Ducatel, (*Manual of Practical Toxicology*, p. 296. Baltimore, 1833,) some French residents of the city of Baltimore collect a variety of the *boletus edulis,* called by them *cèpe,* which they eat without any apprehension.

After all, it would appear, that although there are some vegetables, which seem to be rebellious under any mode of exhibition, yet several of the ordinary vegetables brought to the table, especially those of the farinaceous kind, owe many of their bad effects to the circumstance of their not being well cooked. This is important to be borne in mind, during times of prevalent disease attacking the digestive organs. Perhaps, under such circumstances, the safest plan is to abstain from any except the farinaceous, but if the succulent vegetable—as the cabbage—be taken, it should be young, consequently tender, and unmixed with any substance—as melted butter—which can add to its indigestibility.

Much has been said, since the occurrence of cholera in this country, and in Europe, regarding the qualities of the SUMMER and AUTUMNAL FRUITS, and generally they have been altogether proscribed. In a disease so rife—so fearfully rife—as cholera, coincidences were to be expected, such as that of a person being attacked with cholera, after having eaten fruit—alone, or along with some other article of diet;—and such coincidences, in a period of alarm, have been sufficient to excite a terror against its use. These cases have, however, been mere coincidences. So far as the Author has seen or heard, there is nothing like an invariable sequence, and no occurrence of such coincidences in sufficient frequency to induce us to believe, that the moderate use of ripe fruit, under ordinary precautions, has ever brought on an attack of cholera; accordingly, a reaction took place in many cities and countries, and ripe fruit was not only not discarded, but was recommended to patients labouring under the disease. Some doubts with respect to the propriety of the proscription ought, indeed, to have been suggested by the rarity of such coincidences, compared with the immense multitude of cases of individuals, who, in conformity with the rules of boards of health, or of the officers of eleemosynary establishments, or with the feelings and prejudices of communities or of individuals, had wholly abstained from its use; and still more by the striking fact, that the disease prevailed virulently and extensively in many parts of the north of Europe, during seasons when fruits were scarcely, if at all, attainable. There is, in truth, not the least reason for presuming, that ripe fruits had any thing more to do with the causation of cholera than any other kind of diet, and how easy it might have been to excite equal prejudice, on no more foundation, against any of the common aliments. In the table at the end of this volume, it will be seen, that the ripe, mellow apple was more digestible—in the case of the particular individual experimented upon—than the baked or roasted potato, in the ratio of 545 to 400, and than the boiled in the ratio of 545 to 285; yet potatoes were almost always allowed, and if cholera followed, it was never ascribed to indulging in them; whilst rice, as we have seen, which with us was the diet universally advised, has been supposed by some to have given origin to the disease, and hence the term " rice disease," or *morbus oryzeus,* assigned to it by those individuals.

That strange disease is probably dependent upon a union of endemic and epidemic influences—of the nature of which we know no more than we do of the influences, that lay the foundation to other epidemics—which often requires but a very slight exciting cause to develope it. That such exciting cause may have frequently consisted in indigestible aliment is admitted, but we have not sufficient evidence, that ripe fruit is placed in this category. Unripe fruit has, by all writers, been looked upon as extremely morbific, and we have no doubt it is so; but this is no reason, why the prohibition should extend to a diet so refreshing, and innocuous as the ripe. One writer, indeed, (*American Journal of the Medical Sciences* for August, 1833,) extends an amnesty to vegetable diet in general. " In the prohibition of unripe fruit," he observes, " we entirely accord; but from the sweeping condemnation of fruit and vegetables generally, and the substitution of a diet, consisting chiefly of meat, as has been advised by all health councils, and by many members of the profession, not, however, by our Author (Dr. Hamett,) we must express a most decided dissent. We know nothing more salutary or grateful to the stomach, during the existence of epidemic cholera, than good, fresh, ripe fruits in moderate quantities, daily; nor is there any diet more wholesome at such a period, than one consisting in a good proportion of the various garden vegetables well cooked." "This opinion," he continues, "has been formed from most ample personal experience, and that of very many who adopted our advice, for months, in the largest city of the continent during the most awful ravages of the cholera; and it has been subsequently confirmed by the same manner of life during a month spent in New York city, while the cholera prevailed there." The result of the writer's experience confirms what has been said regarding the want of any thing like an invariable sequence in the case of ripe fruit and the cholera, and, so far as it goes, establishes the wholesomeness of a general vegetable diet. There has been, doubtless, much unfounded prejudice, fostered by, and indeed emanating from, members of the profession, who have embraced the notion, after fancied experience, but too often, perhaps, without full examination: unfortunately, the inconvenience resulting from the opinion has not been confined to the patient, who suffered comparatively little from the privation, but the practices founded upon it embraced so large a mass of the population in every choleric region, that the market gardeners and fruiterers, who are numerous in the neighbourhood of large towns, were ruined by the prohibition, which every where prevailed, and which was not restricted to situations where cholera raged, but extended to cities not visited, and not to be visited, by the epidemic.

The objection to fruits is not new. Arriving at maturity at a period of the year when gastric and intestinal derangements are common, and being often eaten, especially by children, in an unripe state, and in undue quantity, their use has always been esteemed hazardous.

"Cave autumnos fructus
Ne sit tibi luctu"

was a maxim strongly urged by the Schola Salernitana.

The only cautions, necessary in eating the ordinary fruits, are :—to see that they are ripe, and to remove the skins, and seeds, which are totally indigestible, and usually pass through the whole of the intestinal tube unchanged. Something likewise depends upon the texture of the pulp of the fruit. When it is very firm, as in many of the varieties of the *plum* species it often passes the digestive organs unmodified. Dr. Paris considers, that the *orange*, when perfectly ripe, maybe allowed to the most fastidious dyspeptic, —the white or inner skin, as he properly advises, being scrupulously rejected, as it is not more digestible than leather. The recommendation, however, is too general. We have met with many dyspeptics, with whom the saccharine matter of the juice disagrees, occasioning heartburn and flatulence, which it is, indeed, well calculated to induce. The *farinaceous fruits*—as the different varieties of *melon*—are the least digestible of all, and few dyspeptics can partake of them without experiencing more or less inconvenience. The addition of salt and pepper favours their digestibility.

The properties of preserved fruits are like those of the sugar employed in their preservation. A sweeping assertion has been made by some writers on dyspepsia, that " most kinds of preserved fruits, and every thing in the shape of sweetmeats must be carefully shunned." There is no reason for this proscription, except in particular cases. Fruit and sugar, in this form, are infinitely less likely to disagree with the dyspeptic than when they are taken singly, especially if the sugar be in a less concentrated state. We shall see, that the greatest difference occurs in the digestion of sugar, according as it is in a state of concentration, or dissolved in a large quantity of water ;—the former frequently digesting with facility, whilst the latter occasions acidity, heartburn, and most of the signs of indigestion.

## SECTION IV.

Condiments; saline, aromatic, and oily—sugar—salt—salt indispensable—vinegar—pickles—verjuice—capers, &c.—aromatic condiments; much used in torrid climes—oily condiments; butter; oil—preparation of food—object of cookery—roasting—broiling—boiling—baking—frying, &c.—sauces.

It rarely happens in civilized life, that the different aliments are eaten in the way they are presented to us. Besides being frequently subjected to culinary preparation, certain substances, called CONDIMENTS, are often added to them. These substances are employed not simply because they are nutritive,—for many of them possess no such properties,—but because when taken with food capable of nourishing, they promote its digestion, correct any injurious property it may possess, or add to its sapidity. In these respects, they act the part of the *corrigent* in a medicinal prescription. It is not often, that the basis, or main ingredient of a prescription is exactly adapted to fulfil all the views of the practitioner. It may be possessed of obnoxious properties, or it may require to be rendered more palatable; and hence the corrigent is added to the basis;—as in hygiène the condiment is added to the aliment.

Dr. Paris has restricted the term 'condiment' to a substance, incapable, of itself, of nourishing, but which, in concert with our food, promotes its digestion, or corrects some of its deleterious properties,—but this is narrowing the signification too much; for certain articles may with propriety, be regarded, at times, as *aliments*, and, at others, as *condiments*, according as they constitute the basis, or the accessory to a dish;—such are cream, butter, mushrooms, olives, &c., all of which are nutritive. How, too, can Dr. Paris's class of "oily condiments" fall under his definition of a condiment? Oleaginous substances are eminently nutritious.

The *bitter principle*, which exists in grasses, and other plants, appears to be essential to the digestion of the herbivora—by acting as a natural stimulant; and it has been found, that cattle do not thrive upon grasses, which are destitute of this principle. In the "*Hortus gramineus Woburnensis*," by Mr. Sinclair—gardener to the Duke of Bedford—it is stated, that if sheep are fed on yellow turnips, which contain little or no bitter principle, they instinctively seek for, and greedily devour, any provender, which may contain it; and that if they cannot obtain it, they become diseased and die. This bitter principle of vegetables is a good example of the condiments, as defined by Dr. Paris; for it is affirmed to have been proved by many experiments, that it passes through the body, without suffering any diminution in its quantity, or change in its nature; and hence it must be, of itself, incapable of nourishing. We have analogous instances in the charcoal, administered, mixed with fat, for fattening poultry, and in the plan, adopted for the same purpose in some parts of Great Britain,—of giving walnuts, coarsely bruised with the shell, and cramming the animal with this diet.

It is difficult to form any satisfactory classification of condiments. Dr. Paris has divided them into the *saline*, the *spicy* or *aromatic*, and the *oily*; yet it is impossible to bring many substances, that are employed as condiments, under any of these divisions;—sugar, mushrooms, truffles, for example.

Of *sugar*, as a condiment, it is unnecessary to speak, after what has been said of its general nutritive, and digestible properties,— which we have seen to be considerable. It is not, however, in any of its forms very proper for the dyspeptic, especially when taken as an adjunct in small quantities, and in a dilute solution. It is in this way, that tea and coffee very frequently disagree,— turning acid and giving rise to flatulence, distention, and heartburn. Yet very frequently, as has been already remarked, when sugar is taken in large quantity by the same individuals no unpleasant symptoms are the consequence. In this we see an analogy to the ordinary physical differences between weak and concentrated saccharine solutions. Whilst the former speedily run into the vinous and acetous fermentations; the latter will keep for any length of time.

There are some dyspeptics, too, who cannot take the sugar of the cane, and yet can take honey;—but these cases are not many.

*Salt* is the most important of all condiments;—" *aliorum condimentorum condimentum*." It is a natural and agreeable stimulant to the digestive function; is liked by almost every infant; is greedily sought after by wild animals, where it can be obtained in our forests; and by those that are domesticated, is keenly relished when mixed with their ordinary food. In the western part of the United States, there are many salt springs, called *licks*, in consequence of the bison and the deer resorting to them for the purpose of *licking* the earth around them, and it is in the neighbourhood of the tracks to these licks, that the hunter waits,—sure of his game, when the time arrives for its visit to the scene of its enjoyment.

In antiquity, salt was always placed upon the table before any other dish, and was the last to be removed; a custom, which was recommended to be continued by the scholars of Salernum:—

"Sal primo debet poni, non primo reponi,
Omnis mensa malè ponitur absque sale."

The use of salt with the food appears to be of indispensable utility; a diet of unsalted aliment generating disease, chiefly of a cachectic character. Children, who are not allowed a sufficient quantity of this useful condiment, are extremely liable to worms; for whenever the powers of the system, and especially those of the stomach, are enfeebled by the want of proper nourishment, both as respects quality and quantity, these parasites find a nidus in the intestines favourable to their development, and the only way to remove the disposition to their generation is to improve the tone of the system generally, and of the stomach in particular. The use of salt fulfils this indication most effectually, and this is one of the reasons why it has been regarded as an anthelmintic; but its agency is more exerted in preventing, than in removing, worms. The agriculturist is well aware of this anthelmintic property of salt, and it is the main article on which he depends for improving the health of his cattle when affected with bots, flukes, &c. Lord Somerville, in an address to the English Board of Agriculture, refers to a punishment that formerly existed in Holland, and which is illustrative of this subject. " The ancient laws of the country ordained men to be kept on bread alone, *unmixed with salt*, as the severest punishment that could be inflicted upon them in their moist climate. The effect was horrible: these wretched criminals are said to have been devoured by worms engendered in their own stomachs." (Paris, *On Diet*, p. 78.) It is proper to remark, however, that the climate of Holland is extremely favourable to the generation of these parasites; and although it is highly probable that the absence of the salt in the bread aided this effect, the confined air of the prison and the wretched diet allowed the prisoner had probably considerable agency likewise.

If we reflect upon the fact, that every fluid of the body contains common salt, we can more readily understand the importance of a due supply of it in our food; and it is probable, that the free chlorohydric acid, met with in the gastric secretions of the stomach, may arise from its decomposition—in the mysterious chemical changes which take place in that organ through the influence of vitality. It would seem, however, that too large a quantity of this condiment is injurious—a fact which applies to the vegetable as well as to the animal kingdom. In recent times, salt has been employed as a manure, and with excellent effects when sparingly distributed over the surface of the ground; but if too largely used, vegetation is destroyed by it.

*Salted meats,* unless when lightly corned, are more indigestible than fresh. When highly dried, they become more or less coriaceous, and of a texture very unfit for the due action of the gastric secretions. It is probable, however, that the injurious effects, occasioned by over indulgence in salted aliments, have been somewhat exaggerated. The scurvy, when it appeared on long voyages, was at one time presumed to be greatly owing to the use of salted provisions; but experience has shown that a restriction to vegetable diet will produce the same disorder. It is probable, therefore, that the affection, in the case alluded to, was rather owing to restriction to one kind of diet, than to the salt. Dr. Paris, (*Op. cit.* p. 197) suggests, that in appreciating the effects of salted meat as food, it is necessary to bear in mind a chemical fact, which has not hitherto attracted the attention its importance merits. "The salt," he remarks, "thus combined with the animal fibre, ought no longer to be considered as the condiment upon which so much has been said; a chemical combination has taken place, and although it is difficult to explain the nature of the affinities which have been brought into action, or that of the compound to which they have given origin, it is sufficiently evident that the texture of the fibre is so changed as to be less nutritive, as well as less digestible. If we are called upon to produce any chemical evidence in support of such an assertion, we need only relate the experiment of M. Eller, who found, that if salt and water be boiled in a copper vessel, the solution will contain a notable quantity of that metal; whereas, if, instead of heating a simple solution, the salt be previously mixed with beef, bacon or fish, the fluid resulting from it will not contain an atom of copper." " Does not this," he asks, " prove, that the process of salting meat is something more than the mere saturation of the animal fibre with muriate of soda ?"

Certain fish, when salted—as the *anchovy*, *cod*, *haddock*, *herring*, &c.—are used as relishes in the way of condiments. They are stimulating; but the combination of the flesh and salt is very indigestible, and unfit for the dyspeptic.

*Vinegar*, in moderation, is a wholesome condiment, and the extent to which it is employed shows it to be agreeable. Alone, or in the form of *pickles*, it is, in moderation, a useful stimulant to the digestive function. It has been already observed, that free acetic acid is always found in the gastric secretions, and that the solvent property of those secretions is partly owing to this acid. An additional quantity, artificially added, may consequently be occasionally of service. When taken with vegetable substances, it in some degree obviates their tendency to fermentation; and it is said by some writers—by Dr. Paris for example—that fatty and gelatinous substances frequently seem to be rendered more digestible in the stomach by the addition of vinegar; although, he remarks, " it is difficult to offer either a chemical or physiological explanation of the fact." The " fact"—with regard to the fatty substance at least—is, in our opinion, more than doubtful. We have already said that oils undergo very little change in the stomach; nor do they experience any alteration in dilute acetic acid out of that organ.

On fibrin, as we have seen, (page 218) vinegar has a decided action.

When vinegar, or any of the vegetable acids, is taken to excess, it ultimately interferes with the assimilative function, and emaciation is the consequence. " Vinegar," says Dr. Beddoes, " taken frequently, and freely, we know to be destructive to the stomach. When slenderness of waist was particularly in request, many women totally ruined the digestive faculty by vinegar." It is accordingly employed to reduce *embonpoint*.

Verjuice, (*omphacium*,) lemon-juice, capers, &c. are used with the same views as vinegar.

The *aromatic condiments* are very numerous, and may be divided into those that are *tropical* or *exotic*, and those that are *indigenous*. To the former division belong *cinnamon, ginger, cloves*, the different kinds of *pepper, nutmeg, mace* and *pimento* :—to the latter, *lemon* and *orange peel, citron, cumin, aniseed, caraway, coriander, fennel, bay leaves, thyme, sage, mustard, horse-radish, garlic, onion, leek, shallot*, &c. It has been argued by many, that the exotic aromatics, which are mostly stimulant in a high degree, were not intended by nature for the inhabitants of temperate climes. Londe, indeed, affirms, that they ought to be left to the natives of Bengal and India, enervated by their climates; and he asks, with much *naïveté* " why nature has made the allspice grow in both the Indies, if it ought to be eaten in France?" To the question, of what it is natural for us to eat, and what to avoid, reference has already been made. The Creator of the Universe has endowed man with capabilities of converting most of the products of the animal and vegetable kingdom to his sustenance; and it is doubtless as *natural* for him to eat that, which has been furnished by his ingenuity, as that which is presented to him in the state of nature. Otherwise, the culinary art, the great object of which is to make that palatable, digestible and more nutritious, which is deficient in these properties, ought to be abjured. The propriety of this deduction must, indeed, strike every judicious observer, and accordingly Dr. Paris, (*Op. citat.* p. 314) after having made the trite remark, that the exotic spices " were not intended by nature for the inhabitants of temperate climes; they are heating and highly stimulant," expresses his doubts of the validity of the objection to the extent to which it is argued. " I am, however," he remarks, " not anxious to give more weight to this objection than it deserves. Man is no longer the child of nature, nor the passive inhabitant of any particular region; he ranges over every part of the globe, and elicits nourishment from the productions of every climate. It may be, therefore, necessary, that he should accompany the ingestion of foreign aliments with foreign condiment. If we go to the east for tea, there is no reason we should not go to the west for sugar."

The habitual use of such strong stimulants is, doubtless, to be avoided in temperate climes, but their occasional and moderate employment,—especially where the basis of the dish is somewhat difficult of digestion,—is not only harmless to the healthy, and to the dyspeptic, but beneficial. Variety of diet is absolutely necessary for plenary health ; and the digestive function is improved by the occasional ingestion of substances, that excite the stomach within due bounds. We have no doubt, indeed, that if an individual were to accustom himself to the same mild diet for weeks and months together, the digestive function would become gradually enfeebled ;—the same effect being produced upon the stomach, as would be produced on the mental and corporeal powers, by a climate universally the same, that is—devoid of daily vicissitudes and the succession of the seasons, which seem to be wisely bestowed, in order, that animal and vegetable existence may not droop into insignificance.

In India, owing to the heat of the climate, animal food of the grosser kind is not abundantly eaten, whilst rice—a vegetable, possessed of but little stimulating power—forms a chief aliment. The effect of the torrid climate itself is to enervate the whole system, and the digestive functions in particular, and hence the inhabitants fly to hot spices for the temporary stimulation they induce. It is surprising to an inhabitant of the temperate regions of the globe to see the quantities of the hottest spices, that are habitually taken by the Indo-European. Yet such constant over-stimulation of the organ cannot fail to induce debility; and it is this abuse, that we have to guard against, in the employment of aromatic condiments in temperate climes. Their moderate use can be productive of no inconvenience. Yet they are objected to by certain writers on dietetics; who, as Dr. Kitchener has correctly observed, " have merely laid before the public a nonsensical register of the peculiarities of their own palate, and the idiosyncracies of their own constitution." How else can be explained the list of proscriptions in the following doggrel, cited by that writer ?

> " Salt, pepper, and mustard, and vinegar too,
> Are quite as unwholesome as curry, I vow ;
> All lovers of goose, duck, or pig, I'll engage,
> That eat it with onion, salt, pepper, or sage,
> Will find ill effects from't, and therefore no doubt
> Their prudence should tell them—best eat it without.
> But, alas ! these are subjects on which there's no reas'ning,
> For you'll still eat your goose, duck, or pig, with its seas'ning:
> And what is far worse, notwithstanding my puffing,
> You'll make for your hare and your veal a good stuffing ;
> And I fear if a leg of good mutton you boil,
> With sauce of vile capers that mutton you'll spoil ;

> And though as you think, to procure good digestion,
> A mouthful of cheese is the best thing in question;
> 'In Gath do not tell, nor in Askalon blab it,'
> You're strictly forbidden to eat a Welsh rabbit;
> And bread, ' the main staff of our life,' some will call
> No more nor no less than the ' worst thing of all.' "

The veteran author on hygiène—Sir John Sinclair (*Lancet*, Jan. 25, 1834, p. 660,)—at the age of eighty, has strongly recommended *white mustard seed* for the preservation of the health of old people especially. To persons, under sixty, he advises a table-spoonful to be taken at dinner with broth or soup. When swallowed whole, in this quantity, he says it greatly promotes the expulsion of the fæces, but occasionally requires the assistance of an aperient pill at night. When age advances, and health decays, he advises another spoonful of the seed to be taken at breakfast with a little tea or coffee; and he adds;—" to the adoption of this system, thus increasing the quantity as age advances, from one to two table-spoonsful per day, I attribute the excellent health I have enjoyed for such a number of years."

*Butter*, and *oil* constitute the whole of the " oily " class of condiments. Of their nutritive and digestible properties enough has been said already. The former, when not previously exposed to heat, is much more easy of assimilation, than when rendered empyreumatic. *Hot buttered toast* is, consequently, objectionable for the dyspeptic; and melted butter in any form, ought to be carefully avoided. *Oil*, we have seen, when added to salads, although of itself difficult of digestion, diminishes the objections that apply to vegetables eaten in this form. Of the *champignons* and *truffles* enough has been said already.

By far the most important modifications are produced on aliments by the CULINARY PROCESSES to which they are subjected. But few articles of diet are employed in the raw state. Almost all require some preparation to render them more agreeable, more nutritious, or to improve their digestibility.

It would be a curious matter of investigation to trace how far the art of cookery, and the varying extravagance of the table, might be esteemed indicative of the comparative degree of advancement or prosperity of any individual nation, at different periods of its history; but it would lead us away too much from our present object.

In ancient Rome, when she was mistress of the world, and, therefore during the time of her prosperity, and her extravagance, the cook was regarded with unusual honour. The Sicilian cooks were esteemed before all others,—the expression *Siculæ dapes* being a proverbial phrase for a table furnished profusely, and luxuriously. In the time of the first Roman Emperors, enormous salaries were given to the cooks,—upwards of 4,000 dollars being by no means uncommon. Mark Anthony once presented his cook with a whole corporate town or *municipium*, solely because he succeeded in dressing a pudding to the satisfaction of Cleopatra; an example, which the 8th Harry of England—himself of gastronomic celebrity—was not ashamed to imitate,—by parcelling out one of the Crown Manors, as a reward to a lady, who had compounded a pudding to his taste. In modern times, the cook is liberally rewarded for his services. The principal cook, at one of the most celebrated club-houses in London, is stated to have had at one time, a salary of 1500*l*. per annum. "Many cooks in the families of our aristocracy," says a recent English writer, (Truman, *On Food*, p. 107, Lond. 1842,) "have 300*l*. per annum, exclusive of perquisites."

The extravagance of the Roman gourmands almost exceeds the bounds of credibility. According to Nicolaus Peripateticus, Lucullus was the first introducer of this kind of luxury amongst the Romans, and the ordinary expense of his suppers in the Hall of Apollo, was 50,000 drachmæ,—upwards of $7,100. Heliogabalus is said to have given a supper that cost upwards of $107,600; and Caligula one that amounted to the enormous sum of $358,700. The refinements of gourmandise, that occasioned this sottish expenditure can never be rivalled, because the world can never be placed under similar circumstances.

Dr. Paris has made the singular assertion, that "if we inquire into the culinary history of different countries, we shall trace its connexion with the fuel most accessible to them." "This fact," he adds, "readily explains the prevalence of the peculiar species of cookery, which distinguishes the French table, and which has no reference, as some have imagined, to the dietetic theory, or superior refinement of the inhabitants." This idea has been hazarded without due reflection. No two systems of cookery differ more than those of France, and many parts of this country, although the same kind of fuel is equally accessible in both; but the French make a greater use of charcoal, and this may have had some effect in inducing them to discard the larger joints. The truth is, that the essential difference between the modes of cookery, adopted in different countries, is not so much in the boiled, and the roast; in the joint, or the made dish, as it is in the quantity of grease employed, and in the greater or less use of condiments and sauces; and this, like many differences in manners, appears to have had its origin in custom, but how occasioned in the first instance is, at this day, beyond our knowledge.

In our culinary processes, heat is applied either by radiation, or by conduction, so that considerable difference exists in the results. Roasting and broiling are effected in the former way; boiling, baking, and frying in the latter. In roasting, the effects are caused entirely by the rays of heat impinging directly upon the substance, placed at a short distance before the fire; whilst in broiling, the substance is put over the fire, by suspending it in the stream of heated air ascending from the fuel, or by laying it directly on the burning fuel, or on iron bars—as in the common gridiron. In boiling, the caloric is applied through the medium of water, or steam; and in baking, and frying, through the metallic vessel, which is placed immediately over the fire, or through some oily substance in addition,—as in the operation of frying more particularly.

In these various processes, the different organized textures submitted to them are chemically and mechanically modified, as follows:—By *roasting* animal substances, the fibrin is corrugated; the albumen coagulated; the fat melted, and a portion of the water evaporated. The surface becomes brown, and then scorched; and the tendinous parts are rendered softer and gluey. Animal matter loses more by roasting than by boiling;—parting with about one third of its weight; but the greater portion of the nutritive matter is preserved in the gravy. The loss arises from the melting out of the fat, and the evaporation of the water; but the main nutritious portions remain in the meat, whilst in boiling the gelatin is in part removed. Roast meats are hence more nutritive than boiled. It has been computed,—of course only approximately,—that owing to the dissipation of the nutritive juices by boiling, one pound of roast contains as much nourishment as two of boiled meat.

By *broiling*, the surface of the meat is rendered brown, and hard, and thus the evaporation of the juices is prevented, so that a peculiar tenderness, and juiciness is imparted to it. It is the form selected as the most eligible by those, who seek to invigorate themselves by the art of *training*.

By *boiling*, the principles, that are not properly soluble are rendered softer, and more readily acted upon in the stomach. The meat is, however, deprived of most of those principles, that are soluble in hot water; the albumen is coagulated by the heat; and the gelatin, which is not dissolved in the water, is converted into a gelatinous substance. If, therefore, the meat be too long, or too fast boiled, we obtain, where the albumen predominates—as in beef—a hard mass, like an over-boiled egg; or where the gelatin predominates, as in young meats—such as veal—a gelatinous substance, equally difficult of management by the digestive function. The loss, occasioned by boiling, depends partly upon the melting of the fat, but chiefly on the solution of the gelatin and osmazome, which are contained in the soup. Mutton is affirmed to lose about one-fifth; and beef, about one-fourth of its original weight by this process.

*Baking* consists in heating the substance in a confined space, which does not permit the escape of the fumes arising from it: the meat is, therefore, owing to the retention of its juices, more sapid and tender. Baked meats are not, however, so digestible, on account of the greater retention of their oils, which are besides, in an empyreumatic state. In this process, as well as in stewing, the temperature does not exceed $212°$; and therefore the heat is not sufficient to produce browning, or decomposition.

Lastly, *frying* is the most objectionable process of all ;—the heat being generally applied through the medium of boiling oil, or fat, which is thus rendered empyreumatic, and therefore extremely liable to disagree with the stomach.

In all these ways, the meat loses the peculiar nauseous smell and taste, which it possesses when in the raw state, and becomes savory, and grateful to the palate.

Allusion has been made to the loss that takes place in *anima substances*, consequent on the application of heat. This will, of course, be somewhat dependent on the joint, and on the degree of cookery employed. Dr. Roget states, that he has been informed by persons, who salt rounds of beef to sell by retail, after they have been boiled, that they are able to get nineteen pounds of cold boiled beef from twenty-five pounds of raw: but the meat is always rather underdone. The loss, in these cases, by boiling was six in the twenty-five, or about one-fourth. Messrs. Donkin and Gamble boiled in steam fifty-six pounds of captain's salt beef: the meat, when cold, without the bones—which amounted to five pounds six ounces—weighed only thirty-five pounds. In another experiment, one hundred and thirteen pounds of prime mess beef gave nine pounds ten ounces of bones, and forty-seven pounds eight ounces of meat;—and in a third, two hundred and thirteen pounds of mess beef gave thirteen pounds eight ounces of bones, and one hundred and three pounds ten ounces of meat; or, taken in the aggregate, three hundred and seventy-two pounds of salt beef, including bones, furnish, when boiled, one hundred and eighty-six pounds two ounces without bone, being fifty per cent.; or—disregarding the bone altogether—salt meat loses by boiling 44.2 per cwt.

Professor Wallace, of Edinburgh, from a series of very accurate experiments, in a public establishment, deduced the following results:—that in pieces of ten pounds weight, each 100 pounds of beef lost, on an average, by boiling, 26.4; by baking, 30.2; and by roasting, 32.2. Of mutton, the leg lost by boiling, 21.4; the shoulder, by roasting, 31.1; the neck, 32.4; and the loin, 35.9. Hence, it is inferred, that—generally speaking—mutton loses, by boiling, about one-fifth of its original weight, and beef about one-fourth; and that mutton and beef lose, by roasting, about one-third.

*Vegetables* are most commonly boiled or baked; or, if apparently fried or roasted, there is always water present, which prevents the direct action of the fire from penetrating far below the surface. The effect of cookery upon vegetables is to dissolve in the water some of their constituents—such as the mucilage and starch; and to render those, that are not soluble—as the gluten and fibre—softer and more pulpy.

The succulent vegetables, such as cabbage, spinach, &c. should be well boiled; otherwise, they are very difficult of digestion; but with some vegetables, as the potato, the process may be carried too far. A potato, when well boiled, should retain its shape but yet be easily separable. It is overboiled, when, instead of the parts being soft and gelatinous, they are in the form of a dry, insipid powder.

Another effect of heat on certain vegetables is to drive off volatile matters, in which acrimony at times resides in the raw state to such an extent as to render them disagreeable, if not deleterious. The various species of *arum*, for example, when crude, are acrid, and even poisonous; but on being cooked they become mild and wholesome;—the acrimony being resident in a very volatile principle, which is easily dissipated by heat. The onion tribe have their acrimony entirely destroyed by long exposure to heat.

*Fruits* are roasted, baked or stewed, and are thus rendered an agreeable and wholesome aliment, when objections might be urged against them in their raw state. Roasted apples afford a pleasant repast to the sick, and convalescent; and, from their laxative properties, are well adapted for certain dyspeptic cases. Fruit pies are generally wholesome, if the crust be rejected; but if sugar be added, as it generally is in these cases, as well as in dried fruits, the condiment may render that improper which would not have been so, if taken alone.

Another great object of cookery is the addition of *sauces*, which add to the nutritive properties of aliments, or render them more pleasing to the palate. The bases of these are oily or fatty substances, with the juices of the meats themselves, to which different seasonings are added. It is in this department, that the chief art of cookery lies, and that the French excel so greatly all other nations.

Many idle discussions have been indulged regarding the propriety of employing sauces; but in moderation there can be no doubt of their advantage. It has been said, that they induce us to eat more than is necessary; but this abuse ought not to prevent us from making aliments agreeable to the palate, by any addition which does not materially detract from their digestibility. Many of the seasoned sauces, indeed, improve the digestibility of aliments, as has been remarked under the head of condiments. Plutarch affirms, that the ancients knew only two sauces,*—*hunger* and *salt,* and he objects to the use of sauces and seasonings, avouching them to be needless to healthy persons because they never eat but when they are hungry; and unprofitable to the sick, because they ought not to be made hungry, for fear they should eat too much.

There seems, however, to be no reason why the infirm stomachs of invalids should not be allowed some indulgence. "Like other bad instruments," as Dr. Kitchener says, (*Directions for invigorating and prolonging life.*—American edit. p. 176,) "they often want oiling, and screwing, and winding up, and adjusting with the utmost care, to keep them in tolerable order. Although a savory sauce may not be nutritious *per se,* still it is relatively nutritive, as its agreeable flavour promotes the taking of nutritive things, and ensures that diligent attention of the teeth to them, which is the grand foundation of good digestion."

---

\* The word "*sauce*" is, by a common interchange of letters, derived from *salsus,* "salted."

## SECTION V.

Of drinks—physiology of thirst—digestion of liquids—effects of drinking on the digestive function—cold drinks—hot drinks—water; its nutritive properties; different kinds—mode of rendering potable—juices and infusions of animal and vegetable substances; raspberry and strawberry vinegar—lemonade—toast-water—barley and rice water—gruel—tea—coffee; chocolate—cocoa—whey, soda water.

Thus far we have considered the solid food of man. He requires, however, drinks more imperiously even than solids; in consequence of the constant drain of fluid from the system by the various secretions,—the pulmonary, and cutaneous transpiration, the urine, &c.; and of the large proportion, which the fluids, that compose the animal body, bear to the solids.

The necessity for the ingestion of fluids is indicated by thirst, an internal sensation, in its essence resembling hunger, although not referred to precisely the same organs. The desire, however, can be much modified by habit. Whilst some persons require several gallons a day to satisfy their wants; others, who, by resistance, have acquired the habit of using very little liquid, enjoy good health, and do not experience the slightest inconvenience from its privation. This privation, it is obvious, cannot be absolute, or pushed beyond a certain extent. There must always be fluid enough taken to administer to the necessities of the system.

That the sensation of thirst is greatly dependent upon the quantity of fluid circulating in the vessels is shown by the fact, mentioned by Dupuytren, that he succeeded in allaying the thirst of animals, by injecting milk, whey, water, and other fluids into the veins; and Orfila states, that in his toxicological experiments, he frequently allayed, in this way, the excessive thirst of animals, to which he had administered poison, and which were incapable of drinking, owing to the œsophagus having been tied. He found, also, that the blood of animals was more and more deprived of its watery portions, as the abstinence from liquids was more prolonged.

The digestion of liquids differs from that of solids, and the changes, which they experience in the stomach and intestines vary. Some undergo conversion into chyme and chyle; others not. To the latter class belong—water, weak alcoholic fluids, the vegetable acids, &c. Water experiences admixture with the gastric secretions, becomes turbid, and gradually disappears, without undergoing any transformation; part passes into the small intestine; the rest is absorbed directly from the stomach. When any strong alcoholic fluid is taken, the effect is different. Its stimulation causes the stomach to contract, and augments the secretion from the mucous membrane; whilst, at the same time, it coagulates all the albuminous and mucous portions; mixes with the watery part of the mucous and salivary fluids, and rapidly disappears by absorption. The substances, that have been coagulated by the action of alcohol, are afterwards digested like solid food. We can thus understand the good effects of a small quantity of alcohol, taken after certain substances difficult of digestion,—a custom, which has existed from high antiquity, and has physiology in its favour.

Of the liquids, that are capable of being converted into chyme, or chyle, some are so altogether; others in part only. Oil remains longer in the stomach than any other liquid, but it is probably wholly converted into chyle. Milk, as we have seen, coagulates in the stomach, soon after it is received into that organ, after which the clot is digested, and the whey absorbed; so that the coagulation of milk, within certain limits, is a healthy process; yet how often are we not consulted by mothers under great alarm, because an infant has regurgitated the milk in a state of coagulation.

Where the liquid—aqueous or spirituous—holds in suspension the immediate principles of animals or vegetables—as gelatin, albumen, osmazome, sugar, gum, fecula, colouring matter, &c.—a separation takes place in the stomach, between the water, or alcohol, and the substances combined with it. The latter remain in the stomach, and undergo digestion; whilst the aqueous, or spirituous portions are absorbed. The salts united with these fluids, are taken up along with them. In soup, for example, the water and the salts are absorbed, and the gelatin, albumen, fat, and osmazome are digested. Red wine first becomes turbid by admixture with juices formed in, or carried into, the stomach. The albumen of these fluids speedily experiences coagulation, and becomes flocculent; and subsequently, its colouring matter,—entangled, perhaps, with the mucus and albumen,—is deposited on the mucous membrane of the stomach. The aqueous, and alcoholic portions soon disappear.

Liquids reach the small intestine in two forms;—in the state of chyme; and in their unaltered condition. In the former case, they are affected like the chyme obtained from solid food. In the latter case, they experience no essential change, being simply united with the fluids poured into the small intestine—the mucous secretions, the bile, and the pancreatic juice. Their absorption goes on as they proceed; so that very little, if any, attains the large intestine.

It is of importance to bear in mind the different modes in which fluids enter the circulatory system. Those that are converted into chyle are taken up by the chyliferous vessels, which form them into chyle at the moment of their absorption; such as possess the necessary tenuity soak through the coats of the blood-vessels, or pass in by imbibition or *endosmose*. Water—the chief constituent of all drinks—is an essential component of every circulating fluid. We have no evidence, that any action of elaboration takes place on it, whilst experiments have shown that it penetrates most, if not all, animal tissues better than any other fluid whatever; and consequently, passes through them to mix with any of its own solutions. It is probably in this way,—that is by imbibition,—that all venous absorptions are effected; and hence we account for the rapid disappearance of drinks, especially in hot climates, and seasons when the watery portions of the blood have been largely exhaled by transpiration.

The fact of the various tenuous fluids passing into the venous system of the stomach by imbibition explains to us the mode, in which habitual indulgence in spirituous liquors may produce inflammation, and induration of the liver. As the veins of the stomach and small intestines go to form the vena porta; and this vein ramifies like an artery in the substance of the liver, the alcohol must be present in the capillary system throughout that organ, and cannot fail to over-excite those vessels, so as to induce inflammatory irritation, —one of the terminations of which is known to be the deposition of coagulable lymph, followed by induration. This induration interferes with the due circulation of blood through the viscus, and the consequence is the transudation of the more watery parts of that fluid through the coats of the obstructed vessels. Hence ascites so often accompanies induration of the liver in hard drinkers; and it need hardly be added, that dropsy, thus induced may be regarded as generally incurable.

Independently of the appetite for drinks produced by the wants of the system, it arises from conditions of the lining membrane of the stomach, and bowels, occasioned by other causes. A dry, clammy state of the mouth is induced, for example, by certain articles of diet, particularly of the saline kind, or by febrile irritation existing originally in the mucous membrane of the mouth, or produced secondarily by disease elsewhere.

Where the salivary, and other secretions are too sparing to communicate to solid food the due digestive texture, the ingestion of liquids favours the gastric operations; but if they be taken too freely during a meal, the texture is rendered too soft, and the gastric secretions are so much diluted that digestion is more difficult. From this we may infer, that fluids should be taken in moderation; and that an error in quantity, at either extremity of the scale, should be avoided. The desire experienced is the best guide, unless a morbid habit has been induced, and this guide the invalid should follow, without being biassed by the theoretical recommendations of those, who consider that liquids should always be taken during meals, or of those that think they should be universally discarded.

The custom is, in many places, to hand round lemonade, wine, toddy, punch, &c. before dinner; but the valetudinarian had better avoid them. With many dyspeptics these liquids excite immediately an increased secretion of the gastric acids, and heart-burn; and, before the individual sits down to his repast, the stomach is in a very unfit state for the reception of the various articles, that are sent into it at a fashionable dinner party. During fasting, there is no gastric juice in the stomach. It is not secreted until food is present in the organ, or until the desire for food has been experienced for some time, and it will be evident, that admixture with these drinks cannot render it better adapted for the duties it has to accomplish. Perhaps, in all cases, the evil arising from this practice is greater during cold than hot seasons. The perpetual drain of fluids, that takes place from the vessels, during our very hot summers, occasions imbibition through the vessels of the stomach to be so rapid, that before we sit down to dinner, there may be very little fluid remaining in that organ. Every dyspeptic, too, must have felt, that drinking copiously of any fluid, soon after dinner, and whilst digestion is actively going on, has interfered with the process, for reasons similar to those already mentioned; but between the meals of solid food fluid may be taken with much propriety.

It is somewhat amusing to an inhabitant of the warmer regions of this continent to observe the cautions of European dietetical writers, regarding the use of iced drinks, which are so extensively employed here, and almost universally with thorough impunity. It is remarked by one of the most respectable of those writers, that "persons disposed to dyspepsia, frequently require fluids to be raised to the temperature of the body:" "for the stomach," it is said, "not having sufficient vital energy to establish the reaction which the sudden impression of cold produces in a healthy condition, falls into a state of collapse, and is consequently unable to proceed in the performance of its requisite duties," and the remark is said to "apply particularly to the residents of hot climates." This can rarely, however, happen. The Author resided for nine years in a country situation, where, during the summer season, every one—from the infant on its first legs to the aged individual—used ice, whenever he was disposed, during the summer, and yet he does not recollect a solitary instance of the kind of collapse alluded to. Occasionally, a person may be met with, who experiences gastrodynia after its employment, but the cases are exceedingly rare. Iced drinks have this very important advantage, that, however thirsty a person may be, he cannot load the stomach so much as by the use of spring water at the ordinary temperature; and there is great reason for the belief, that the injurious effects of cold fluids, taken during the summer season, are more dependent upon the quantity than upon the temperature. Some years ago, it was very common, in Virginia, for the labourers in the harvest field to be killed by drinking copiously of spring water, whilst overheated; and in our cities the deaths, from this cause, are annually numerous; but, since the custom has prevailed in Virginia of supplying the labourers liberally with ice, cases of death are very unfrequent. When a fatal event occurs from drinking water at the ordinary temperature, the quantity taken is so great as to distend the stomach, and apparently death is partly produced by the sudden impression made upon the pneumogastric nerves distributed to that organ, or upon the ganglionic nerves, in a manner somewhat analogous perhaps to the cases of sudden death, produced by slight blows on the epigastric region, of which so many examples are on record.

Hot liquors, when received into the stomach, stimulate the exhalants of the lining membrane to increased secretion, whilst they augment the action of the muscular coat. In this way, a drink of very hot water may aid digestion, when food, difficult of digestion, has been taken, or when the powers of the stomach are enfeebled; but its habitual use cannot fail, like that of other stimulants, to be followed by a corresponding degree of debility.

The fact of pain in the teeth following the ingestion of cold or hot water, when these organs are tender or carious, has led to the belief, that such temperatures are unfavourable to the teeth. This, however, is more than doubtful. It is not easy to explain why teeth become carious. When they are removed from the body, they require powerful chemical agents to destroy them, and, in this respect, they are probably similarly circumstanced when in the body. Various causes of an extraneous character have, notwithstanding, been assigned. (See the Author's *Practice of Medicine*, 2nd edit. i. 44, Philad. 1844.) But there is great reason for the belief, that extraneous agents have little effect in the production of caries; and that the decay commences beneath the enamel; for this hard envelope of the teeth may be broken away so as to expose the bony part, and unless the fracture extends to the cavity of the tooth, there will be no tooth-ache, and, if there be no internal disposition to caries, the tooth may remain sound for life. These deductions are corroborated by the well known fact, that persons of unhealthy habit, and of particular districts, are infinitely more liable to dental caries than others. There are parts of southern France, and the remark is applicable to portions of every country, where it is extremely rare to see a good set of teeth.

If the teeth are decayed internally, and yet there is no caries visible externally, hot or cold fluids, taken into the mouth, may excite much pain in them; in the same manner as they do, when the teeth have been filed so much, that but a thin shell of bone protects the dental cavity; but in no other way probably do they affect these organs.

WATER.—In discussing the various properties of different liquids, the arguments, regarding the "natural," have been extended to them, and it has been contended, that water is the most natural drink, and that all others, which are the products of art, ought to be avoided. The remarks already made, regarding the most natural food of man, are equally appropriate here. Water is doubtless sufficient for all the purposes of man, provided it possesses the proper qualities. So is a very limited range of animal or vegetable food, but this is no reason why he should not have recourse to variety. The question, whether there ever was a time when man confined himself to the simple banquet, provided for him by the bounteous hand of nature—"his food the fruits, his drink the crystal well"—and whether it be not his duty to recur to it was at one time much agitated, and was not worthy of being revived.

Allusion has already been made (page 184) to the question, whether water be indispensable to animals; and, in favour of the negative view, it has been affirmed, that the rabbit, and the sheep can live a long time, if not altogether, without this fluid. There would seem, however, to be some deception here as their vegetable food is succulent, and therefore consists largely of water. Redi—the Italian naturalist—instituted a series of experiments to ascertain how long animals can live without food. Of a number of capons, which he kept without either solid or liquid food, not one survived the ninth day; but one, to which he allowed water, did not die until the twentieth day. Pouteau allowed some of his patients nothing but water for several weeks, without their falling off materially, and the histories of shipwrecked mariners demonstrate with what little food man can subsist, provided he has a sufficient allowance of water; whilst, without water, or a substitute, no quantity of solid food can support him beyond a few days.

Much stress is generally laid, in estimating the salubrity of places, on the qualities of the water with which it is supplied; although it is probable, that this exerts but a limited agency. It was at one time supposed, that the inhabitants of countries situate at the foot of lofty mountains are particularly liable to diseases of the glandular system—especially of the thyroid gland, constituting *goïtre* or bronchocele; and that these diseases are occasioned by drinking the snow water, perpetually descending from the icy summits; but the knowledge of the fact, that the same diseases prevail at the base of lofty mountains, whose tops are never clad with snow, dispelled the illusion. We frequently observe persons, who have been accustomed to drink water, that has percolated through a free stone formation, affected with bowel complaints when they visit a region of lime-stone formation,—and conversely; but the effect is usually temporary; and it is probable, that the presence of foreign matters, unless they are to such an extent as to constitute mineral waters, has no permanent influence on human health. Dr. Paris says, that hard water—that is, water containing sulphate of lime—" has certainly a tendency to produce disease in the spleen of certain animals, especially in sheep," and that this is the case on the eastern side of the island of Minorca, as we are informed by Cleghorn. The difficulties in proving that such disease is owing to any impregnation in the water are obvious. The affection is probably endemic; and, like most endemic diseases, in its origin inscrutable. The same may be said of the elephantiasis, endemial in Egypt, and which was, of old, ascribed to the impure water of the Nile. The qualities of water, as met with under ordinary circumstances, are well compared by Celsus. " Aqua levissima pluvialis est; deinde fontana; tum ex flumine; tum ex puteo; post hæc ex nive, aut glacie; gravior his ex lacû: gravissima ex palude."

*Rain Water*, when collected at a distance from houses or other elevated objects, is the purest natural water, and has the least specific gravity: but, when collected in large towns, it contains impurities, carried down from the smoky atmosphere, or washed from the roofs of houses. The bodies, which it usually holds in solution, are carbonic acid, and minute traces of the carbonate of lime and of chloride of calcium. Carbonate of ammonia is another ingredient; it is derived from the putrefaction of nitrogenized substances, and it is owing to its presence, that rain water has a softer feel than distilled water. According to Liebig (*Organic Chemistry, in its Application to Agriculture and Philosophy*, Lond. 1842,) atmospheric ammonia furnishes the nitrogen of plants. It is rarely used for drinking, as it possesses much of the mawkish quality of distilled water; for which, indeed, it is used as a substitute.

*Spring Water*, in addition to the substances detected in rain water, generally contains more or less sulphate of lime. When this is to such an extent as to curdle soap, the water is said to be *hard;* if not, *soft*. It differs, of course, according to the formation through which it passes. Soft water is superior to hard for domestic, and medicinal purposes, dissolving vegetable matters more readily, and not endangering the decomposition of mineral substances to any extent. The taste of persons differs much in respect to spring water; some preferring the hard; others the soft. Animals perhaps universally choose the soft; and horses appear to like it as well when muddy as when clear. President Jefferson, indeed, expressed to the Author the opinion, from his own observations, that they preferred it.

*River Water* is derived from the conflux of numerous springs and rain water. It is generally pretty pure; and is the variety with which most large towns are principally supplied. In its course, it loses some of the air, which gives to spring water its taste, and is consequently more vapid. The water of some of the rivers, that supply large towns, is remarkably turbid, and into it all the filth is discharged. The Thames water is so full of animal and vegetable matters, that it requires to stand for some time before it deposites them; and it is scarcely potable on long voyages, until it has undergone the kind of self-purification, mentioned under another head. At one time, the English metropolis was almost wholly supplied with this impure water of the Thames, but the large water works at London Bridge have been discontinued, and the water is now obtained from other sources. It is a common remark, that the excellence of the London porter is dependent upon its being made from the water of the Thames; but it seems that it is never used for this purpose. To brew porter to perfection, it must be made in large quantities, and this appears to be the great secret of the signal success of the extensive breweries of London.

*Well water* is essentially the same as spring water, but liable to impregnation, owing to the land springs filtering through the sides, and conveying impurities into it. This may be prevented, in very deep wells, by lining them with cast iron cylinders. The water, under such circumstances, contains no impregnation, except what it derives from the formations through which the main spring passes. Dr. Percival affirms, that bricks harden the softest water, and give it an aluminous impregnation. The old wells must, therefore, furnish much purer water than the more recent, as the soluble particles of the walls are gradually washed away. The briskness, and sapidity of this and other water is owing to the air, and carbonic acid mixed with it.

Allusion has been made to the fancied unwholesomeness of *snow water*. It resembles rain water—being in truth only frozen rain—and is equally salubrious. The same characters belong to the water from melted ice. It is thoroughly wholesome, and is drunk, during the summer season, wherever the climate will admit of its being collected, and preserved at a moderate expense. In this form, it is a luxury—almost a *necessary*—in the middle states of this country more particularly—where there is not a tavern on the road—on the eastern side of the Blue ridge—that does not furnish ice to the traveller in any abundance. When the sea-water freezes, the ice—it has been imagined—does not contain the salts. This, however, would seem to be erroneous. The product of the freezing of sea-water is an imperfect sort of ice, porous, incompact, and imperfectly diaphanous. It consists of spicular shoots, or thin flakes, which retain within their interstices the stronger brine. This saline ice never, therefore, yields pure water; yet if the strong brine contained within it be first suffered to drain off slowly, the loose mass that remains will melt into a brackish liquid, which in some cases may be deemed potable. (Professor Jameson, in *Narrative of Discovery and Adventure in the Polar Seas and Regions*, Amer. edit., p. 29. New York, 1831.)

*Lake water* is composed of rain, spring, and river water, and is likely to be impure from decayed animal and vegetable matter. A great deal, however, will depend upon the magnitude of the collection, and the degree of stagnation. Water, taken from stagnant ponds and ditches, is especially unwholesome;—the animal, and vegetable matters, contained in them, being—during the summer, and autumnal seasons, particularly—in a state of decomposition. In such a condition, it can scarcely fail to be unwholesome, and is said, by hygienic writers, to be productive of affections of the stomach and bowels. Dr. Paris affirms, that he has known endemic diarrhœa arise from such a circumstance; and similar testimony is afforded by others (Cheyne, in *Dublin Hospital Reports,* iii. 11.) Yet the water of the Thames, when inclosed in tanks, and undergoing the decomposition, which has been described before, is drunk by the numerous crews of the British men of war, without much, if any, effect upon their health; and Mr. Chadwick, as the result of his sanitary inquiries (*Report to her Majesty's Principal Secretary of State for the Home Department,* &c., p. 77, Lond. 1842,) infers, that water containing animal matter, " which is the most feared, appears to be less frequently injurious than that which is the clearest, namely, spring water,—from the latter being oftener impregnated with animal substances; but there are instances of ill health produced by both descriptions of water."

*Marsh water* is the most impure of all, as a general rule—being more stagnant than lake water, and, of course, more loaded with decomposing animal and vegetable matters.

In the conveyance of water, it is not unimportant to attend to the materials of which the pipes are made. Cast iron and wood are those generally employed, and with propriety, as they can communicate no deleterious properties to the water;—not so, when lead and copper are the vehicles. Many instances are on record of disease having been induced by particles of these metals dissolved in the water; a result still more likely to happen, if the water contain an unusual quantity of carbonic acid. Dr. Lambe, in his " Researches into the Properties of Spring Water," &c., mentions that the proprietor of a well ordered his plumber to make the lead of a pump of double the thickness of the metal usually employed on such occasions, to save the charge of repairs; because he had observed that the water was so " hard," as he termed it, that it corroded the lead very soon. Lead is known to be an active poison, and this destruction of the metal could not fail to communicate noxious properties to the water passing through it.

It would appear, that the greatest danger is to be apprehended from the purest waters, provided they contain—as by the by they always do—atmospheric air. It is owing to its saline impregnation, that water, kept in leaden cisterns, or flowing through leaden pipes, is so rarely injurious. The investigations of Dr.

Christison, (*Transactions of the Royal Society of Edinburgh*, vol. xv. pt. 2, p. 271,) led him to infer, that leaden pipes ought not to be used for conveying water, at least where the distance is considerable, without a careful examination of the water;—that the risk of a dangerous impregnation with lead is greatest—as before observed—from the purest waters;—that water which tarnishes polished lead, when left at rest upon it in a glass vessel for a few hours, cannot be safely transmitted through leaden pipes without certain precautions; and conversely, that it is probable, although not yet established, that if polished lead remain untarnished, or nearly so, for twenty-four hours in a glass of water, the water may be safely conducted through leaden pipes;—that water, which contains less than about $\frac{1}{8000}$th of salts in solution, cannot be safely conducted in leaden pipes without certain precautions; and that even this proportion will prove insufficient to prevent corrosion, unless a considerable part of the saline matter consists of carbonates and sulphates, especially of the former; and that so large a proportion as $\frac{1}{4000}$th, probably even a considerably larger proportion, will be insufficient if the salts, in solution, be in a great measure muriates;—and that when the water is judged to be of a kind, which is likely to attack leaden pipes, or when it actually flows through them impregnated with lead, a remedy may be found, either in leaving the pipes full of water and at rest for three or four months, or by substituting for the water a weak solution of phosphate of soda, in the proportion of about $\frac{1}{25000}$th part,—the object being to form, whilst the water is at rest, a fine film of mixed carbonate and phosphate of lead, which shall adhere so firmly as not to be swept away when the water is allowed to flow, and which will serve as a lining to prevent the contact of the running water with the metal. (Pereira, *Treatise on Food and Diet*, &c., Amer. edit. by Dr. C. A. Lee, p. 49. New York, 1843.)

Where water is foul, in consequence of gross mechanical impurities mixed with it, it may be filtered through an artificial bed of sand and gravel, as the purest waters naturally are. Filters are also made of porous stone, gravel, &c., which separate the animal, vegetable, and insoluble mineral substances suspended in it, and make it potable, when it would not otherwise be so. To render the water of marshes and ponds potable, it has been advised to boil them, under the idea that the boiling temperature will render the organic matters innoxious, and disengage the unwholesome gaseous principles, which they may contain. To improve them still farther, they may be agitated, so as to restore the air they have lost by boiling, and be then filtered through sand, or charcoal. It has been proposed to add to such water a small quantity of chlorine, or of one of the chlorides; but a quantity, sufficient to destroy the foulness of the fluid, can hardly fail to communicate a taste and smell, disagreeable to most individuals.

Another mode of preserving water from corruption, and of purifying it when corrupted, is by passing it through coarsely powdered charcoal;—forming one layer of the filter, for example, of charcoal, and the other of sand; sprinkling powdered charcoal into the water, until the evidences of decomposition are removed, and then filtering it. A plan, recommended by Lowitz to preserve water, is,—to be in the first place extremely attentive to the cleanness of the casks, rubbing them first with sand, and afterwards with powdered charcoal; then putting into each common sized cask, filled with water, about six or eight pounds of powdered charcoal, and a sufficient quantity of sulphuric acid to communicate to it a slight acidity, and stirring the charcoal from time to time, so as to mix it with the water. When about to be used, it must be filtered through a linen bag, containing a little powdered charcoal.

When the object is to purify water already corrupted, charcoal powder is gradually added until the offensive odour is no longer exhaled: a small quantity is then filtered through paper or linen, to see whether it passes clear; and if not, charcoal is added so long as it is turbid. When sulphuric acid is employed, it must be put into the cask, before using the charcoal, in sufficient quantity to communicate a slight degree of acidity, but if the water be intended for boiling vegetables, common salt may be substituted for the acid. All these operations, according to Lowitz, may be performed in five or six minutes. The charcoal may be used over and over again. It is only necessary to dry it, or—what is better—to expose it to considerable heat in close vessels, and to pulverize it anew. It considerably weakens the taste of the sulphuric acid, probably by deoxygenizing it, and reducing it to the state of sulphur. Two drops of the acid communicate to four ounces of water a marked taste of acidity, but this is almost entirely destroyed by the addition of the charcoal.

In the fine establishment of the *Quai des Célestins* in Paris, enormous quantities of river water are purified by so arranging the apparatus, that the fluid passes first through sponges, which deprive it of the coarse foreign substances, after which it is made to percolate through powdered charcoal; and, lastly,—to restore the air it has lost during filtration, it is made to fall, under the form of rain, from a height, into a large wooden reservoir, 14 or 15 feet broad. Berthollet recommended a similar plan for the preservation of fresh water on long voyages. This consisted in strongly charring the interior of the water casks before filling them, and the plan has been found by Kruzenstern and others to be successful. In the ships of war of some nations, however, the tanks are of iron, and, therefore, the charcoal cannot be employed in this shape. Powdered charcoal will have to be thrown into them. It is affirmed, indeed, that when the water, employed in the navy was carried there in casks, it became putrid and offensive owing to the vegetable admixture; and that the substitution of iron tanks for the casks has remedied the evil, so that the water can now be kept for any length of time, without becoming offensive either to the palate or the nose. The metal becomes oxidized, and the oxide of iron, thus formed, mixes with the water, but, by its weight and insolubility, it soon falls, at least for the most part, to the bottom; and should a small portion remain suspended, and be drunk, it can have no injurious effect, but may possibly prove beneficial. (Pereira, *edit. cit.* p. 234.)

A patent has been recently taken out by Professor Clarke, of Aberdeen, for the purification of water. It is said to consist in the addition of lime, which unites with the excess of carbonic acid in the water, and forms carbonate of lime: this precipitates along with the carbonate of lime held previously in solution in the water. The effect of the process is similar to that of boiling water; but, as remarked by Dr. Pereira, it has no effect on the sulphate of lime of common water, and, therefore, can have little or no influence in rendering hard water soft.

Whenever water is unusually contaminated it may be boiled, filtered, and agitated in the manner already described. There are many valetudinarians, and some whole nations—as the Chinese—

who never drink water that has not been boiled. The process is, however, unnecessary, unless under the circumstances referred to, or where the water appears to contain supercarbonate of lime, which is soluble. Long ebullition drives off the superabundant carbonic acid, and carbonate of lime, being insoluble, is deposited in the vessel.

Distillation frees fresh or salt water from all its impurities—organic and inorganic. Distilled water is, however, extremely vapid by reason of the privation of its air,—a deficiency, which may be supplied in the way already described. The fluid, obtained from the distillation of sea water, is said to be disagreeable, in consequence of some matters passing over in distillation, which render it brackish; but still, on voyages, where the supply of fresh water is consumed, it may form a useful succedaneum. As the hardness of water is dependent upon the sulphate of lime dissolved in it, filtration can have no effect upon it; but the addition of an alkaline carbonate—in the proportion of from ten to fifteen grains to every pint—twenty-four hours before it is used, will decompose not only it but all the earthy salts.

Another division of drinks comprises the JUICES AND INFUSIONS OF ANIMAL AND VEGETABLE SUBSTANCES.

There are many cooling drinks, made by adding sugar, or acidulous or mucilaginous syrups, to water. Emulsive drinks are also made from many of the kernels, especially from the almond. The qualities of these beverages are dependent upon those of the water, and the particular substance united with it. The saccharine solutions, as well as the acidulous—*raspberry* and *strawberry vinegar, lemonade,* &c.—are apt to induce heartburn and flatulence in those of feeble digestive powers.

*Toast water* is a beverage used by those who fancy—and there are such—that cold water disagrees with them. Dr. Kitchener, strangely asserts, in the teeth of daily experience, that " cold water, fresh drawn from a well, cannot be drunk without danger." Toast water is made by browning a crust of bread, or a biscuit, and immersing it in a jug of boiling water. By this process, it would appear to take up a small portion of gum and starch. Toasted oatcake, and toasted oatmeal, have been used for the same purpose. Dr. Kitchener affirms, that a roll of fresh, thin cut, lemon peel, or dried orange peel, infused with the bread, is a grateful addition, and that the whole forms a very refreshing summer drink. It is so generally employed in sickness, that it can scarcely be regarded as a common beverage for the healthy. The same may be said of *barley water* and *rice water*. The former is usually made from " pearl barley,"—that is, barley deprived of its cuticle, which contains an acrid resin. Pearl barley consists chiefly of fecula, with some mucilage, gluten and sugar, which water partly extracts by decoction. Barley or rice water speedily runs into the acetous fermentation, if left to itself, and is apt to disagree with one of weak digestive function. Its flavour is improved by the addition of lemon juice, lemon peel, and sugar candy.

*Gruel* is made from decorticated oats, to which the name *groats* is given. When these are boiled, they yield their starch to the water, and form a bland, and nutritious compound. The rules, given by Dr. Kitchener for the formation of gruel, are as follows: " Ask those who are to eat if they like it thick or thin; if the latter, mix well together by degrees, in a pint basin, one table-spoonful of oatmeal with three of cold water; if the former, two spoonsful. Have ready in the stewpan a pint of boiling water or milk. Pour this by degrees to the oatmeal you have mixed with the cold water: return it into the stewpan: set it on the fire; and let it boil for five minutes, stirring it all the time to prevent the oatmeal from burning at the bottom of the stewpan: skim and strain it through a hair sieve." To convert this into *caudle*, add a little ale, wine or brandy with sugar. This forms a celebrated diet for the parturient female in Great Britain.

Gruel may be made in the same manner from the meal of Indian corn: and to augment its nutrient properties, broth, or milk may be substituted for the water.

" Plain gruel, " says Kitchener, ( *Op. cit.* p. 204,) " is one of the best breakfasts and suppers that we can recommend to the rational epicure,—is the most comforting soother of an irritable stomach, and particularly acceptable to it after a hard day's work of intemperate feasting; when the addition of half an ounce of butter, and a teaspoonful of Epsom salt will give it an aperient quality, which will assist the principal viscera to get rid of their burden."

Perhaps these as well as the following liquid preparations scarcely ought to be classed under the head of drinks. They have been so, however, by writers on dietetics, and we cannot describe their properties more conveniently than in this place.

The word *tea* is now applied, in many cases, synonymously with infusion. Thus we say " beef tea, sage tea, balm tea," &c. The word was, however, originally restricted to the tea plant and afterwards to its infusion, and became gradually extended in its signification, in a way of which we have many examples in philology.

The tea plant is a native of China and Japan, and has been cultivated, and in general use, in those countries, from remote antiquity. It was unknown in Europe until the middle of the seventeenth century, when a small quantity was first imported by the Dutch; and, in 1664, the English East India Company imported two pounds and two ounces, as a present to the king. At this day, it has become an article of such commercial importance to China, as to employ more than 50,000 tons of shipping in its transportation from Canton. Yet so great is the home consumption, that, it is said, were Europeans and Americans to abandon the commerce altogether, the price would not be materially diminished in China.

There are two principal kinds of tea imported into this country, and Great Britain—the *black,* and the *green.* The *black* teas, beginning with the lowest qualities, are *bohea, congo, campo, souchong, pouchong* and *pekoe ;* the *green* teas are, *twankay, hyson skin, young hyson, hyson, imperial,* and *gunpowder*. In the year 1800, the annual consumption in England, according to the "*Encyclopædia Americana,*" was somewhat above 20,000,000 pounds; since which time it has been gradually declining, owing to increase of duty, and to the monopoly of the English East India Company. The consumption, about fifteen years ago, was estimated at about 25,000,000 pounds, which for a population of sixteen and a half millions, gives but one pound nine ounces per head, whilst in 1800 it was one pound thirteen and a half ounces. Owing, it would seem, to this monopoly, the prices of tea are higher; the qualities inferior, and the varieties fewer in England than on the continent of Europe, or in the United States. The following table drawn up about 1830, will enable us to form some idea of the proportionate quantity of tea, consumed at that time by various nations. The difference it will be observed is great. In this country, the consumption has remained nearly stationary for some years, whilst that of coffee has rapidly augmented.

|  |  | Pounds. |
|---|---|---|
| Russia (almost all black) | - - - | 5,563,444 |
| Holland | - . - - | 2,700,000 |
| France | - - - - - - | 230,000 |
| Importations into Hamburg | - - - | 1,500,000 to 2,000,000 |
| do " Venice and Trieste | - - | 700 |
| United States | - . - - | 6,000,000 to 8,000,000 |
| England, &c | - - . - - | 25,000,000 |

Nothing can be more discrepant than the views, that have been entertained regarding the properties of tea. Whilst some have esteemed it a poison,—although, they must admit, a slow one,—others have extolled it, not only as a valuable alimentary, but an excellent therapeutical agent. The plant consists of mucilage, extractive, resin, gallic and tannic acids; so that it is possessed of astringency, especially the green variety. In addition to this—with some constitutions particularly—it produces narcotic effects,—vigilance, restlessness, &c., although these symptoms are not frequently observed where its use is habitual, unless it is taken in too strong an infusion, or—in a more dilute state—in too great quantity.

In inquiring into the dietetic virtues of tea, it is important to recollect the ordinary additions. These are hot water, sugar, and milk. In this shape, it is unquestionably stimulant, and nutrient; but is apt to disagree with the dyspeptic, by reason of the sugar contained in it. Without the sugar, the stimulant effect of the hot fluid might be beneficial. As a meal—taken at the usual period of four or five hours after dinner—it is devoid of all objection, and furnishes a due supply of fluid aliment; but, if taken so early after dinner as to interfere with the digestion of solid food, its use is objectionable, for reasons before stated, and which apply to drinks in general.

As a proof of the prevalent discrepancy regarding the effects of tea upon the system, it may be observed, that whilst some regard it as a stimulant—and this is the general belief—others think it a sedative; and, that whilst the majority esteem the green teas to be more narcotic, and therefore, it is conceived, more noxious, Tourtelle gives the preference to them over the bohea.

It is interesting to bear in mind, connected with this hygienic question, the discrepancy in the customs of different countries, and of different parts of the same country. Thus, whilst black tea is most commonly used in Great Britain, and in this city (Philadelphia;) green tea is more used in France, and in Virginia. Nor has the Author, except in rare cases, observed the latter to disagree; yet Dr. C. A. Lee (Appendix to Amer. edit. of Pereira, *On Food and Diet*, p. 298) is "satisfied that green tea does not, in any case, form a salubrious beverage to persons in health, and should give place to milk, milk and water, black tea, milk and sugar, which, taken tepid, form very agreeable and healthy drinks."

When employed in moderation, the particular variety may be wholly left to the taste of the consumer.

Tea is sometimes made from the leaves of the sage—once so much vaunted; from the balm—*melissa*—and, in some of the country parts of the United States, from the *laurus sassafras*. In Paraguay, the infusion of the mattee—*Ilex Paraguensis* is highly esteemed, and is by many preferred to the Chinese tea. The observations, made on the latter, are equally applicable to the infusion of those vegetables.

*Coffee*—the seed of an evergreen, cultivated in hot climates—was not known in England until about the time tea was introduced there. It was imported about the middle of the sixteenth century into Constantinople, and it would appear, that, in 1652, Daniel Edwards, a Turkey merchant, took to England with him a Greek servant, named Pasqua, who understood the methods of roasting coffee, and making it into a beverage. This man first publicly sold coffee in England, and kept a house for that purpose.

The best coffee is obtained from Mocha, on the Red Sea. It is termed Mocha, and Turkey coffee. The next in esteem is raised in Java, and the East Indies; whilst the lowest priced is obtained from the West Indies and Brazil. In this country, the Java coffee is chiefly used; but many prefer the green coffee from the West Indies, which is, in the general opinion, far inferior.

The quantity of coffee annually supplied by Arabia, was supposed many years ago to be upwards of 14,000,000 of pounds. Before the commencement of the French revolution, the island of Saint Domingo alone exported more than 70,000,000 of pounds, per annum; and at the present day such is the fertility of that island, that coffee enough is said to be raised there to greatly reduce the price in all parts of the civilized world.

Coffee is generally drunk throughout the continent of Europe. In France, it is in universal request, and is prepared better perhaps than in any neighbouring country. In England, tea is a more common drink. In the year 1827, there were imported into the United States 50,051,986 pounds, of which 21,697,789 pounds were exported. In the same year, England imported 47,938,047 pounds, of which she exported 29,475,690 pounds.

The following table exhibits the imports and exports of coffee, with the quantity left for consumption or exportation during the years 1837, 1838, 1839 and 1840. (Hazard's *Commercial and Statistical Register*, and *American Almanac* for 1842.)

| Years. | Imports. | Exports. | Left for Consumption. |
|---|---|---|---|
| 1837 | 88.140.403 | 12.096.332 | 76.044.071 |
| 1838 | 88.139.720 | 5.267.087 | 82.871.633 |
| 1839 | 106.196.992 | 6.824.475 | 99.872.517 |
| 1840 | 94.996.095 | 8.698.334 | 86.297.761 |

The amount of coffee consumed from 1834 to 1840, according to the population of 1840, would allow to each individual in the United States $4\frac{7}{10}$ pounds per annum.

The following rules for judging of the quality of coffee, and for preparing it for use, are contained in a paper, communicated by professor Emmett, of the University of Virginia, to the "*Virginia Literary Museum.*" *First.* The raw coffee should be round, and small grained; free from dirt, and of a light colour. It should have no appearance of mouldiness, and be quite free from any strong smell. It should not be long kept in sacks with other provisions, as there is no substance more apt to obtain strong, and disagreeable odours from the presence of its neighbours. Rum injures it; and Miller even goes so far as to state, that a few bags of pepper, on board a ship from India, upon one occasion spoiled the whole cargo. *Secondly.* When the grains are large, flat and of a green colour, they should be kept on hand, in a dry situation, a long time before they are used.  *Thirdly.*  The roasting of coffee is a difficult operation for the housekeeper.  When carried far enough, an aromatic oil is formed by the heat, and forces itself out upon the surface of the grains, giving them a glossy appearance, and an odour, which is considered to increase their perfection.  Too little torrefaction prevents the aroma from appearing; too much completely volatilizes it, leaving nothing but a flat bitter taste.  The heat should be strong, and the operation as brief as possible, without burning the grains.  The roaster should be close or well covered all the time,* and in order to improve the looks, and flavour, a small piece of butter may be added to the coffee whilst parching.  *Fourthly.*  When thus prepared, coffee may be preserved for use in large quantities, without losing much of its freshness; provided the vessels containing it, be kept well covered.  *Fifthly.*  An infusion of coffee is better than a decoction, simply because the heat, in the last case, being stronger and more lasting, drives off more of the aromatic oil.  It is better, therefore, to grind the coffee very fine, and then to expose it, by means of a bag or strainer, to the action of boiling water, than to boil it for any length of time.

Coffee, when infused and taken hot, with milk and sugar, acquires the same properties from those additions that tea does.  In this state, it is usually taken for breakfast, and at tea time in England, and in this country; but the afternoon meal in France is generally devoid of milk.  Almost all the Mohammedans drink coffee at least twice a day, and without sugar.  The Turks drink coffee at all times of the day, and present it to visiters, both in the forenoon and afternoon; and the opium eater lives almost wholly on coffee and opium.

Coffee has been the favourite beverage of many distinguished persons.  Frederick the Great, and Napoleon drank it freely, and Leibnitz, and Voltaire, were equally fond of it.  It has been considered to possess the power of counteracting the effects of narcotics, and this is the cause why it is so largely used by those, who indulge in opium.  Coffee has been styled an " intellectual" drink, and hence it has been, and is, a favourite beverage with the literary and scientific; yet when first introduced into Europe, it—as well as tea—

---

\* It is proper to remark, however, that in Asia, where the coffee is excellent, open pans or tin plates are used, and if the time allows, a boy is employed to pick out every bean, when it has attained the right degree of brownness.

was strongly abused by the medical faculty. Fontanelle's physician proscribed it as deleterious, but the poet properly reminded him, that twenty-four years had elapsed since he first commenced the use of the *poison*. (Prof. Emmett, *loc. citat.*) The poison, in his case, must have been unusually tardy in its operation, as he lived upwards of a century. In 1708, much about the same period, a barber named Farr, was presented by the inquest of St. Dunstan's in the west, in London, " for making and selling a sort of liquor, called ' coffee,' to the great nuisance and prejudice of the neighbourhood.

We have remarked, that the infusion of coffee has been regarded as possessing the power of counteracting the effects of narcotics; and on many persons it has an antisoporific influence, when taken strong, and about the usual period for sleep; hence it is had recourse to by those, who are desirous of nocturnal study. It is manifestly tonic, and somewhat stimulating, and for all these reasons it has received the epithet " intellectual."

Coffee, when taken hot, in small quantity, and soon after dinner —as is the custom with the French—aids digestion, and is therefore proper for the dyspeptic. There are persons, however, with whom the feeble tonic powers of the coffee do not so well counteract the tendency to fermentation in the sugar added to it, as the astringent properties of tea. Whilst labouring under a severe attack of dyspepsia, the Author could not take coffee in this form, without the supervention of heartburn, flatulence, &c., whilst he could take tea with comparative impunity.

The French are in the habit of employing a strong infusion of coffee as a therapeutical agent, where a light tonic is demanded.

It appears from recent investigations of organic chemists, that *theine*, the peculiar principle of tea, and *caffeine*, the principle of coffee, are identical. " We shall never certainly," says Dr. Liebig, " be able to discover how men were led to the use of the hot infusion of the leaves of a certain shrub (tea,) or of a decoction of certain roasted seeds (coffee.) Some cause there must be, which would explain how the practice has become a necessary of life to whole nations. But it is surely still more remarkable, that the beneficial effects of both plants on the health must be ascribed to one and the same substance, the presence of which in two vegetables, belonging to different natural families, and the produce of different quarters of the globe, could hardly have presented itself to the boldest imagination. Yet recent researches have shown in such a manner as to exclude all doubt, that caffeine, the peculiar principle of coffee, and theine, that of tea, are in all respects, identical:—" and he adds,—" Without entering minutely into the medicinal action of caffeine (theine) it will surely appear a most striking fact, even if we were to deny its influence on the process of secretion, that this substance, with the addition of oxygen, and the elements of water, can yield taurine, the nitrogenized compound peculiar to bile." (*Animal Chemistry*, edit. cit. p. 169.)

Numerous articles have been recommended as substitutes for coffee. About fifty or sixty years ago, a deception was practised upon the Parisians, by mixing ground and roasted acorns with the genuine coffee powder. Fashion led the way, and the person, who hit upon the lucky thought, is reported to have realized a fortune. Endeavours have often been made, in France, to discover a substitute for foreign coffee. M. Pajot Descharmes states, that the seeds of the *forest broom* answer the purpose extremely well, according to the opinion of one, who had used them for twelve years. It is also affirmed, that for many years these seeds have been substituted for coffee in that part of Holland, which borders on Germany. In other parts; in the Netherlands, and in France, the root of the wild succory—*cichorium intybus*—is used instead of, and mixed with, coffee; and the Author has never observed any deterioration from the admixture: it certainly produces no injurious effects upon the health. So common is the employment of this root for the purpose indicated, that it has become an article of export from Liège. Certain beans and lupines have been used for the same purpose. In Great Britain, rye has been extensively employed. Dillenius gives an account of substitutes made with peas, beans, and kidney beans; but, he says, that made of rye comes nearest to true coffee. Hunt's " economical breakfast powder," is a spurious coffee, which is nothing more than roasted rye. Grape seeds, yellow water-flag seeds, yellow potatoes, peas, beans, burdock, barley, sunflower seeds, beach nuts, almonds salsify root, &c. have been substituted, but they are all far inferior to the genuine article.

*Chocolate* is a kind of cake or hard paste, the basis of which is the pulp of the cacao or chocolate nut, the production of a West India and South American tree,—the *theobroma cacao* or cacao tree. Previously to being formed into chocolate, the nuts are generally toasted, or parched over the fire in an iron vessel, after which their thin outer covering is easily separated. The kernel is then pounded in a mortar, and subsequently ground on a smooth, warm stone. Sometimes a little arnotta is added; and, with the aid of water, the whole is formed into a paste. This is put, whilst hot, into tin moulds, in which it congeals in a short time; and in this state it is the chocolate of the shops. Chocolate, thus prepared, is called, in France, *chocolat de santé*. It is sometimes aromatized by the addition of pepper, cinnamon, cloves, vanilla, &c. The *chocolat à la vanille* contains three ounces of vanilla, and two of cinnamon to twenty pounds of common chocolate. Dr. Paris asserts, that the vanilla is a substance very liable to disagree with the stomach, and to produce a train of nervous symptoms. This too general censure can only have been founded on some idiosyncrasy. The vanilla is a common ingredient for flavouring ice-cream, &c. in the United States, and it has never fallen to our lot to observe the consequences mentioned by Dr. Paris. Morin, (*Manuel d' Hygiène*, p. 67, Paris, 1827,) gives a decided preference to the chocolate aromatized by vanilla, or cinnamon, over the *chocolat de santé*, or, as he terms it, the *chocolat des ignorans*, from its being a compound of indigestible substances. Chocolate is indeed, very unfit for the dyspeptic. It contains a fecula, charged with concrete oil, mixed with a bitter brown matter, more or less aromatic, which is torrefied in the preparation of the chocolate; and it is of course more or less digestible, according to the greater or less degree of this torrefaction, and the greater or less quantity of the fatty or oily matter.

*Cocoa* is employed as a substitute for chocolate. It contains less nutritive matter, and therefore is more readily digested. The oily matter is in much smaller quantity; and it possesses some astringency, which adapts it for those of relaxed bowels.

Of *whey*, as a drink, mention has already been made. (Page 244.)

There are some other drinks, occasionally employed, the properties of which will be obvious from the admixture. *Imperial* is one of these. It is a solution of cream of tartar, flavoured with lemon peel, and resembles lemonade.

*Soda water* is a fashionable drink, and when solid food is not undergoing digestion in the stomach, it is an agreeable beverage. Its qualities are dependent upon the carbonic acid or fixed air it contains, which is a pleasant stimulus to the digestive function, and is often employed, when the action of the stomach has been enfeebled by a previous debauch: hence its use in the morning with hard drinkers. It may be prepared artificially, by dissolving half a drachm of carbonate of soda, and twenty-five grains of tartaric acid in separate half tumblerfuls of water, adding the two together, and drinking the mixture whilst in a state of effervescence. The preparation, however, is different from genuine soda water, which is a feeble solution of soda, impregnated with carbonic acid,—the resulting compound, in the other case, being a tartrate, instead of a carbonate of soda. With those who are predisposed to calculous depositions of a phosphatic kind, alkaline soda water is an improper drink.

## SECTION VI.

Simple fermented liquors—bad effects of their abuse—wines—their sensible, and chemical properties—proportion of alcohol in different fermented liquors—brisk wines—Burgundy wines—claret wines—Oporto wines—Spanish wines—Madeira wines—wines of the Rhine, and Moselle—sweet wines—cider—malt liquors—distilled fermented liquors—liqueurs.

On the subject of SIMPLE, or DISTILLED, FERMENTED LIQUORS, the observations we have to make are exclusively of a medical—not of a moral—nature. Every philanthropist must deplore the mischief daily induced by the abuse of these substances, and ardently desire the success of those excellent societies, whose object is to interfere with the pernicious practice of dram drinking, which has prevailed so extensively in this country, and in most others;—for there is hardly a people, that has not discovered some mode of producing alcohol. Too often, however, in their laudable enthusiasm, the writers on the great subject of temperance have quitted the strong moral basis on which the abuse of ardent spirit rests, and have attempted to show, upon data totally inadequate, the physical evils, that result from the occasional moderate use, not only of ardent spirits, but of wine, and almost every variety of fermented liquor.

A writer in the "*American Almanac*," for 1830—founding his deductions on some kind of evidence obtained in Boston—asserts, that not less than between 30,000 and 40,000 persons die annually in the United States from the use of alcohol;—that the bills of mortality of the city of Boston, for the two previous years, give on an average fifty deaths, " occasioned so directly by intemperance, as to be entered under names of disease to which none but drunkards fall victims;" and supposing, " that, on an average throughout our country, the deaths from intemperance bear about the same proportion to the whole number, that they do in Boston," he estimates the *direct* victims to the use of ardent spirits to be annually, in the United States, 10,000. The "names of disease" are not given. We are, therefore, left in the dark. Allusion, however, is doubtless made to the " mania a potû," " mania e temulentiâ"— " delirium tremens;" but it appears scarcely within the verge of possibility, that 10,000 persons should die annually in the United States from delirium tremens, which is not a very fatal affection. Of 84 cases, treated during the years 1840–1841, in the women's lunatic asylum of the Philadelphia Hospital, which is under the Author's charge for six months of the year, but one died. (*Practice of Medicine*, 2d, edit. ii. 279. Philadelphia, 1844.)

Professor Hitchcock, of Amherst college, in some lectures on diet, regimen and employment, delivered to the students of that college, in spring term 1830, estimates at from 30,000 to 50,000 the annual number of those—above twenty years of age—who die prematurely, in consequence of the use of these substances. It is probable, that these estimates are far beyond the amount of the mischief, extensive and revolting as it unquestionably is. On the precise amount of deaths, produced by the indirect action of ardent spirit, our data are especially defective. There is not a disease, so induced, but admits of other causes; and here is an insurmountable source of perplexity in forming any estimate, other than what is founded on mere guess-work. The evil, resulting from the abuse of ardent spirit—and indeed of some of the simple fermented liquors, in which the spirit is in a state of combination with other substances—is of sufficient magnitude. It requires no amplification. To any point that demands correction or modification, the estimate or the language of hyperbole is injurious, inasmuch as it does not induce unhesitating assent. The temperance societies, established through our land, and from the example of this country, in many parts of Great Britain, have rendered important service. Moderation—the never failing attendant on good sense—has already modified, and will continue to modify, some of the asperities, and impracticable parts of their original constitution: unnecessary self-privation and rigour will gain few proselytes, and so far defeat the praise-worthy intentions of many of their founders. The attempt to proscribe the use of wine is one of those objectionable ultra projects, which—to say the least of it—is injudicious, because unfeasible. Excessive indulgence, or abuse, is unquestionably to be deprecated—moderate *use*, even if habitual, except in particular constitutions, we may safely pronounce to be devoid of every noxious influence.

On this subject some pertinent remarks have been indulged in by Dr. Paris. (*Op. cit.* p. 268.) " Volumes," says he, " have been written to prove, that spirit, in every form, is not only unnecessary to those who are in health, but that it has been the prolific source of the most painful, and fatal diseases to which man is subject; in short that Epimetheus himself did not, by opening the box of Pandora, commit a greater act of hostility against our nature, than the discoverer of fermented liquors. Every apartment, it is said, devoted to the circulation of the glass, may be regarded as a temple set apart for the performance of human sacrifices; and that they ought to be fitted up, like the ancient temples of Egypt, in a manner to show the real atrocity of the superstition that is carried on within their walls. This is mere rant and nonsense; a striking specimen of the fallacy of reasoning against the *use* of a custom from its *abuse*. There exists no evidence to prove, that a temperate use of good wine, when taken at seasonable hours, has ever proved injurious to healthy adults. In youth, and still more in infancy, the stimulus, which it imparts to the stomach, is undoubtedly injurious; but there are exceptions even to this general rule. The occasional use of *diluted* wine has improved the health of a child, by imparting vigour to a torpid stomach. We ought, however, to consider it rather as a medicine than as a luxury." " Without entering farther," he adds, " into the discussion of a question, which has called so many opponents into the field, it may be observed, that, whatever opinion we may have formed, as to the evils or advantages consequent upon the invention of wine, we are not called upon as physicians to defend it: our object is to direct remedies for the cure of those diseases, which assail man as we find him in the habits of society, not as he might have been had he continued to derive his nourishment from the roots of the earth, and his drink from its springs. As these habits, says Dr. Philip, are such, that more or less alcohol is necessary to support the usual vigour of the greater number of people, even in health, nothing could be more injudicious than wholly to deprive them of it when they are already weakened by disease, unless it could be shown, that even a moderate use of it essentially adds to their disease, which, in dyspeptics, is by no means the case. My own experience coincides with that of Dr. W. Philip. In cases where the venous stimulant has been withdrawn, I have generally witnessed an aggravation of the dyspeptic symptoms, accompanied with severe depression of spirits: like Sinbad in the Arabian tale, the patient has borne a weight on his shoulders, which he has in vain attempted to throw off, until the fermented juice of the grape enabled him to triumph over his enemy."

The experience of every one must be in favour of the last observation of Dr. Paris. In all cases, it is important to avoid any sudden alteration of inveterate habits. Delirium tremens is a common consequence of the sudden relinquishment of the use of fermented liquor or opium, and, in times of pestilence, many an individual has fallen a victim to the sudden abstraction of stimuli to which his system has been long accustomed. Hence the propriety of Hoffman's second rule of health, which he borrowed from Hippocrates. (*Aphorism.* 50. sect. ii.)—"Ne subito muta assueta, quia consuetudo est altera natura." (*Septem Leges Sanitatis*, in Hoffm. *Dissert.* iii. decad. 2.)

> "Pliant nature more or less demands
> As custom forms her; and all sudden change
> She hates of habit, even from bad to good.
> If faults in life, or new emergencies
> From habits urge you, by long time confirmed,
> Slow must the change arise, and stage by stage,
> Slow as the stealing progress of the year."
>
> ARMSTRONG.

WINE.—Although the term *wine* is more strictly, and especially, applied to the fermented juice of the grape, it is used for any liquor that has become spirituous by fermentation. The presence of tartar—the bitartrate of potassa—has been regarded as the circumstance by which the grape is most strongly distinguished from all other fruits, that have been applied to the art of wine making. Its juice, moreover, contains within itself all the principles essential to vinification, in such a proportion and state of balance as to enable it, at once, to undergo a regular, and complete fermentation, whereas the juices of other fruits require artificial additions for the purpose. It has been observed, that all those wines which contain an excess of malic acid are of bad quality; hence the great defect, inherent in our domestic wines, and which causes them to partake of the properties of cider; the malic acid always predominating in our indigenous fruits.

All wines are produced from the juice of the grape, called "must." They may be divided into the *red*, and the *white*. The red are made from the must of black grapes, fermented with the envelope of their stones; the white from white grapes, or else from the must of black grapes, fermented without the envelope. In order to obtain them foaming, (*mousseux*,) they must be bottled before the fermentation is finished. Carbonic acid is then formed, and not being able to escape, in consequence of the pressure to which it is subjected, it remains in solution in the wine; but as soon as the cork is drawn, the carbonic acid assumes in part the gaseous state, and escapes from the wine, causing it to be brisk and foaming. This is the character of the wines of Champagne. The sweet wines are those that contain undecomposed sugar, either owing to too much saccharine matter being present in the must, or to the addition of sugar causing the quantity of saccharine matter to be greater than what is necessary for the fermentation. Muscat is a wine of this character.

All wines, when subjected to analysis, afford nearly the same products. They contain much water; alcohol, in variable quantity; a little mucilage; tannic acid; a blue colouring matter which becomes red, when it unites with acids; a yellow colouring matter; bitartrate of potassa; tartrate of lime; acetic acid; and, at times, other salts,—as the chloride of sodium, and the sulphate of potassa. It is to the alcohol, that they owe their strength; the more abundant it is, the more generous is the wine. From the mucilage they derive no remarkable properties: it probably, under particular circumstances, renders them ropy. The tannic acid gives them a kind of roughness, and the power of being clarified by a solution of glue or of white of egg. It unites with the gelatin or albumen of these substances, and is precipitated with them, carrying down, at the same time, all the matters held in suspension. The bitartrate of potassa, and the acetic acid give them tartness,—so that wines acquire additional value by keeping, not only because their principles undergo modifications in their combinations, but because tartar is deposited.

The grapes of warm countries being very saccharine, the wines, formed from them, are generous, and rich in alcohol, whilst they contain scarcely any acid: on the other hand, the wines of cold countries are sour, and by no means strong; but they may be improved by adding chalk, and saccharine matter to the must. The chalk neutralizes the acid, and the saccharine matter augments the quantity of alcohol. It must not, however, as Thénard has properly remarked, (*Traité de Chimie*, p. i. liv. i. chap. v.) be always inferred, that a wine is better in proportion as it is more generous, or more rich in spirit. Some of the Burgundy wines, of good quality, yield scarcely more spirit than those of the neighbourhood of Paris, and much less than those of the south, yet there is a signal difference between them. This difference, he thinks, cannot be attributed to the mucilage, or the tannic acid, but probably belongs to a substance, which has hitherto escaped the researches of the chemist, and which forms the *bouquet*, supposed by some chemists to be of an oily nature, but which they have not been able to separate.

This *bouquet* is peculiar to each species, and enables us to distinguish them from each other. In sweet, and half fermented wines, it appears to be derived immediately from the fruit, as in those made from the Frontignan, and Muscat grapes; but, in the more perfect wines, as claret, and Burgundy, it has no resemblance to the natural flavour of the fruit, but is altogether the result of the vinous process.

Some wines are artificially flavoured by the addition of extraneous substances, as almonds—in the case of Madeira and Sherry—to which—it is said—they are indebted for their nutty flavour. Among the ancients, it was the custom to give a resinous flavour to wines by the introduction of turpentine into the casks,—a practice, which is said still to prevail in modern Greece. The most important ingredient in wines, in a hygienic point of view, is the alcohol, and the form of combination in which it exists. The researches of the chemist, on this subject, have led to singular results, and have shown, that wines are not intoxicating in an exact ratio with the alcohol they contain; and hence that the addition of other matters may materially modify the action of the alcohol on the nervous system. When, with the view of appreciating the amount of alcohol in wines, it was separated by distillation, it was attempted to show, that in those cases, in which an unexpected amount was discovered, the elements of the alcohol might have existed in the wine, and that they might have become combined, during the process of distillation, so that although the elements might be present in a greater quantity than in wines more intoxicating, a larger amount of free alcohol was contained in the latter. Rouelle and Fabbroni, indeed, affirmed, that alcohol was not completely formed in these cases, until the temperature was raised to the point of distillation; but Gay Lussac overturned this hypothesis, by separating the alcohol by distillation, at the temperature of 66° Fahrenheit; and, by the aid of a vacuum, it has been accomplished at 56°. The most complete demonstration, however, of the independent existence of alcohol in wines was furnished by the experiments of Mr. Brande. By precipitating the colouring matter, and some other elements of the wine, by the subacetate of lead, and saturating the clear liquor by subcarbonate of potassa he separated the alcohol without any elevation of temperature. In this way, he succeeded in forming a table of the quantity of spirit in various wines, and in other simple, as well as distilled, liquors. In referring, however, to the estimates of Mr. Brande, as contained in the following table, it is proper to bear in mind, that many of the wines are prepared expressly for the London market, and are more brandied than the same varieties sold in the United States. This is strikingly the case with Port. Dr. Henderson, too, has remarked, that some of the wines analyzed by Mr. Brande were mixed with a considerable quantity of adventitious alcohol. His additions and corrections have the letter H affixed.

*Proportion of Alcohol, S. G. 0.825, in one hundred parts by measure of the following wines, and malt and spirituous liquors.*

| | |
|---|---|
| 1. Lissa,............26.47 | Red Madeira,............18.40 |
| do............24.35 | Average,............20.35 |
| Average,............(a)25.41 | 16. Cape Muscat,............18.25 |
| 2. Raisin Wine,............26.40 | 17. Cape Madeira,............22.94 |
| do............25.77 | do............20.50 |
| do............23.20 | do............18.11 |
| Average,............25.12 | Average,............20.51 |
| 3. Marsala,............26.03 | 18. Grape Wine,............18.11 |
| do............25.05 | 19. Calcavella,............19.20 |
| Average,............(b)25.09 | do............18.10 |
| 4. Port—average of six kinds,............23.48 | Average,............18.65 |
| do.—highest,............25.83 | 20. Vidonia,............19.25 |
| do.—lowest,............21.40 | 21. Alba Flora,............17.26 |
| 5. Madeira,............24.42 | 22. Malaga,............17.26 |
| do............23.93 | 23. White Hermitage,............17.43 |
| do. (Sercial,)............21.45 | 24. Roussillon,............19.00 |
| do............19.24 | do............17.26 |
| Average,............22.27 | Average,............18.13 |
| 6. Currant Wine,............20.55 | 25. Claret,............17.11 |
| 7. Sherry,............19.81 | do............16.32 |
| do............19.83 | do............14.08 |
| do............18.79 | do............12.91 |
| do............18.25 | Average,............(d)15.10 |
| Average............19.17 | 26. Malmsey Madeira,............16.40 |
| 8. Teneriffe,............19.79 | 27. Lunel,............15.52 |
| 9. Colares,............19.75 | 28. Scheraaz,............15.52 |
| 10. Lachryma Christi,............19.70 | 29. Syracuse,............15.28 |
| 11. Constantia—white,............19.75 | 30. Sauterne,............14.22 |
| red,............(c)18.92 | 31. Burgundy,............16.60 |
| 12. Lisbon,............18.94 | do............15.22 |
| 13. Malaga,............18.94 | do............14.53 |
| 14. Bucellas,............18.49 | do............11.95 |
| 15. Red Madeira,............22.30 | Average,............14.57 |

(a) 15.90 H.    (b) 18.40 H.    (c) 14.50 H.    (d) 12.91 H.

| | | | |
|---|---|---|---|
| 32. Hock, | 14.37 | 42. Orange Wine—average of six samples made by a London Manufacturer, | 11.26 |
| do. | 13.00 | | |
| do. (old in cask,) | 8.88 | | |
| Average, | 12.08 | 43. Tokay, | 9.88 |
| Rudesheimer, (1811) | H. 10.72 | 44. Elder Wine, | 9.87 |
| do. (1800) | H. 12.22 | 45. Rhenish Wine, | H. 8.71 |
| Average, | H. 11.47 | 46. Cider—highest average, | 9.87 |
| Johannisberger, | H. 8.71 | lowest, | 5.21 |
| 33. Nice, | 14.63 | 47. Perry—average of 4 samples, | 7.26 |
| 34. Barsac, | 13.86 | 48. Mead, | 7.32 |
| 35. Tent, | 13.30 | 49. Ale, (Burton,) | 8.88 |
| 36. Champagne, (still,) | 13.80 | do. (Edinburgh,) | 6.20 |
| do. (sparkling,) | 12.80 | do. (Dorchester,) | 5.56 |
| do. (red,) | 12.56 | Average, | 6.87 |
| do. | 11.30 | 50. Brown Stout, | 6.80 |
| Average, | 12.61 | 51. London Porter, (average,) | 4.20 |
| 37. Red Hermitage, | 12.32 | do. Small Beer, (average,) | 1.28 |
| 38. Vin de grave, | 13.94 | 52. Brandy, | 53.39 |
| do. | 12.80 | 53. Rum, | 53.68 |
| Average, | 13.37 | 54. Gin, | 51.60 |
| 39. Frontignac, | 12.79 | 55. Scotch Whisky, | 54.32 |
| 40. Cote Rotie, | 12.32 | 56. Irish do. | 53.90 |
| 41. Gooseberry Wine, | 11.84 | | |

Where brandy is added to wine, there is more or less uncombined spirit, but this does not bear an exact ratio to the quantity added, because a renewed fermentation is excited by the vintner, which assimilates and combines a portion of the spirit with the wine—an operation which is called "fretting in." The addition of spirit cannot but be injurious in a hygienic respect, as the evils —hepatic and others—that are consequent upon the use of ardent spirit cannot fail to attend upon the habitual use of such wines. Where the alcohol exists in combination with the other ingredients of the wine, although the compound may give occasion to gouty and other affections, in which disorder of the digestive organs forms a part, the evils that follow the use of alcoholic liquors are not to apt to be induced.

When the stronger wines are kept for some time, a change occurs, which is regarded by the wine drinkers as very favourable to them. Red wine gradually deposits a quantity of tartar, in combination with extractive and colouring matter, which forms what is called the *crust;* so that a considerable portion of that which is more likely to disagree with the stomach, is thus removed. It is probable, that a more intimate admixture takes place in the bottle, between the alcohol and the other constituents, so that its action becomes more disguised; for the wine loses its strong character, and is less intoxicating. There can be no doubt of the improvement of the flavour of Madeira by a voyage or two to the East Indies; but the chemist has never succeeded in detecting the chemical change that it has undergone in such case. The lighter wines, as a general rule, are not as much improved by motion and age as the stronger; and some of them, as Burgundy, are so delicate, that the agitation produced by a voyage even across the British channel will often spoil them.

Let us now inquire briefly into the dietetic qualities of various sorts of wines.

1. *Brisk wines.*—Of late years, in this country, sparkling Rhenish and Moselle wines, and Rivesaltes, have been introduced; but many of them have gone out of fashion, and, after all, it must be admitted, that champagne is the chief of the class. Brisk wines intoxicate speedily; probably in consequence of the carbonic acid in which they abound, and the volatile state in which their alcohol is held; so that the alcohol, in this way, is applied at once, and in a very divided state, to a large extent of nervous surface. For this reason, the excitement is of a more lively, and transitory character, than that which is caused by any other species of wine, and the subsequent exhaustion less. Experiments have shown, that carbonic acid gas is powerfully penetrant, and hence we can understand, why it should readily pass, along with the alcohol combined with it, through the coats of the vessels of the abdominal venous system by imbibition.

Dr. Paris thinks, that independently of the alcohol, thus held in solution in the carbonic acid, it is probable that some active aromatic matter is volatilized together with it; which he conceives, may account for the peculiar effects produced on some persons by champagne.

Brisk wines are very apt to disagree with the gouty, probably from exciting gastric derangement; and there are many persons, who are unable to take champagne without the supervention of headach on the same or the following day. It would seem, that gout is by no means frequent in the province in which this wine is made; experience seems, however, to show, that its use is noxious to the gouty, and the dyspeptic; yet the Author has repeatedly remarked, that gouty individuals have been able to take five or six glasses of champagne with impunity when a single glass had disordered their digestive function;—probably owing to the stimulant effect of the larger quantity preventing the derangement, that a smaller quantity of the beverage was wont to induce. Sparkling Muscat or Rivesaltes is perhaps the most objectionable of the class, and it is now scarcely used in this country.

2. *Burgundy Wines.*—These are of two kinds—*red* and *white*—but they are not so much used in the United States. Their *bouquet* is peculiar, and powerful; and they generally affect the nervous system more than some wines, that contain a larger quantity of alcohol; hence it has been supposed, that they hold, dissolved, some unknown principle of great activity.—The average per centage of alcohol is, by the table, 14.57. They are more heady (*capiteux*) than claret, which according to the analysis of Mr. Brande contains more spirit. They have been employed in disorders, in which stimulant and subastringent tonics seemed to be indicated; and the same observation applies to the wines of the Rhone, and to the lighter red wines of Spain and Portugal.

3. *Claret Wines* are more generally drunk, especially in the warmer regions of the globe, than any other European wines. They are well fermented, and contain less aroma, and spirit, but more astringency, than the produce of the Burgundy vineyards. They do not excite intoxication as readily as most other wines, and hence are less stimulant, and better fitted for daily use. " They have, indeed," says Dr. Henderson—in his valuable " *History of Wines*"—" been condemned by some writers as productive of gout, but, I apprehend, without much reason. That with those people, who are in the practice of soaking large quantities of port, and madeira, an occasional debauch in claret may bring on a gouty paroxysm, is very possible; but the effect is to be ascribed chiefly to the transition from a strong brandied wine to a lighter beverage,—a transition almost always followed by greater or less derangement of the digestive organs. Besides, we must recollect that the liquor, which passes under the denomination of claret, is generally a compounded wine. It is therefore unfair to impute to the wines of the Bordelais those mischiefs, which, if they do arise in the manner alleged, are probably, in most instances, occasioned by the admixture of other vintages of less wholesome quality."

4. The *Wines of Oporto*,—called "*port*"—and especially that which is prepared for the British market, abound in astringency, and their intrinsic potency is largely increased by the brandy added to them prior to exportation. Owing to their astringency, they are preferred as a tonic in diseases where such agency is

deemed necessary. Their habitual use is more apt, perhaps, to induce gout than any other kind of wine, and they are very apt to disagree with the dyspeptic :—owing, it has been presumed, to the gallic acid which they contain. On this account, the wines of Alicant, and Rota have been recommended in preference, where astringents are needed, and where the port might disagree, as they contain more tannin, and less acid. The excitement, induced by port wine, is of a more sluggish character, than that which follows the use of the purer French wines, and it does not enliven the fancy to the same extent.

5. *Spanish Wines.*—These and particularly the *Sacks*, *(secco,* Spanish ; *sec,* French; "dry") or dry wines were at one time greatly drunk in England, both dietetically, and medicinally. The older English writers speak of *sherris sack*, meaning sherry, and of *Canary sack*, or the dry wines of the Canaries. The wines of Xeres (*sherry*) are still extremely fashionable, and there is, perhaps, no wine more agreeable, and more wholesome than pale sherry, duly mellowed by age. It is almost totally free from acidity, and therefore best adapted to the dyspeptic, and gouty. It is, perhaps, the least variable wine in its properties, and hence the *vinum album Hispanicum* is the only wine recommended in the British Pharmacopœias.

6. The *Madeira Wines* are, in this country, preferred to all others ; and, when not too acidulous, they are perhaps as wholesome as any others. There are many dyspeptics, however, who can take sherry with impunity, and who are compelled to abstain from madeira. With such, Sicily madeira, which contains less acid, and is slightly bitter, can frequently be drunk, when the real madeira cannot, but it is an infinitely inferior wine. The same may be said of Cape madeira.

7. The *light wines of the Rhine,* and *Moselle* are much less spirituous, and heady than those we have described. There is, however, free acid in them, which causes them to disagree with some stomachs. In the countries where they are produced, they are frequently prescribed with a view to their presumed diuretic properties. Dr. Henderson affirms, that in certain species of fever, accompanied by a low pulse, and great nervous exhaustion, they have been found to possess considerable efficacy, and may be given with more safety than most other kinds. They are also said

to be of service—like most acid, and subacid substances—in diminishing obesity.

8. *Sweet wines* contain the largest proportion of extractive, and saccharine matter, but by no means the least quantity of ardent spirit, notwithstanding the assertion of Dr. Paris to the contrary. A reference to Mr. Brande's table will show, that the Constantia, Muscat, and Lunel are not low in the scale; but the quantity of spirit is disguised by the free sugar, or that which remains unchanged during the process of vinification; hence they ought to be regarded as mixtures of wine, and sugar: accordingly, whatever arrests the progress of fermentation must have a tendency to produce a sweet wine. Thus, boiling the *must*, or drying the fruit— by partially separating the natural leaven, and dissipating the water—occasions this result, as is exemplified by the manufacture of the wine of Cyprus, the *vino cotto* of the Italians (*vinum coctum* of the ancients, *vin cuit;*) by that of Frontignac; the rich and luscious wines of Canary, and of Constantia: the celebrated Tokay —*vino tinto* (Tent of Hungary); the Italian *montefiascone*, the Persian *scheraaz*, and the Malmsey wines of the Archipelago. The ancients had a better opinion of the qualities of the sweet wines, than of the drier, or more fully fermented,—an opinion, which we of the present day can hardly suppose to have been founded on experience. The free sugar, which they contain, renders them extremely unfit for the dyspeptic; and scarcely any one of feeble digestive powers can drink them with impunity. They are only fit to be used as agreeable cordials. Among the Greeks and Romans, the sweet wines were those most commonly in use; and in preparing them, the ancients often inspissated them until they became of the consistence of honey, or even thicker, in which form they constituted the *vina cocta* of the latter people. Before being drunk they were diluted with water.

The following table, of the quantity of wines, imported into the United States for the year ending September, 1829, will indicate the relative amount of the various kinds used at that time in this country.

## DOMESTIC WINES. 317

|  | Gallons. |
|---|---|
| Madeira, | 282,660 |
| Burgundy, Champagne, Rhenish, and Tokay, | 23,562 |
| Sherry and Saint Lucar, | 62,689 |
| Wines of Portugal and Sicily, | 352,350 |
| ———— Teneriffe and Azores . | 61,467 |
| Claret, &c. in bottles or cases, | 356,332 |
| Other wines, not in bottles or cases, | 1,838,251 |
| Gallons, | 2,977,311 |

The wines, that are made by the house-keeper—including the ordinary domestic or home-made wines of this country and of Great Britain—contain so much free saccharine matter, that they are extremely apt to disagree with the stomach of the dyspeptic, and of those of feeble digestive powers. It rarely happens, that domestic wines are fully fermented, and if they are, they are so inferior to the foreign, that the end is not equal to the labour. As this country produces the indigenous grape in so much luxuriance, it has been supposed, that it would be well adapted for the manufacture of good wine. Many experiments have, however, been made in various parts of the United States, but none have been completely successful. Families, experienced in the art, from France and Italy, have settled here for the express purpose, but every attempt has in a great measure failed. There is a wine, made in North Carolina, called the *Scuppernong*, which has been highly extolled. We have tasted but one sample, which was worthy of the epithet "good," and this had the flavour of madeira wine, probably in consequence of the indigenous wine having been placed on madeira lees, which is not unfrequently the case. It is extremely difficult to pronounce upon the precise climate and soil, which will be favourable to the production of the proper grape. On some of the small hills of Germany, and elsewhere, which are celebrated for the excellence of their wines, a slight difference of exposure and soil occasions the greatest diversity in the product; so that the land, in one case, will sell for many hundred dollars per acre more than in the other. The effect produced by difference of soil and climate is also signally evinced by the fact, often proved, that if the vine, that produces the Hochheimer, at Hochheim on the Maine, be transplanted to the banks of the Moselle, it produces the Moselle wine; if to certain parts of France, the *Vin de Grave;* if to Portugal, the

Bucellas, and if to the Cape of Good Hope, the wine has the characteristic Cape *smaak* (smack.)

*Cider*, the product of the fermentation of apple juice; and *perry*, of the juice of the pear, resemble each other, in properties. When very sweet, they are apt to disagree, especially with those of weak digestive powers; but many dyspeptics are able to drink hard cider with impunity, and even with advantage. Hard cider is a favourite drink with the New-Englanders. In the middle and southern states, the sweet cider is generally preferred. The crab cider of the south resembles champagne in its properties, and is sometimes almost equal to it; whilst its feebler character enables it to serve as a delightful beverage, especially during the warmth of summer.

MALT LIQUORS.—These, in some shape, are employed as a beverage in most countries. The Egyptians, according to Herodotus, understood the art of making a fermented liquor from barley; and such a drink, according to Tacitus, was much used by the ancient Germans. Malt liquors differ from wines chiefly in the following points:—they contain a much greater proportion of nutritive matter, and less of spirit, but they have in addition a peculiar bitter, and narcotic principle, derived from the hop. At one time, a strong prejudice existed against the hop, but it is now allowed to be a most valuable ingredient. Without it, indeed, or some substitute—and none is equivalent—the ale would not keep, especially that intended for the warmer climates; and, accordingly, the *pale ale*, destined for the India market, is always made intensely bitter with the hop. Independently of the flavour and tonic properties, which hops communicate, they precipitate, by means of their astringent principle, the vegetable mucilage, and thus remove from the beer the active principle of its fermentation; consequently, without hops, malt liquors would have to be drunk either new, and ropy,—or old and sour. (Paris, *Treatise on Diet*, 5th. edit. p. 287. Lond. 1837.)

It would seem, that the extractive matter, furnished by malt, is highly nutritive, if we judge from the appearance of the draymen and coal-heavers of the British metropolis, who are allowed porter in great quantities;—the common daily allowance, in some establishments, being a gallon. When used to this extent, however, a degree of polyæmia or plethora is induced, which although it may sufficiently demonstrate the nutritive qualities of the beverage, is not a healthy condition. In the system of "training,"—to be described hereafter,—and which consists in raising the powers of the pugilist or the pedestrian to the full extent of which he is capable, mild, home-brewed ale is recommended for drink,—about three pints per day. It is in consequence of its nutritive properties that ale has been called by Dr. Kitchener, '*liquid bread.*' " Home-brewed beer," says that eccentric writer, " is the most invigorating drink. It is, indeed gentle reader! notwithstanding a foolish fashion has barbarously banished the natural beverage of Great Britain, as *extremely ungenteel.*" (*Op. citat.* p. 27.)

The usual division of malt liquors is into porter, ale, and table or small beer. The two first resemble each other in strength, and in dietetic virtues. The latter, are weaker but possessed of all the properties of the other to a less extent.

None of these drinks digest very readily with the dyspeptic: the extractive is apt to run into the acetous fermentation, particularly in the case of small beer, and to produce flatulence, and heartburn; but to those, that are accustomed to their use, and with whom they do not disagree, even the stronger kinds are wholesome; and happy, Dr. Paris has observed, is that country, whose labouring class prefer such a beverage to the mischievous potations of ardent spirit. Still, when taken in too great quantity, they induce positive mischief. There is a body of men, employed on the Thames, whose business is to raise ballast from the bottom of the river. As this can be done only when the tide is ebbing, their hours of labour are regulated by that circumstance; and, consequently, vary through every period of the night and day. They work under great exposure to inclemencies of weather: their occupation requires great bodily exertion, occasioning profuse sweating, and much exhaustion. In consideration of this their allowance of liquor is very large; each man—it is affirmed by Dr. William Budd (Tweedie's *Library of Medicine*, 2nd Amer. edit. iii. 587, Philad. 1842) drinks from two to three gallons of porter daily, and generally a considerable quantity of spirit besides. This immoderate consumption of liquor forms the only exception, so far as relates to food, which these men offer to the lower classes in London. Gout is remarkably frequent among them, and although not a numerous body, many of them are every year admitted into the Seamen's Hospital ship affected with that disease. This, as related by Dr. Budd, is a very interesting fact, and seems to show, that no amount of bodily exertion is adequate to counteract the influence of such large doses of porter;—the exposure to wet and changes of temperature probably favouring its operation.

The remarks, already indulged, will have shown how detrimental the constant abuse of SPIRITUOUS LIQUORS must be to the liver, and to the functions of the stomach, and intestines in general. There is hardly, indeed, a faculty—mental or corporeal—but is made to totter under the stimulation, excited in it by the pernicious habits of the dram drinker. Objectionable, however, as its constant use or abuse must be, it cannot be presumed, that the occasional employment of diluted spirit can be productive of all the physical evils that have been ascribed to it. We have already remarked, that man requires variety of food, and that he exhibits the characteristics of health more strongly under such circumstances, than when restricted to one kind of aliment. In like manner, the transient and occasional stimulation, caused by ardent spirit properly diluted, and not in too great a quantity, may arouse the organs to a more vigorous discharge of their functions, instead of causing mischievous results. We have referred to the effect produced on the action and secretions of the stomach by a small quantity of alcohol, taken after an aliment difficult of digestion, and to the mode in which it occasions beneficial effects; but, except in such cases, or as an occasional beverage, the use of ardent spirits, especially the daily use, ought to be avoided.

Dr. Beaumont found, that the free use of ardent spirits, wine, beer, or any intoxicating liquor, when continued for some days, invariably produced erythematic and aphthous patches in the villous lining of the stomach. He found, however, that eating voraciously, or to excess; swallowing food coarsely masticated, or too fast; the introduction of solid pieces of meat suspended by cords into the stomach, or by muslin bags of aliment, secured in the same way, almost invariably produced similar effects if repeated a number of times in close succession. These morbid changes were seldom indicated by any ordinary symptoms or special sensations, and could not, in most cases, have been anticipated: their existence was only ascertained by actual ocular observation on the individual with the fistulous opening into the stomach more than once referred to. Dr. Beaumont adds, " In the case of the subject of these experiments, inflammation certainly does exist, to a considerable extent, even in an *apparent* state of health—greater than could have been believed to comport with the due operations of the gastric functions." (*Experiments and Observations on the Gastric Juice,* &c., p. 240. Plattsburg, 1833.)

Alcohol, in its state of purity, is identical, whatever may be the substance whence it is extracted; but as it is never taken pure, it preserves the flavour of the bodies—or rather a flavour derived from the bodies—whence it is obtained. Hence the difference between brandy, rum, whisky, gin, kirschwasser, arrack, &c.

*Liqueurs* consist of spirit, in which certain aromatic substances are macerated. They, of course, possess the united properties of the alcohol, and the aromatics. As, however, a large quantity of sugar is added to them, the alcohol is somewhat masked, and does not produce equal inconvenience. They are handed round at many tables immediately after dinner, or breakfast, and can scarcely be noxious in the small dose in which they are usually administered. Some of them are impregnated with narcotics, which, of course, add to the noxious qualities of the spirit. When ardent spirit is mixed with sugar and lemon juice, it forms " punch," one of the most agreeable, but unwholesome forms in which alcohol is taken. It is almost a poison to many dyspeptics; yet a modern writer on hygiène, (Dr. J. Johnson, in *A Treatise on Derangements of the Liver,* &c. American Edit. p. 204,) asserts, that acids correct, in a great degree, the deleterious effects of spirituous liquors. The result of our experience is the very opposite to this.

## SECTION VII.

*Alimentary regimen best adapted for man—evils of too great a quantity of food—proper number of meals—sudden changes of regimen unwholesome—regimen must vary according to different circumstances—best regimen for developing the full powers—training—how practically effected—tobacco—history of its introduction—its effects on the functions—snuffing—smoking—chewing.*

Having canvassed the special qualities of the various substances employed for human sustenance, it is time to inquire briefly into the alimentary regimen, best adapted for the health of man. Here we have to pay regard, not only to the due quality of the solid and liquid food, but to the quantity employed. This, unless a morbid habit has been induced, will be best learned by attending to the earliest intimations of satiety; provided the repast be made from a single dish. When there are many, an artificial appetite is apt to be excited, which leads to intemperance—for there may obviously be intemperance in solid, as well as in liquid aliment; and this is one of the strong objections to the system of loading the table with so many tempting dishes, as is the custom at the dinners of the wealthy, in most parts of the globe. "I have already," observes Dr. Paris, (*Op. cit.*) " alluded to the mischief, which arises from the too-prevailing fashion of introducing at our meals an almost indefinite succession of incompatible dishes. The stomach being distended with soup, the digestion of which, from the very nature of the operations, which are necessary for its completion, would in itself be a sufficient labour for that organ, is next tempted with fish, rendered indigestible from its sauces; then, with flesh and fowl: the vegetable world, as an intelligent reviewer has observed, is ransacked from the *cryptogamia* upwards; and to this miscellaneous aggregate are added the pernicious pasticcios of the pastry cook, and the complex combinations of the confectioner. All these evils, and many more, have those who move in the ordinary society of the present day to contend with. It is not to one or two good dishes, even abundantly indulged in, but to the overloading the stomach, that such strong objections are to be urged: nine persons in ten eat as much soup and fish as would amply suffice for a meal, and as far as soup and fish are concerned, would rise from the table, not only satisfied but saturated. A new stimulus appears in the form of stewed beef, or *côtelettes à la suprême:* then comes a Bayonne or Westphalia ham, or a pickled tongue, or some anomalous salted, but proportionately indigestible, dish, and of each of these enough for a single meal. But this is not all: game follows; and to this again succeed the sweets, and a quantity of cheese. The whole is crowned with a variety of flatulent fruits, and indigestible knick-knacks, included under the name of dessert, in which we must not forget to notice a mountain of sponge cake. Thus then it is, that the stomach is made to receive, not one full meal, but a succession of meals, rapidly following each other, and vying in their miscellaneous and pernicious nature with the ingredients of Macbeth's caldron. Need the philosopher, then, any longer wonder at the increasing number and severity of dyspeptic complaints, with their long train of maladies, amongst the higher classes of society."

It is impossible to indicate accurately the quantity of food proper for each individual. Children, and those in the age of adolescence, when every thing is undergoing development, require more *nourishment* than the adult, or the aged. Yet the latter, especially when far advanced in life, appear to demand a larger quantity of *food* than the former. The assimilative organs in them perform their office but imperfectly, and tardily, and a much smaller proportion of nutritive matter is separated;—hence it is that more of the raw material is necessary.

For the reason already assigned, it will be understood why children, and young persons bear abstinence so badly, and why, as has been graphically represented by Dante, (*Inferno,* Canto xxxiii.,) Count Ugolino della Gherardescha should have seen his sons successively expire before him of hunger.

We elsewhere have pointed out the advantages, in a hygienic respect, of employing a variety of aliments;—a circumstance, which, as Magendie remarks, is indicated to us by our instinct, as well as by the changes, that attend upon the seasons,—as respects the nature and kind of alimentary substances. But one or two dishes should be used, and these should be dressed as simply as possible.

Much has been said with regard to the proper number of meals, and the intervals that ought to elapse between them. Regularity in the periods ought certainly to be observed. They should be as nearly equidistant as practicable, and at such intervals, that one digestion may be completed before the materials are furnished for another. The digestive process is not always accomplished in the same time by different individuals, or by the same individual at different periods. It rarely, however, requires more than five or six hours. *Breakfast, dinner*, and *tea*, are the meals usually taken with us, and where they are made to fall at regular and sufficient intervals, no more are necessary. " Early breakfast,"—says a recent writer, (Dr. Johnson, *Op. cit.*, &c., p. 201,) " dinner as near the middle of the day as fashion or folly, or pride, will permit—a pretty hearty tea or coffee in the evening about six o'clock, and no supper, will be found the most salutary code which the physician can lay down." He adds, however,—" there are many constitutions where even in valetudinary health, a *little* animal food for supper both agrees well, and contributes to repose. Here the practice then is not detrimental." The number of meals must, however, be regulated by the age. Children eat more frequently than adults with impunity, and even with advantage, but it is important that they should not take too much at a time; and, in this way, digestion may be readily accomplished, as the quantity of food may not exceed the powers of the stomach.

As a general rule, the evening repast should be light, especially when we retire to rest soon afterwards. When the stomach is loaded, the circulation is interfered with, and the brain receives irregular impressions, which give occasion to painful and distressing dreams, nightmare, and—when in a higher degree—to somnambulism. Hence it is that in civic life, where plethora is apt to be induced by continued full living, apoplexy so frequently follows a surfeit at supper.

Every sudden change in regimen is unwholesome. Food, containing but little nutriment, and not markedly wholesome, may agree better, when we are accustomed to its use, than that which is more wholesome. Whenever, therefore, epidemic sickness prevails, a change in regimen should be made gradually, for fear that the new circumstances, under which the individual may be placed, may occasion so great a change in the economy as to render him more liable to an accession of disease, (page 308.) These observations, however, do not apply to the constant mutations in diet, that occur during the exercise of social intercourse. Where persons are

## ALIMENTARY REGIMEN.

careful in the quantity of their aliment, and sedulously avoid undue stimulation from simple and distilled fermented liquors, the influence upon both mind and body by the dietetic changes, adopted in social life, are not only harmless but beneficial. Monotony does not agree with the feeble, and the valetudinary; and in those of good health the condition is confirmed by the varied diet, and entertainment afforded by society. It has been the custom, in times of spreading sickness, to advise, that social entertainments should be neglected, and such advice would be most rational were it to be presumed, that they must necessarily degenerate into mere Bacchanalian orgies; but if excesses be not committed, the cheerfulness and hilarity, which such intercourse engenders, may steel the system against the intrusion of morbific agents as effectually as any other plan that could be devised.

The alimentary regimen should be regulated, as far as practicable, by the constitution, and especially by the gastric powers of the individual. The robust, and the vigorous require a different diet from the weak, and the valetudinary. Regard should be had to difference of pursuits. Literary persons, and such as are compelled to lead a sedentary life, should eat less than those who are engaged in laborious, and fatiguing occupations; and their food should be lighter, and more delicate. The same may be said of the civic and the rural resident,—especially of him, who has been accustomed to all the luxuries attendant upon high life in towns, and him, who has been doomed to the fatiguing operations of the farm. The coarse, and compact food, which the latter could digest with facility, would be invincible by the gastric powers of the former; and conversely, the regimen of the citizen would be unfit to maintain the hardihood, and vigour of the rustic.

The delicate, the sickly, and all whose digestive powers are feeble, require more care in their dietetic observances. The qualities of different kinds of aliment that have already been pointed out may guide them in their choice. They should shun those that are difficult of digestion, and let their regimen be substantial, but light, and taken in small quantities several times during the day. When no idiosyncrasy contra-indicates its use, milk in various forms of preparation is an excellent diet. This, with good bread, forms a compound of both animal, and vegetable food. Meat, especially the more digestible kinds, should be eaten in moderation, but the more indigestible varieties of vegetables and fruits should be carefully avoided. Climate and season likewise suggest some variation. Animal food appears to agree better in northern climates and in the colder seasons, whilst the use of vegetables seems more appropriate to warm climates and seasons. Much of this, however, is an affair of habit. It is important, too, in taking our meals, that the process should not be too rapidly accomplished, and that care should be taken to duly masticate and insalivate the food. Where it is "bolted," or swallowed in large mouthfuls, digestion is not as speedily accomplished; the texture of the solid is not sufficiently softened, and as the gastric secretions have to act from circumference to centre, the solution is not as readily effected. The French have a proverb on this subject, which, like all proverbs,—to use the language of Sir Thomas Browne on another subject—"are founded on some bottom of reason:"—"*Viande bien machée est à demi digérée.*"—"Meat well chewed is half digested." Dr. Beaumont—as before remarked—found, that eating voraciously or to excess, and swallowing food imperfectly masticated, or too fast, produced the same erythematic and aphthous patches on the villous coat of the stomach, as the free use of ardent spirits, wine, beer, or any intoxicating liquor, continued for some days.

There are many other topics, connected with the history of alimentary substances, which are usually discussed by dietetical writers. They are mostly, however, of minor importance, and embrace an attention to minutiæ, which is unnecessary, and therefore passed over here. Situate as man is in civilized life, there are numerous habits—dietetic and others—to which he is addicted from his very infancy, and which become so inveterate as to constitute second nature. These it is scarcely requisite to canvass.

It has been an interesting investigation with the *hygienist*,—as the French have not inappropriately termed the physician, who is engaged in inquiring into the influence of extrinsic and intrinsic agencies on man, and into the means best adapted for preventing the injurious effects of such agencies,—to determine upon the kind of management, calculated for developing the full powers of the system, or for screwing up the different functions to their full height. This is well exhibited by the experimental results of the system of TRAINING for athletic exercises, and especially for pedestrianism, and pugilism, which has long been made an object of special study, is practised as an art, by many persons out of the profession, and is guided by rules, and by experience not unworthy the attention of the physician.

It has, indeed, been properly remarked by a hygienic writer, that the advantages of the training system are not confined to pedestrians and pugilists; but that they extend to every man; and that were training generally introduced instead of medicine, for the prevention and cure of diseases, its beneficial consequences might promote happiness, and prolong life.

"Our health, vigour and activity," says one of the most experienced trainers and pedestrains—Captain Barclay—"must depend upon regimen, and exercise; or, in other words, upon the observance of those rules, which constitute the theory of the training process. It has been made a question, whether training produces a *lasting*, or only a *temporary* effect on the constitution. It is undeniable, that if a man be brought to a better condition,—if corpulency, and the impurities of his body disappear,—and if his wind and strength be improved, by any process whatever, his good state of health will continue until some derangement of his frame shall take place from accidental or natural causes. If he shall relapse into intemperance, or neglect the means of preserving his health, either by omitting to take the necessary exercise, or by indulging in debilitating propensities, he must expect such encroachments to be made on his constitution as must soon unhinge his system. But if he shall observe a different plan—the beneficial effects of the training process will remain until the gradual decay of his natural functions shall, in mature old age, intimate the approach of his dissolution."

Such views are certainly philosophical, and have been so regarded; and it has been suggested, that a similar plan might be adopted with considerable advantage to animate, and strengthen enfeebled constitutions—prevent gout—reduce corpulency—cure nervous and chronic weakness, hypochondriac, and bilious disorders, &c.—and to increase the enjoyment, as well as prolong the duration of feeble life, for which medicine, unassisted by diet and regimen, affords but trifling and transient relief. (Kitchener, *Op. cit.* p. 10.)

The cardinal rules, adopted in the system of training, are:—to go to bed early;—to rise early;—to take as much exercise as practicable in the open air, without inducing fatigue;—to eat and drink moderately of plain nutritious aliment; and especially to keep the mind occupied and serene.

In the work just cited, Dr. Kitchener has given a brief sketch of the usual method of training persons for athletic exercises, which he says has received the entire approbation of Mr. Jackson, teacher of sparring, and of several professors, and experienced amateurs. The alimentary canal is cleansed by a gentle emetic, followed by two or three mild purgatives, administered at intervals. They are directed to eat beef and mutton, rather *under* than *over* done— for reasons laid down in another chapter. (See page 276.) No seasoning or sauce is allowed; broiled meat is preferred to either roast or boiled; and stale bread or biscuit is enjoined. Neither veal, lamb, pork, fish, milk, butter, cheese, pudding, pastry, nor vegetables are permitted; chiefly because they are not considered to be as easily assimilated, or to furnish as much rich chyle as the diet selected. The animal food must not be salted; but the restriction to fresh meat is said not to be absolute.

If the athlete be a civic resident he is sent into the country;— the necessity of breathing a pure air, and the strictest temperance being uniformly and rigorously insisted upon by all trainers. Mild home-brewed ale is recommended for drink—about three pints per day, taken at breakfast, and dinner, and a little at supper,—not in draughts, but in small quantities, alternately with the solid food. They, who do not like beer, are allowed wine and water,—red wine being preferred to white, and not more than half a pint, or four or five common sized wine glasses being permitted after dinner, and none after supper. In no case are spirits, however diluted, permitted.

Eight hours' sleep are considered to be usually necessary; but this is properly regulated by the previous habits of the person. They, who require very active exercise, need a longer period of repose.

The breakfast consists of meat, and is taken at eight o'clock, and the dinner at two. Supper is not recommended, but they are allowed a little cold meat about eight o'clock, and take a walk after, between that time and ten, when they go to bed.

Captain Barclay, during his celebrated walk of 1,000 miles in 1,000 successive hours lived as follows.—He breakfasted after returning from his walk, at five in the morning. He ate a roasted fowl, and drank a pint of strong ale, and then took two cups of tea, with bread and butter. His lunch was at twelve; and it consisted, on alternate days, of beef-steaks and mutton chops,—of which he ate a considerable quantity. He dined at six, either on roast beef, or mutton chops,—his drink being porter and two or three glasses of wine; and he supped at eleven on cold fowl. He ate such vegetables as were in season, and the quantity of animal food he consumed daily was from five to six pounds.

The time which is found to be requisite for communicating the full powers by training, depends greatly upon the previous habits, and age of the individual. If in the vigour of life—between twenty and thirty-five—a month or two is generally found sufficient. "By this mode of proceeding, for two or three months," says Dr. Kitchener, (*Op. cit.* p. 17,) " the constitution of the human frame becomes greatly improved, and the courage proportionately increased: a person who was breathless, and panting on the least exertion, and had a certain share of those nervous and bilious complaints, which are occasionally the companions of all who reside in great cities, becomes enabled to run with ease and fleetness. The restorative process having proceeded with healthful regularity, every part of the constitution is effectively invigorated, and a man feels so conscious of the actual augmentation of all his powers, both bodily and mental, that he will undertake with alacrity a task, which, before, he shrank from encountering."

The great principles on which this practice is founded will be readily understood by a reference to the different chapters that compose this work.

---

There are certain customs, connected with the gastric functions, that cannot well be passed by, without a brief notice, especially as, by some, they are presumed to be of injurious tendency, whilst by others they are looked upon as not only harmless but salutary.

We allude particularly to those that consist in the use of TOBACCO, —an extraordinary plant, "which," as Dr. Paris has remarked, (In the Historical Introduction to his *Pharmacologia*,) notwithstanding its powers of fascination has suffered romantic vicissitudes in its fame and character: it has been successively opposed and commended by physicians—condemned and eulogized by priests and kings—and proscribed and protected by governments; whilst at length this insignificant production of a little island,* or an obscure district, has succeeded in diffusing itself through every climate, and in subjecting the inhabitants of every country to its dominion. The Arab cultivates it in the burning desert— the Laplander, and Esquimaux risk their lives to procure a refreshment so delicious in their wintry solitude;—the seaman, grant him but this luxury, and he will endure with cheerfulness every other privation, and defy the fury of the raging elements; and in the higher walks of civilized society, at the shrine of fashion, in the palace, and in the cottage, the fascinating influence of this singular plant commands an equal tribute of devotion and attachment."

The employment of tobacco prevailed on this continent long before its discovery by Europeans. It is, indeed, utterly impossible to form the slightest idea of the period when it was first introduced. Tradition does not afford us any clue. Humboldt asserts, that it has been cultivated from time immemorial by the natives on the Orinoco, and it was used all over the continent of South America at the time of the Spanish conquest.

Tobacco is said to have been first smoked in the presence of Europeans, in 1518, on the occasion of an interview between Grisalva—a Spaniard—and the casique of Tobasco or Tabaco; and it was noticed by Cortes in Yucatan in the following year. The first time it was sent to Europe was probably in 1559, by Her-

---

* It is not likely, by the way, that the plant derived its name from the island Tobago. The specific name *Tabacum*, as well as *Tabaco*, the name of a province of Yucatan, and *Tobago*—the island—were probably taken from *tabac*, the name of the instrument or reed which was used by the Americans in smoking the leaf. An old writer, Joshua Sylvester, sportively refers it to *Bacchus!*—

"*Tobacco*, as Τω Βακχω one would say,
To cup god *Bacchus* dedicated ay."

nandez de Toledo, when Jean Nicot was French ambassador at the court of Lisbon, who transmitted or carried either the seed, or the plant to Catharine de Medicis. From these circumstances it acquired the name *Herba Reginæ, Nicotiana,* and the *Embassador's Herb.* Very early, before 1589, the cardinal Santa Croce—returning from his nunciature in Portugal—took the tobacco along with him to Italy ; hence the herb was called *Santa Croce,* and the exploit was considered to shed as much lustre on the Santa Croce family as the deed of his progenitor in carrying back to Italy the wood of the true cross. The virtues, at that time hyperbolically ascribed to the plant, are enumerated in some Latin verses by Castor Duranti, of which the following version is given by M. des Maizeaux, in Bayle's *Dictionary,* v. 26. Lond. 1738.

> Nomine quo Sancte Crucis herba vocatur, ocellis,
> Subvenit, et sanat plagas, et vulnera jungit,
> &c. &c. &c.

> "The herb, which borrows Santa Croce's name,
> Sore eyes relieves, and healeth wounds ; the same
> Discusses the king's evil, and removes
> Cancers and boils ; a remedy it proves
> For burns and scalds, repels the nauseous itch,
> And straight recovers from convulsion fits.
> It cleanses, dries, binds up, and maketh warm :
> The head ache, tooth ache, colic, like a charm
> It easeth soon ; an ancient cough relieves,
> And to the reins, and milt, and stomach gives
> Quick riddance from the pains which each endures;
> Next the dire wounds of poisoned arrows cures ;
> All bruises heals, and when the gums are sore,
> It makes them sound, and healthy as before.
> Sleep it procures, our anxious sorrows lays,
> And with new flesh the naked bone arrays.
> No herb hath greater power to rectify
> All the disorders in the breast that lie,
> Or in the lungs. Herb of immortal fame !
> Which hither first by Santa Croce came,
> When he, (his time of nunciature expired)
> Back from the court of Portugal retired;
> Even as his predecessors, great and good,
> Brought home the cross, whose consecrated wood
> All Christendom now with its presence blesses ;
> And still the illustrious family possesses
> The name of Santa Croce, rightly given,
> Since they in all respects resemble Heaven,

Procure as much as mortal men can do,
The welfare of our souls, and bodies too."

It is not certain at what precise period tobacco was introduced into England, but the example of Sir Walter Raleigh, who was very fond of it, was soon followed, and to him must be assigned the *credit* of first causing its use to be general. The nauseating effects, which it induced,—with the waste of time, and the considerable expenditure of money, gave occasion to much opposition on the part of several of the rulers of Europe. In the *Counterblaste to Tobacco*, by King James the First, it is affirmed, that many persons expended as much as 500 pounds per annum in the purchase of the article;—a heavy sum in those days. "Tobacco, divine, rare, super-excellent Tobacco," says quaint old Burton,—"which goes far beyond all their panaceas, potable gold, and philosophers stones, a soverain remedy to all diseases. A good vomit, I confess, a vertuous herb, if it be well qualified, opportunely taken, and medicinally used; but as it is commonly abused by most men which take it as tinkers do ale, it is a plague, a mischief, a violent purger of goods, lands and health; hellish, divelish and damned Tobacco, the ruine and overthrowe of body and soul." (*Anatomy of Melancholy*, pt. 2, sec. 4, mem. 2, subsec. 2.)

At the latter end of the 16th century, its use appears to have extended to all classes. In the *Tobacco-Battered*, of Joshua Sylvester, we have the following apostrophe. (Cited in *Lond. Med. and Phys. Journal* for Dec. 1810, p. 445.)

"O Great Tobacco! greater than Great Can,
Great Turk, Great Tartar, or Great Tamerlane:
With Vultur's wings thou hast (and swifter yet
Than an Hungarian Ague, English Sweat)
Through all degrees flown far, nigh, up and down,
From Court to Cart; from Count to Country Clown,
Not scorning Scullions, Cobblers, Colliers,
Jakes-farmers, Fidlers, Ostlers, Oysterers,
Roagues, Gypsies, Players, Panders, Punks; and all
What common Scums in common Sewers fall.
For all as *Vassals*, at thy neck are bent,
And breathe by thee as their new *Element*.

So prevalent and injurious was its abuse, that Elizabeth published an edict against its indulgence. James imposed severe pecuniary fines to abolish its use, and Charles—his successor—continued them. "It had, however," says Dr. A. T. Thomson, (*Elements of Materia Medica and Therapeutics*, vol. ii p. 119,) "a royal opponent in James the First, who published a philippic against it,—the "Counterblaste to Tobacco," in which he remarks, that smoking is a custom " loathsome to the eye, hateful to the nose, harmeful to the braine, dangerous to the lungs; and, in the black, stinking fume thereof, nearest resembling the horrible Stygian smoake of the pit that is bottomless ;" (*Apophthegms of King James*, 1671,) a sentiment in which although some might accord, yet from which many would strongly dissent. The same monarch proposed as a banquet for the devil,—a loin of pork, and a poll of ling and mustard, with a pipe of tobacco for digestion: he endeavoured to abolish its use by a heavy penalty, and enacted that no planter in Virginia should cultivate more than one hundred pounds of it; but the advantage derived to his revenue from its importation soon produced the abolition of these restrictions. An edict had been previously published against its use in the time of Elizabeth, in which the reason for prohibiting it is stated to be—a fear lest Englishmen should become, like the barbarians from whom its use was derived;—" Anglorum corpora in barbarorum naturam degenerasse, quum iidem ac barbari delectentur." (*Annal. Eliz.* p. 143.) But it was not in England alone, that war was waged against this American herb: in the sixteenth century, (1590) Shah Abbas prohibited the use of tobacco in Persia; but, as the punishment was penal, many of his subjects, rather than discontinue smoking, fled to the mountains: in 1624, Urban VIII. excommunicated all snuff-takers who committed the heinous sin of taking a pinch in church: in 1653, all smokers in the Canton of Appenzel were cited before the council, and punished: in the year 34 of the same century, the Russians, whose peasantry now smoke all day long, were forbidden to smoke under the penalty of having the nose cut off; and Amurath VII. also rendered it a capital offence. In Russia, indeed, the animosity against the use of tobacco, in any form, was so great, that a particular tribunal was instituted for punishing smokers—the *Chambre au Tabac:* it was not abolished until the middle of the eighteenth century. So late as 1690, Innocent XII. excommunicated all who took snuff in St. Peter's church;

and in Constantinople, where the use of tobacco in every form is now as common almost as eating, every Turk who was found smoking was conducted in ridicule through the streets, with a pipe transfixed through his nose, and seated on an ass with his face towards the tail : one reason for which was, that it was supposed the use of tobacco rendered the men impotent; and certainly if taken in excess, such a result is likely to follow from its use. But like many other bad customs, tobacco triumphed over all its opponents; and it has become almost universal. Not only in Europe, but even in the islands of the Pacific, where it was introduced by Europeans, its use is carried to the most ridiculous excess. "In the Sandwich Islands," says Kotzebue, in the Narrative of his Voyage of Discovery, " it is so generally used, that children smoke before they learn to walk : and grown up people have carried the practice to such an excess, that they have fallen down senseless, and often died in consequence."

The use, or rather the abuse, of tobacco has so many disagreeable concomitants, that—independently of its real effects—numerous others, of a more questionable kind, have been ascribed to it.

It is certainly, when taken in the necessary quantity, a most virulent poison, belonging to the acro-narcotic class, or to those, that chiefly act on the nervous system, and on the lining membrane of the alimentary canal. Every part of the plant possesses activity, but the properties appear to reside in an acrid, alkaline principle, and an essential oil to which that principle adheres with great obstinacy. Its poisonous effects are exhibited to a slight degree in those who commence its use incautiously. It produces nausea, and often deadly sickness and vomiting, with vertigo, and sometimes somnolency; and these results supervene, even if the plant be merely applied to an abraded surface.

It has been a common remark, that they who are engaged in the manufacture of tobacco are exposed to numerous infirmities, produced by the deleterious influence of the narcotic exhalations from the plant; and Ramazzini asserts, that even the horses, employed in the tobacco mills, are most powerfully affected by the particles of tobacco. It is probable, that the mischief,—if any result,—is produced more by the small particles diffused in the air in one of the processes—that of snuff making—than from any narcotic influence of the plant; and hence we could comprehend that snuff-grinders might, like millers, glass-cutters, &c., be exposed to lung affections, owing to the fine particles entering the lungs during inspiration, and exciting obstructions in those organs. (Parent Duchatelet, *Annales d'Hygiène*, &c. p. 1.) Yet even the operation of snuff-making, it is asserted, is not positively unwholesome, in this or in any other manner. From a report, recently presented to the Minister of Public Works, of France, it appears, that the manufacture of tobacco is not only not deleterious, but that those engaged in it are less subject than others to the prevalent epidemics, and even to phthisis itself. M. Simeon, who states this as a fact, (*Annales d' Hygiène Publique*, Oct. 1843) is of opinion, that the exemption of the workmen from disease may be ascribed to the narcotic property of the tobacco; and is desirous of attracting the attention of the physician to the subject to determine whether advantage might not be taken of such a virtue—provided it be possessed by the plant—for the alleviation or prevention of disease. In the manufactories of snuff in France, in which 5,000 persons are employed, the workmen seem to become habituated to the atmosphere; to be neither liable to peculiar diseases, nor to disease generally, and to live, on an average, as long as other tradesmen. Yet the prejudice on this subject was at one time so strong, that it was declared to be necessary for public salubrity, that the manufactories of tobacco should be removed out of large towns, on account of their unhealthiness.

When tobacco is used, in any shape, to excess, it blunts the sensibility, not only of the organs with which it comes in contact, but of the whole nervous system; or it induces so great a susceptibility to impressions, that existence becomes painful.

*Snuffing* is perhaps the least injurious mode of employing it. In Russia and Persia, the penalty of death was formerly attached to the use of tobacco, in every form, except that of snuff, and for this the nose—the offending member—was cut off; yet we are told, that the Persians were so much attached to its use, that it was common for them to expatriate themselves when no longer permitted to indulge in it at home.

The prevalence of the habit in his time was thus satirized by Samuel Wesley.

> " To such a height with some is fashion grown,
> They feed their very nostrils with a spoon.

> One, and but one degree is wanting yet,
> To make our senseless luxury complete;
> Some choice regale, useless as snuff and dear,
> To feed the mazy windings of the ear."

Like other habits its use becomes "second nature," so that the greatest distress arises from its privation; and in the nervous individual the whole economy may be deranged from this cause. M. Mérat (Art. *Tabac,* in *Dictionnaire des Sciences Médicales*) has given a *ne plus ultra* case of this kind! "I recollect," says he, "about twenty years ago, while gathering simples in the forest of Fontainbleau, I met a man stretched on the ground, who seemed to me to be dead, but on approaching him he asked in a feeble voice if I had any snuff. On my replying in the negative, he sank back almost in a state of insensibility. He remained in this state until I brought a person to him, who gave him several pinches, after which he informed us, that he had set out on his journey that morning, supposing that he had his snuff-box along with him, but he soon found he had left it behind; that he had travelled as long as he was able, till at length, overcome by distress, he found it impossible to proceed farther, and without my timely aid he would certainly have perished." This we say is a *ne plus ultra* case. It is, however, inconceivable how much distress is experienced, when the habit is interrupted from any cause; unless by sickness, in which the desire for it often passes away for the time, but recurs on the restoration of health. Yet, during the suspension of its use in these cases, it has appeared to us, that many nervous symptoms have supervened, which could be fairly referred to that cause.

Snuff-taking, in excess, is apt to induce dyspepsia. The snuff passes down into the pharynx, and thence into the stomach, so that large quantities will occasionally be evacuated by vomiting; and it is not uncommon to find snuff in the matter expectorated by coughing;—the snuff and mucus distilling from the posterior nares, and producing cough by which they are ejected from the mouth.

One of the greatest inconveniences, resulting from snuffing, is its obtunding effects upon the olfactory nerves, which it renders totally unfit for the appreciation of the more delicate odours; whilst by closing up the tortuous passages through the anterior, and posterior nostrils, and the nasal cavities, it renders the voice disagreeably nasal, so that all public speakers should avoid its use to this extent. It has been, however, a favourite practice with some of the greatest ornaments of the stage, without producing any injury to the voice. With such it may be presumed, the use did not amount to an injurious abuse. When taken so as to affect the voice, not only is the nasal twang manifest, but, owing to the air of inspiration being drawn almost wholly through the mouth,—in consequence of the diminished size, or absolute occlusion of the nasal passages, a disagreeable kind of snoring accompanies inspiration.

*Smoking* was perhaps the earliest form in which tobacco was employed. It is practised in two ways—either with the cigar, or drawn through a pipe—the effects being essentially the same in both, although differing somewhat according to the strength, or character of the tobacco used.

When tobacco is smoked by those not habituated to it, it gently stimulates the pulmonary mucous membrane, and, by augmenting the mucous secretion, acts as an expectorant: in such it is apt to produce, even in a very small quantity, its peculiar narcotic effects;—nausea, vomiting, vertigo, general indisposition, &c. Tobacco contains two main active principles, a peculiar oily-like alkaloid, called *nicotina* or *nicotia;* and a camphoraceous volatile oil, termed *nicotianin, concrete volatile oil of tobacco,* and *tobacco camphor,* both of which act violently on the economy, but not in the same manner. The latter rises with the smoke, enters the bronchial tubes, and, through the medium of the nerves distributed to the pulmonary vessels, affects the circulating system; and if it be in large quantity, and the individual unaccustomed to its use, it may paralyze the heart, and render it totally unfit to persevere in its functions. Such has been the case where smoking has been indulged to excess.

As it is chiefly the nicotianin, which enters the lungs during smoking,—or rather, as the first and main effects are produced by it, the poisonous influence is not perhaps as powerfully exhibited as in chewing, where both the nicotianin and the nicotia must necessarily come in contact with the lining membrane of the mouth; but it is, in its results, a more cleanly and less offensive form of employing the herb, and is therefore more followed by the better classes in many countries. It does not affect the breath, or the teeth so much as chewing, but still sufficiently to require, that proper attention should be paid to them, and to the interior of the mouth. " As the smoker," says M. Deslandes, (*Manuel d' Hygiène*, p. 423,) " makes a chimney of his mouth, his teeth become black, and fuliginous; and his breath acquires a detestable odour. Hence, cleanliness, and the preservation of the teeth require, that the mouth should be washed after smoking."

*Chewing* is perhaps the most offensive form in which tobacco is employed, inasmuch as it is liable to both moral and physical objections; whilst the discharge of the salivary fluid—so useful an agent in digestion—cannot fail to enter occasionally into the causation of dyspepsia.

Tobacco, in this mode of employment, produces the same effects upon the system as smoking; and, when indulged to excess, is equally prejudicial: except, however, in such cases it is doubtful whether it be very pernicious. On commencing its use, the brain and nervous system are deranged by it, but these effects soon disappear, and when the pipe or the *quid* is used in moderation, no indisposition is experienced, and the system becomes habituated to its employment. When, however, indulgence becomes abuse, the nerves become unstrung:—stupor; indisposition to mental or corporeal exertion; tremors; nausea; and the whole tribe of dyspeptic complaints supervene, and the victim of intemperate indulgence finds his existence burdensome to himself, as well as to those around him. Within the last few years, the Author has met with more than one individual in the unhappy condition just depicted,—a condition resembling greatly the affection to which the habitual drunkard is liable, when the quantity of his wonted stimulus is withdrawn.

A common notion prevails, that the use of tobacco, by chewing or smoking, prevents the impression of miasmata—animal as well as terrestrial—but there does not appear to be much foundation for the belief. The impression, made by these morbific agents, is not upon the nervous expansions of the nose and mouth that are concerned in sensation. They probably enter the blood-vessels by traversing the mucous membrane of the air passages, and produce their effect upon the nervous system, either through the nervous ramifications distributed to the blood-vessels, or upon the great nervous centres through the medium of the circulation. In neither way could tobacco probably act as a prophylactic; and no harm would perhaps arise were its use to be altogether abandoned. A few months before Dr. Franklin's death, he declared to one of his friends, that he had never used tobacco in the course of his long life, and that he was disposed to think that there was not much advantage to be derived from it, for he had never known a man that used it, who advised him to follow his example. (*American Quarterly Review*, vol. ix p. 136.)

The following Table exhibits the quantity of tobacco exported to different countries from the United States during the years 1837, 1838, 1839 and 1840. (*American Almanac*, for 1842.)

| Years. | England. | France. | Holland. | Germany. | To all other countries. | Total. |
|---|---|---|---|---|---|---|
|  | hhds. | hhds. | hhds. | hhds. | hhds. |  |
| 1837 | 20.723 | 9.110 | 22.739 | 28.863 | 18.797 | 100.232 |
| 1838 | 24.312 | 15.511 | 17.558 | 25.571 | 17.641 | 100.593 |
| 1839 | 30.068 | 9.574 | 12.273 | 14.303 | 12.777 | 78.995 |
| 1840 | 26.255 | 15.640 | 29.534 | 25.649 | 22.406 | 119.484 |

# CHAPTER III.

### CLOTHING.

Substances used for clothing—wool—silk—hair—down, &c.—influence of the colour, shape, pressure, &c. of vestments—of individual vestments—particular applications, and precautions—adaptation of clothing to temperature, &c.

We have elsewhere remarked, that the human body, in our climates, and indeed we may say in every climate—a few days in the summer excepted—is exhaling caloric. During the winter season, in temperate climates, the expenditure is of course great, and hence clothing is required, partly for the purpose of preserving our own heat in proximity with the body, and partly to prevent the impressions of extraneous heat, or cold,—particularly of the latter.

The substances, that are used for clothing—the *Res vestiariæ*—are animal or vegetable. The animal matters are wool, silk, and hair, or down; the vegetable—linen and cotton chiefly.

The best clothing to protect us from external heat or cold is one that is a bad conductor of caloric; in other words, one that does not permit the matter of heat to pass readily through it. Substances, whose temperature is below that of the human body, and which conduct heat rapidly, appear to us colder than such as transmit it more imperfectly. Thus, a piece of iron, and a woollen night-cap may be at the same temperature, as indicated by the thermometer, yet the iron feels much the colder of the two, because it conducts the caloric it receives from us rapidly into its interior, and then abstracts more from us; whilst the outer portions of the woollen night-cap receive their charge of caloric from us, but they conduct it so slowly into the interior, that less is abstracted, and accordingly the night-cap feels to us the warmer article of the two.

From this it is manifest, that the article of clothing, which is the worst conductor of caloric, or which refuses most to receive, and to transmit the matter of heat, is the warmest; because the caloric, given off by our bodies, is in this way retained at the surface of the skin. This is the case with woollen articles. For the same reasons, it can be readily conceived, that if the external temperature be greater than that of the human body, these same articles of clothing will be adapted for preventing the intrusion of caloric. Accordingly, a woollen night-cap would protect us better from the scorching rays of the sun than an iron helmet of equal thickness, especially if blackened. If polished, the calorific rays would be mainly reflected, but if obscured by black paint,—owing to the more ready transmission, the caloric would pass through in such quantity as to scorch the head, whilst the interior of the night-cap might be scarcely hotter than the body. We can hence understand, why the Spaniard, and the Oriental should throw their woollen mantles over them, when they have to expose themselves to the rays of a vertical sun.

The mode, in which stuffs are woven, has some effect in rendering them better or worse conductors of caloric. Those, whose tissue is loose and porous, and includes air in its interstices, and which might seem, in the first instance, well adapted for permitting the escape of caloric, are actually worse conductors than closer stuffs, although there may be the same quantity of material in each;—a fact, which was proved by Count Rumford. This is owing to air being a bad conductor of caloric, and hence we can understand, why furs, long napped woollens, &c. are so advantageously used as clothing in the colder regions of the globe; and why carded wool, or cotton, inclosed in silk or calico, forms an article of clothing, or a bed covering commonly called a "comfort," which will retain much more heat around the body, than a closer tissue of the like weight, made of the same materials. It will be understood, also, that a freshly carded blanket is much warmer than one, which has been so long used, that the nap is worn off.

There is another circumstance, which interferes with the warmth of cloth-stuffs. This is the greater or less facility with which they imbibe, or give off moisture. Linen, for example, imbibes the moisture from the body with great rapidity, and parts with it readily. It, consequently, is cooler than cotton, or woollen, which imbibe moisture more slowly; give it off more tardily; and can contain a considerable quantity of moisture without its being sensible.

A knowledge of these properties will guide us in the choice of the materials for clothing, adapted to different climates, seasons, sexes, ages, &c.

Cloths, formed of hemp or linen, are good conductors of caloric, and therefore cool. They readily imbibe, and part with humidity, and when wet they are better conductors of caloric than when dry. They are, therefore, not well adapted for cool climates, and seasons. Cotton is a worse conductor of caloric, and absorbs and retains a portion of the perspiration. It is, consequently, a warmer clothing; whilst wool is, as we have seen, a very bad conductor of caloric, and never allows the matter of perspiration to escape to such an extent as to cause a powerful sensation of cold.

M. Londe (*Nouveaux Elémens d' Hygiène*, vol. ii. p. 356) asserts, that the use of woollen next the skin is one of the most precious means, that therapeutics possesses. His remarks might have been extended, with much propriety, to hygiène. In the cold and temperate regions of the globe, it forms one of the best protections to the body, both against the impression of cold, and the vicissitudes to which certain countries are liable. " Flannel next the skin," says Sir Geo. Lefevre (*Thermal Comfort*, Amer. edit., p. 32. New York, 1844,) "in the shape of waistcoat and drawers, should be worn at all times in the autumn and winter, and far into the spring. There are several kinds of fleecy hosiery, as there are of great-coats, and these may be adapted to different seasons. The lighter kind should be worn in the autumn and spring, and the thicker flannel in winter. As regards the chest, a very light kind of woollen waistcoat should not be dispensed with even in the dog-days; a cotton jacket may be substituted in very hot weather, but something more than the common shirt is necessary to absorb the moisture generated by heat, which, remaining unabsorbed upon the cooling of the body, generates cold by evaporation, particularly upon exposure to a draft of air, and this is prejudicial to tender lungs." "It is a habit," he adds, "with many to wear their flannels in bed, which is by no means advisable, unless under circumstances where chamber warmth cannot be commanded, and even then it is better to heap additional covers on the bed than to wear flannel next the skin at night. It loses half its daily advantage by this nocturnal use, and unless where there is confirmed disease and risk of accession of cold from partial removal of the bed-clothes during sleep, it should always be dispensed with. The body rises more refreshed and more invigorated from having been enveloped with linen than when cased in flannel for so many hours successively. It is a more comfortable sensation to sponge the chest with vinegar and water, and then to put on a dry flannel jacket, than to take a damp one off and put it on again, for there is no class whose means are ample enough to command a large wardrobe or permit of daily changes. It is of more importance to keep the feet warm; and woollen socks should be worn during the night, when there is a tendency to cold feet in the severer seasons. Invalids often complain of being kept awake and suffering actual pain from cold feet, and nothing can be more injurious than the effect of such abstraction of warmth to delicate people. Warm socks or full length woollen stockings should be always worn in such cases. If there is no tendency to cold feet, they may be dispensed with, and advantageously; for it is conducive to good health, that the body should, during sleep, be free from all unnecessary confinement in shape of tight clothing or bandages."

The Author has worn a flannel jacket for many years through the summer, and does not think, that he has suffered more from heat than when he was accustomed to dispense with it during that season; whilst the inconveniences, resulting from the upper cotton, or woollen clothes becoming soaked with the perspiration have been avoided. He has thought, too, that with many infants, under two years of age, the tendency to bowel affections, during the summer and autumnal months, has been obviated by having a flannel bandage next the skin. M. Londe has a strange notion, that it is the source of the greater part of human infirmities—at least of all those, for the cure of which it is the most potent agent —and chiefly because it tends "to render us," he affirms, "susceptible, impressible and accessible to the slightest causes of disease;" but the objection appears to us to be equally applicable to any, and every variety of, clothing. It is owing to our clothing, and to the use of flannel in particular, that we can bear, with comparative impunity, the irregular and unlooked for vicissitudes,—thermometrical as well as hygrometrical,—to which we are constantly subjected. M. Londe's dread, indeed, of the *flanelle Angloise* must be regarded as almost morbid. To an inhabitant of the United States, accustomed as many are, and as all ought to be, to use it during the colder seasons, the following cautions appear ludicrous. " I repeat," says he, " and I cannot too often repeat,—be careful not to abuse this valuable agent. How many blisters, cauteries, and moxas may it not prevent in the long run, if we are not prematurely prodigal of it; and to what an ' arsenal' of these agents shall we not be compelled to have recourse, and often in vain, for having prematurely, and unnecessarily used a flannel jacket."

By those who believe that endemic, epidemic, and even contagious influences are exerted on the skin, and thence on the rest of the system, it has been strongly advised to case the frame in flannel, and warm clothing. It has even been attempted to show, that the ancient Romans suffered less from malarious disease, chiefly because they were always enveloped in warm woollen dresses. Brocchi ascribes the immunity of the sheep, and cattle, which feed night and day in the Campagna di Roma, to the protection afforded them by their wool; and Patissier affirms, that warm woollen clothing has been found effectual in preserving the health of labourers, digging and excavating drains, and canals in marshy grounds, where, previous to the employment of these precautions, the mortality from fever was very considerable; (A. Combe, *Principles of Physiology*, &c.—Amer. edit. p. 55.) but although these facts exhibit the utility of such clothing, in strengthening the resistance of the body against the usual effects of malarious and other influences, they by no means establish, that the skin is the channel, through which diseases, produced by a specific poison, affect the frame.

The utility of wearing flannel next the skin—as a hygienic measure—in warm, as well as in cold climates, is said to be so well understood, that in the British army, and navy, the practice is strongly insisted upon. Dr. Combe asserts, that Captain Murray, late of her Britannic majesty's ship Valorous, told him, that he was so strongly impressed, from former experience, with a sense of the efficacy of the protection, afforded by the constant use of flannel next the skin, that when, on his arrival in England, in December, 1823, after two years' service amidst the icebergs of the coast of Labrador, the ship was ordered to sail immediately for the West Indies, he ordered the purser to draw two extra flannel shirts, and pairs of draws for each man, and instituted a regular daily inspection, to see that they were worn. These precautions are stated to have been followed by the most happy results. He proceeded to his station with a crew of one hundred and fifty men; visited almost every island in the West Indies, and many of the ports on the Gulf of Mexico; and, notwithstanding the sudden transition from extreme climates, returned to England without the loss of a single man, or having any sick on board on his arrival. In the letter, in which Captain Murray communicates these facts to Dr. Combe, he adds, that every precaution was used, by lighting stoves between decks, and scrubbing with hot sand, to insure the most thorough dryness, and every means put in practice to promote cheerfulness among the men. When in command of the Recruit gun brig, which lay about nine weeks at Vera Cruz, the same means preserved the health of his crew, when the other ships of war, anchored around him, lost from twenty to fifty men each. "That the superior health," says Dr. Combe, (*Ibid.* p. 72,) "enjoyed by the crew of the Valorous, was attributed chiefly to the means employed by their humane, and intelligent commander, is shown by the analogy of the Recruit: for although constant communication was kept up between the latter, and the other ships in which sickness prevailed, and all were exposed to the same external causes of disease, yet no case of sickness occurred on board the Recruit. Facts like these are truly instructive, by proving how far man possesses the power of protecting himself from injury, when he has received necessary instruction, and chooses to adapt his conduct to his situation."

The aged and the infirm are particularly benefited by the use of flannel. To the rheumatic it is almost indispensable, as well as to those, who are liable to catarrh, or are predisposed to serious pulmonary disease. Such persons ought to be literally cased in flannel, as soon as the weather is so cold, as to be uncomfortable to them.

The first application of flannel to the skin often excites almost insupportable irritation, but this generally goes off in a short time,

Should the itching be intolerable, cotton or linen may be placed next the skin, and flannel over it, but this is by no means an equivalent.

*Silk is a bad conductor of caloric, but it is scarcely ever applied next the skin, except in the case of stockings, and very generally cotton stockings are placed under. It is an excellent envelope, where it is desirable to augment the thickness of vestments without adding much to their weight; as where carded, or batted, cotton is placed between pieces of silk.

Lastly :—Furs—peltry in general—are the warmest clothing materials of all, when put next the skin; but, as they are frequently used, they are inservient rather to ornament than warmth. In northern countries, they are universally worn with the latter view.

They who are familiar with the laws of the radiation and conduction of luminous heat will be aware that they are much influenced by the colour of clothing. White colours reflect the calorific rays, which are absorbed by the black. Franklin, with his ordinary penetration, and ingenuity, exhibited this, by placing pieces of cloth of different colours on snow, in the sun. Underneath the white cloth no snow was melted; under the black a considerable quantity. The colours, used in his experiments, were black, deep blue, lighter blue, green, purple, red, yellow, white, and othe colours, or shades of colour. In a few hours, the black had sunk so much as to be out of the reach of the sun's rays; the dark blue almost as low; the lighter blue not quite so much as the dark; and the other shades of colour less as their tint was lighter; while the white cloth remained on the surface of the snow. An experiment—similar to Franklin's but with coloured metals—was made by Sir Humphry Davy. He took six pieces of copper, (each an inch square, and two lines thick,) of equal weight and density, and coloured one of the surfaces white, one yellow, one red, one green, one blue, and one black. On the centre of the under surfaces was placed a portion of a mixture of oil and wax, which became fluid at 76°. The plates were then attached to a board painted white, and the coloured surfaces of all the pieces equally exposed to the direct rays of the sun. The result was, that the cerate on the black plate first began to melt; then that on the blue; next the green, and red; and lastly the yellow. The square, coated with white, was scarcely affected by the heat, although the black had completely melted.

Some experiments performed by Dr. Stark, of Edinburgh, (*Edinburgh Philosophical Journal*, for July, 1834,) strikingly agree with those referred to above, although instituted on bodies of very different qualities. Various experiments, instituted by the Author's friend, Professor A. D. Bache, (*Journal of the Franklin Institute* for Nov. 1835, p. 291) seem to show, however, that the supposed influence of colour on the absorption and radiation of non-luminous heat remains to be demonstrated; and lead to the inference, that provided the person be not exposed to the sun, the particular colour of the clothing is not of real importance. In the transmission, however, of luminous heat, it will be manifest, that white is least adapted. When we are exposed to the direct rays of the sun, the external temperature being so much higher than that of the body, no caloric can escape from us, but we experience no inconvenience from this cause, compared with what would result from the heat of the sun's rays, provided the colour were such as to readily allow of their passage:—hence the colour of white is in such case cooler than black. We can thus understand, that owing to the greater absorbing power of the skin of the dark races, they may suffer less from excessive solar heat than the white, and this is, perhaps, the main use of the rete mucosum or black pigment. To ascertain, whether such were the fact, Sir Edward Home (*Lectures on Comparative Anatomy*, iii. 217, Lond. 1823) made the following experiment. He exposed the back of his hand to the sun at 12 o'clock with a thermometer attached to it, another thermometer being placed upon a table with the same exposure. The temperature indicated by that on his hand, was 90°; by the other 102°. In forty-five minutes, blisters arose, and coagulable lymph was thrown out. The pain was very severe. In a second experiment, he exposed his face, eyelids, and the back of his hand to water heated to 120°; in a few minutes, they became painful, and when the heat was farther increased, he was unable to bear it; but no blisters were produced. In a third experiment, he exposed the backs of both hands, with a thermometer upon each, to the sun's rays. The one hand was uncovered; the other had a covering of black cloth, under which the ball of the thermometer was placed. After ten mimutes, the degree of heat of each thermometer, and the appearance of the skin were examined. This was repeated at three different times. The first time the thermometer under the cloth stood at 91°, the other thermometer at 85°; the second time they indicated respectively 94° and 91°; and the third time 106° and 98°. In every one of these trials, the skin that was uncovered was scorched, whilst the other had not suffered in the slightest degree. From all his experiments, Sir Everard concludes, that the power of the sun's rays to scorch the skin of animals is destroyed when applied to a black surface; although the absolute heat, in consequence of the absorption of the rays, is greater.

There is another point, connected with the colour of clothes, which is not without its hygienic importance.

The sense of smell sufficiently indicates, that when pieces of cloth, of different colours, are exposed to the odorous particles, emanating from bodies, some absorb a larger amount of odours than others; but no accurate comparative deductions could be formed from the evidence furnished by this sense. Dr. Stark (*Loc. citat.*) has ingeniously subjected the vapour of camphor to different coloured substances, and has afforded evidence of the particular attraction of colour for odours, resting on ocular, as well as on mathematical demonstration; from which it would appear, that the darkest colours—as black and dark blue—absorb twice as much as white; and he infers, that in times of contagious diseases black is the worst colour that could be worn. "If it be thus certain," he remarks, "that odorous emanations have not only a particular affinity for different substances, but that the colour of these substances materially affects their absorbing, or radiating quality, the knowledge of these facts may afford useful hints for the preservation of the general health, during the prevalence of contagious diseases. From their minute division, and vast range of action, latent poisonous exhalations or effluvia, inappreciable by the balance, may no doubt exist to a dangerous extent, without being evident to the sense of smell. But in most cases it will be found that, when contagious diseases prevail to such extent, the emanations from the sick will, if attended to, give the surest indications of the contamination of the surrounding air. Besides, even if we allow, that infectious emanations have no necessary connexion with odours, the experiments will afford the strongest possible presumption, that the emanations of an infectious nature in common with odours, vapours, and emanations generally, are emitted on the one hand, and on the other received, according to the same general laws:"—and he concludes:—" Next, therefore, to keeping the walls of hospitals, prisons, or apartments occupied by a number of individuals, of a white colour, I should suggest that the bedsteads, tables, seats, &c. should be painted white, and that the dresses of the nurses and hospital attendants should be of a light colour. A regulation of this kind would possess the double advantage of enabling cleanliness to be enforced, at the same time that it presented the least absorbent surface to the emanations of disease. On the same principle it would appear that physicians and others, by dressing in *black*, have unluckily chosen the colour of all others most absorbent of odorous and other exhalations, and of course the most dangerous to themselves and patients. Facts have been mentioned, which make it next to certain, that contagious diseases may be communicated to a third person through the medium of one who has been exposed to contagion, but himself not affected; and in fact the circumstance of infectious effluvia being capable of being carried by medical men from one patient to another, I should conceive one of the means by which such diseases are propagatad in the ill-ventilated and dirty habitations of the poor exposed to their influence. Even in my own very limited experience, I think I have observed some melancholy instances of the effect of *black dress* in absorbing the hurtful emanations of fever patients in a public hospital; and many facts are incidentally noticed by medical writers and referred to other causes, which I should not hesitate to ascribe chiefly to exposure of this nature. Not to mention individual cases, in the sessions held at Oxford in July, 1577, there arose amidst the people such a damp that almost all were smothered. Lord Bacon attributes this effect to the smell of the jail, where the prisoners had been close and nastily kept; and mentions it having occurred twice or thrice in his time, when both the judges that sat upon jail, and numbers of those who attended the business, or were present sickened and died. A similar occurrence, related by Sir John Pringle, happened at the Old Bailey sessions in 1750, when four of the judges were attacked and died, together with two other of the counsel, one of the under sheriffs, several of the jury, and others, to the amount of about forty in the whole. My explanation of the peculiar fatality of these emanations to the judges, counsel, and jurors, was the peculiar attraction of their official black for the putrid effluvium, as Sir John calls it; and the escape of two of the judges who sat on one side of the Lord Mayor, to the current of air that was in the room not sending the baneful odours in their direction.

Even if it be admitted, that certain of the deductions of Dr. Stark may be questioned, there can, then, be no doubt of the greater attraction of some colours than of others for odorous, and probably for miasmatic, emanations.

The shape of clothing has likewise its influence on the economy. Clothes, that are made very large, and permit the air contained within them to be easily renewed, are better adapted for warm seasons and climates, than those that are narrower and closer, and prevent the ready escape of the air they contain, which is of course raised to the temperature of the body. The latter are to be preferred in cold climates and seasons. The Turks, Persians, &c., afford us examples of the first kind of clothing; the northern Europeans, and the Esquimaux, of the latter: indeed, the clothes of the greater part of European nations are intended to keep off cold, and are, therefore, made upon the latter principle. Independently, however, of temperature, the shape of clothing has an effect by the greater or less pressure exerted by it on certain parts;—according as the course of the circulating fluids is impeded, as by the cravat or stock when too tightly applied;—or according as respiration and digestion are retarded by articles, that prevent the due expansion of the thoracic, and abdominal cavities—as by tight corsets. The injury here, however, is produced by too great pressure. A gentle pressure, especially in the case of those whose abdomen is pendulous, favours the functions of the viscera and ,facilitates digestion. At other times, compression is employed with the view of aiding the action of organs, as where a bandage is put round the loins to admit of greater muscular exertion. Whenever a considerable effort is required, the force is largely concentrated in the lumbar muscles; the pelvis is the fixed point—the centre of action—and the application of a bandage around the loins acts much like the aponeuroses, that surround muscles, and prevent the displacement of their fasciculi, during energetic contraction.

Lastly,—the effect of any kind of clothing can only be exerted upon the part to which it is applied. Most articles of clothing leave certain parts of the body uncovered, and whether this be favourable to health or not becomes a matter of question. In this, however, as in every analogous case, we are greatly influenced by habit; and the danger usually arises from not rigidly adhering to custom; that is, from occasionally covering a part, and at others leaving it exposed, without due cause.

After these general observations, it will not be necessary to dwell long on individual vestments. The flannel jacket—and, indeed, every vestment, which comes in contact with the skin—should be changed before it becomes largely imbued with the sebaceous matter, that constantly exudes from it. Twice a week, under ordinary circumstances, may be sufficient; and once a week is perhaps as frequent as is customary. The neck of the ordinary shirt or chemise—whether it be made of linen or cotton—should be so wide as not to press upon the external jugular veins, and thus retard the return of blood from the head, whilst its passage to the brain by the deep seated arteries is unimpeded. Cerebral congestion, and apoplexy, may be produced by such compression. The cravat —an article of dress peculiar to the moderns—requires the observance of the same cautions. It is still discarded by people of different climates—the Orientals, Poles, Kalmucks, and various Tartar tribes—but is largely used in Europe, and on this continent. It was first introduced into France in 1660, by a regiment of Croats, and was hence called a 'croate,' afterwards a 'cravat'. In the first instance, the cravat was formed of silk, muslin, or cotton, but it has now almost given place to the stock. When this is very firm, and tightly buckled on, it interferes so much with the circulation as to render the face suffused and bloated; and the retardation of the circulation is, at times, to such an extent as to cause hemorrhage from the nose, and occasionally turgescence of, or effusion of blood from, the encephalic vessels, preceded by heaviness, vertigo, tinnitus aurium, &c., especially if the effects of compression be favoured by stooping, which facilitates the flow of blood to the head, whilst it impedes its return; or if the head be suddenly turned round, so as to augment the pressure on the vessels of the neck.

Besides these inconveniences, M. Londe remarks, that he has known the constriction of the cravat occasion tumefaction of the maxillary glands in many youths; and Baron Percy has seen the military stock, ordered by an ignorant officer for the purpose of giving the appearance of *embonpoint*, cause ulcerations, callosities, hoarseness, and malposition of the lower jaw.

There is another point, connected with the cravat or stock, which is of hygienic moment. Unless great care is taken to keep the neck covered, serious affections are apt to result;—especially if the cravat or stock be taken off when the person is much heated. A regiment of infantry, according to Baron Percy, being on their march, in hot and stormy weather, the soldiers became heated, and out of breath. The Colonel permitted them to take off their stocks. Soon afterwards, they entered a gorge of the Vosges, exposed to the north-west wind, without covering the neck. On the following day, seventy-three soldiers were sent to the hospital,—the greater part attacked with inflammatory sore throat; and, in a few days, more than three hundred others were taken sick, apparently from the same exposure.

In singing or declaiming, the cravat should be loose, as well as during sleep. In the last case, indeed, it had better be removed, as injurious pressure can scarcely be prevented, unless it is made of very soft materials.

The cincture or girdle is used by very fat individuals,—in whom the weight of fat prevents the abdominal muscles from giving due support to the viscera, and thus occasions imperfect digestion. It is employed, likewise, by such as have to exert great muscular effort, for the purpose of supporting the sacro-lumbar muscles, as already mentioned. The surgeon, and the accoucheur, prescribe it to give the same support, whenever any large evacuation has taken place from the cavity of the abdomen; but it is obvious, that, if too tightly girded, it may interfere with the functions both of the thoracic and abdominal viscera, and may favour the production of hernia in such as are predisposed to it.

Stockings are of comparatively modern introduction. They were unknown to the ancients. Custom has rendered them indispensable to the adult; and in many countries, where they are worn in after life, they are dispensed with in childhood. There is a singular sympathy between the state of the cutaneous functions of the feet and of other parts. Every one is aware of the danger of exposing the feet to cold and moisture; and of the numerous ailments, that are apt to follow it. The knowledge of this physiological fact should induce great attention to those parts of the body in unusual atmospheric vicissitudes. In infancy, many a child is preserved from serious disease by the employment of the simple precaution of keeping the feet warm and dry; and there are but few adults, who would not suffer by aberrations from such precautions. They, who are liable to attacks of rheumatism, or to catarrh, should be especially careful on this head; and, whenever the temperature is such as to appear to them to require it, they should put on their woollen hosiery.

The invention of garters necessarily followed that of stockings. The only inconveniences, likely to result from them, is when they are constantly worn too tight. They then compress the superficial veins of the leg, and may excite varices. The best kind of garter is the elastic; and less injurious compression is exerted when it is worn above, than below, the knee.

With regard to the ordinary vestments; pantaloons, trowsers, breeches, waistcoats, coats, mantles, robes, &c. it is only necessary to say, that they should not exert any partial, or injurious compression. It is hardly requisite to lay down rules for the use of an additional coat. The feelings are the best guides in these cases, and no one should neglect their monitions. Dr. Kitchener asserts, that the desire of appearing young and hearty often prevents old men from wearing great coats, and other defences against the vicissitudes of the weather; but that after the age of forty, when the renovating powers of our machinery decline rapidly, all avoidable exposures to cold, &c. are acts of extreme folly. "Although the want of warm clothing," says Dr. Edwards, (*On Physical Agents*, &c. p. 267,) " is actually felt, it is often declined from a wish to reserve it for an advanced age. But it frequently happens, that this very precaution is the cause of preventing that age from being attained."

Shoes and boots should be made so large as not to induce unequal and undue pressure, which is the great cause of corns and bunyons. The material of the upper part should be soft, for the like reason. Clogs are worn in many countries, when the person is out of doors, to keep the feet dry; but in this country over-shoes are more used. These are generally made of elastic gum. They should only be worn out of doors: otherwise, they cease to have any protective influence; and, moreover, they prevent the escape of the moisture from the feet themselves, and may hence be injurious without such precaution.

Braces or supports for the trowsers have been much objected to. It has been said, that, by passing over the shoulders, they interfere with the action of respiration; and one writer has asserted that they favour hernia. These objections seem to be altogether gratuitous. It is impossible, that they could lay the foundation for hernia more than—or as much as—the tight waistband, for which they were substituted.

There is one article of female apparel to which we must refer, as occasionally productive of mischief, and therefore properly stigmatized by writers on hygiène. We allude to the corset, which was doubtless introduced for the purpose of displaying the general contour, and preventing undue compression, and displacement by the more external articles of clothing. It has, however, been much abused,—being occasionally applied so tight as to force the development of organs from the parts which it compresses towards the upper and lower portions of the trunk; to interfere with respiration and digestion; and at times to press so injuriously upon the false pelvis—the expanded ilia—as to interfere with the safety of parturition: the proper action of the different muscles is cramped, and the gait becomes stiff, awkward, and unnatural. The late Dr. Godman—who wrote an essay " on tight lacing," which is contained in the volume of " Essays," published since his decease—has recommended the following plain, and judicious general rules regarding the use of this fashionable article of apparel. 1st. Corsets should be made of smooth, soft, elastic materials. 2dly. They should be accurately fitted, and modified to suit the peculiarities of figure of each wearer. 3dly. No other stiffening should be used but that of quilting or padding; the bones, steel, &c. should be left to the deformed or diseased, for whom they were originally intended. 4thly. Corsets should never be drawn so tight as to impede regular natural breathing,—as under all circumstances, the improvement of figure is insufficient to compensate for the air of awkward restraint caused by such lacing. 5thly. They should never be worn, either loosely or tightly, during the hours appropriated to sleep, as by impeding respiration, and accumulating the heat of the system improperly, they invariably injure. 6thly. The corset for young persons should be of the simplest character, and worn in the lightest and easiest manner, allowing their lungs full play, and giving the form its full opportunity for expansion.

A few remarks are necessary regarding particular applications, and precautions. The ridiculous custom of swathing infants, or of bandaging them from head to foot, is now almost abolished;—perhaps wholly so in this country. M. Londe refers to a case, in France, which he himself witnessed, and the cause for which, according to the father, was the fear lest, without swathing, the infant might break its back (*casser les reins*.) The rule, now adopted with children, is—to clothe them sufficiently to protect them from cold; to have the different vestments made in such a manner as to exert no constriction, but, on the contrary, to allow of the free use of the extremities; and, at an early age especially—and, indeed, always—to change them as soon as they are imbued with moisture; for nothing is more prejudicial than to permit wet clothes to dry upon the body. The attention to sufficient clothing is especially necessary soon after birth, when the powers of calorification are not as completely established as they are subsequently. Many an infant perishes from the attempts to harden it by exposing it too freely to a cold temperature before it is capable of resisting the depressing influence.

Of the necessity for those advanced in life—in their second childhood—to take due care of themselves, as respects additional clothing, enough has already been said. The same general precautions, too, that apply to man may be transferred to the female; but there are particular circumstances in which she is placed, that demand special cares, and attention.

It need hardly be said, that if firm, and tightly laced corsets are injurious to the unimpregnated female, they must be still more so during pregnancy. A certain degree of support is neccessary for the abdomen, but the busk and the whalebone had better be avoided, notwithstanding it is the custom, with females in Great Britain, to wear them through the whole term of utero-gestation.

It will be equally obvious, that if tight garters be prejudicial at other times, they must be yet more so in this condition, when the return of blood by the abdominal veins, which communicate with those of the lower extremities, is impeded by the pressure of the gravid uterus. For some time after delivery, a bandage ought to be applied to the abdomen to compensate, in some degree, for the loss of that compression of the viscera, which is produced in the previous months by the uterus, and its contents.

From what has been already remarked, it is not requisite to dwell on the following general precautions, the importance of which is obvious. Wet clothes should not be suffered to dry slowly on the body, especially by exposure to a current of air, which gives occasion to rapid evaporation, and consequent refrigeration. In all such cases, dry clothing should be substituted, and the skin be well dried, and rubbed; or if this be impracticable, the wet garments had better be dried on the body by artificial heat. If we are compelled to be exposed to a draught of air, especially when heated, as where the wind enters through a broken window, or through some crevice, the part with which the air comes in contact should be carefully covered. We could not *à priori* suppose, that any serious mischief could result from so trifling an exposure; but experience has sufficiently shown, that such is frequently the case; and that there is greater danger where the capillary action of a small portion of the body is irregularly modified, than when the same morbific agent is directed over an extensive surface, or over the whole of the body. This fact has given occasion to a proverbial remark with the Spaniards, which may be thus rendered:—

> "If cold wind reach you through a hole,
> Go make your will, and mind your soul."

The invalid must be especially careful to suit the quantity and quality of his clothes to the temperature, and not to quit his winter clothing too soon. It was a cautious saying of the distinguished Boerhaave, that we ought to put off our winter's clothing on midsummer's day; and put it on again the day after. It is impossible to indicate any fixed period of the year when the change should be accomplished, but considerable caution is required on the part of every one, and especially of those, that are liable to pulmonary, abdominal, or neuralgic affections. It is incumbent, likewise, on all to be careful, that the clean clothing is always well aired. Many have lost their lives by an inattention to this circumstance. In some parts of Scotland, the caution on this head is carried to a ridiculous, and disgusting extent. If a patient of the poorer classes be ordered a change of linen, the physician may find that a relation or friend has worn it for some time, to insure its being well aired! In such a state, it is of course totally unfit to serve as a *change*,—in cases of typhus fever, for example in which such change is most commonly directed. There is, moreover, this striking objection to the use of clothing,—especially of under clothing, which has been worn by others,—that diseases of a loathsome nature may, in this way, be communicated.

# CHAPTER IV.

### BATHING AND MINERAL SPRINGS.

Ancient baths—different kinds of baths—functions of the cutaneous envelope—effects of bathing on the functions of the skin—cold bath—warm bath—hot bath—tepid bath—sea bathing—manner of bathing—time of bathing—duration of the bath—vapour bath—shower bath—affusion—ablution—douche—foot bath—practices accessary to bathing—flagellation—friction—shampooing—kneading—anointing—mineral springs.

OF other appliances to the skin we shall consider, next in order, the hygienic properties of different kinds of baths,—a luxury of universal adoption with the ancients, and more used with certain nations of Europe at the present day than with us. We need not dwell on the grandeur, and excellency of the ancient bathing establishments, of which those of the Romans were pre-eminent:—on the magnificence of their *thermæ*, *bagnios* or hot baths, which were provided with all varieties:—the *frigidarium* or cold bath;—the *caldarium* or hot,—the *tepidarium* or tepid;—the *vaporarium* or vapour bath; with the *apoditerium*, or undressing room; the *unctuarium* or perfuming room; and the numerous attendants;—the *balneator*, who had the management of the bath;—the *capsarii*, slaves who took charge of the clothes of the bathers:—the *aliptæ* or anointers, and the *unguentarii*, who took care of the unguents. All these were abundantly characteristic of the splendour of the imperial city, when she was " terrarum domina gentiumque:"—

> " The mistress of the world, the seat of empire,
> The nurse of heroes, the delight of gods;
> That humbled the proud tyrants of the earth,
> And set the nations free."

At this day, the large cities of the world—in all its divisions—are provided with these necessary establishments for cleanliness, and comfort, but the nations of continental Europe excel us greatly in this respect.

Bathing may be regarded as the immersion or stay, for a longer or shorter period, of the whole, or a part of the body in some medium. Usually, this medium is water at different temperatures; and various names are given to the bath, according to the medium, the extent of surface to which it is applied, and the temperature. A " general bath" is one in which the whole body is plunged except the head. A " hip bath," *coxæluvium*, one in which the lower part of the trunk, and upper part of the thighs are immersed. The " hand bath" *manuluvium*, is a bath for the hands :— the " foot bath," *pediluvium*, a bath for the feet ; the " head bath," *capituluvium*, a bath for the head : the " half bath" or *semicupium*, is for half the body; the " shower bath" is made to fall like a shower upon the body ; a " dry bath" is made of ashes, sand, &c. and the " warm air bath," by its name, sufficiently indicates its nature. Moreover, the " electric bath," which is given by placing the person upon an insulated stool,—communicating by means of a metallic wire, with the principal conductor of the electrical machine in action,—is sometimes employed,—as well as the " animal bath," which consists in wrapping an animal, recently killed, or its skin, around the body, or some part of it. These last baths are more used, however, for therapeutical, than for hygienic purposes.

On inquiring into the effects of baths upon the economy, it is well to glance at the functions of the cutaneous envelope, to which they are of necessity applied.

When the human body is surrounded by the rare, and elastic medium, in which it is ordinarily placed, the secretory organs of the skin are constantly throwing off a considerable amount of fluid, in the form of insensible perspiration. This, according to the experiments of Lavoisier and Saguin, is, on the average, about eleven grains per minute; but it varies in quantity, according to the external temperature, the degree of previous exertion, &c., and according to the state of health of the individual. We know, likewise, that an extensive sympathy exists between the skin and the mucous membranes—so that if the functions of the one be much modified, the other is apt to sympathize. Hence, the frequency of cutaneous affections, dependent upon gastric, or intestinal irritation, and conversely. But the mucous membranes do not alone exhibit this consent of parts. There is scarcely an organ in the body that may not be affected by undue, or irregular action, excited in some portion of the capillary system of the skin. Now, the chief general effects of bathing are to modify the condition of the cutaneous system, and, through it, of other parts of the economy. It is, in the first place obvious, that most baths form an atmosphere, if we may so term it, around the body, which is heavier, and denser than air; and as water is a better conductor of caloric than air, the former, although at the same temperature, appears to us hotter or colder than the latter. The same degree of cutaneous transpiration, consequently, cannot take place in the denser medium; and the trifling aeration, that occurs at the surface of the body, is prevented: the action of the capillary vessels is also modified according to the temperature; and the sympathetic effects, produced on distant organs, vary in like manner. The same may be said of the sensations occasioned by baths at different temperatures, which react more or less, through the great nervous centres, on the whole economy.

Some have presumed, that baths furnish more or less water to the system by absorption, but this is apocryphal. We have elsewhere shown it to be sufficiently demonstrated, that cuticular absorption rarely happens, and that when it does it cannot be to a great extent; and farther, that it is effected more readily in some parts than in others, and by some agents than by others. (*Human Physiology*, 5th edit. i, 643. Philad. 1844.)

Again, bathing certainly produces a local action upon the skin with which the fluid comes in contact,—rendering it soft, supple; and, where the immersion is prolonged, blanched, and rugous. This is doubtless caused by mere imbibition of the water. According, also, to the temperature of the fluid, the blood is repelled from, or solicited into, the vessels. The more particular effects produced on the economy will, however, be best understood by considering each variety of bath distinctly.

The *cold bath*, physiologically considered, has been regarded by some as extending from the medium temperature of a climate, or from the temperature of the springs—which nearly corresponds to this—downwards. Now as the medium temperature of Philadelphia is about 53°.5 of Fahrenheit, and as the heat of the the body is nearly 100°, the sudden application of a fluid at that temperature,—either in the common, or shower bath,—is succeeded by all those feelings, that indicate the sudden abstraction of heat. A general chill or shivering succeeds; or, in other words, a *shock* is experienced : the skin is pale, and shrunken, in consequence of the blood no longer filling the cutaneous capillaries, and the papillæ are distinct, communicating the roughness to the surface that has been called the 'goose-skin'—*cutis anserina*—and by the French, *chair de poule:* the cutaneous exhalation is greatly diminished; the intellectual manifestations are rendered dull; the whole nervous system has its action depressed; and the same may be said of the circulatory system. It has been denied by some, that the blood surchanges the internal organs; but it seems obvious, that if the cutaneous capillaries be devoid of blood, the fluid, which previously circulated in them, must be directed elsewhere. This, however, is not probably the main cause of the torpor of the great cerebral centres, which is apparent in such cases. It would rather seem, that the sudden, and even the gradual application of cold to the surface has the immediate effect of diminishing the nervous and vascular activity on the surface of the body; and that this effect is extended by sympathy to every part of the nervous and vascular systems.

So far, then, the cold bath acts as a sedative agent; but, after stepping out of the bath, a different train of phenomena succeeds— the order being somewhat modified, according as the bath has been taken in an open stream, or in a collection of fresh water, or in the sea, or in a close and warm apartment; and according as there may have been, in the first of these cases, much or little air stirring. In a warm chamber, the transition from the bath to the warmer air of the apartment rather abstracts from the sedation that has been produced, especially if the body be speedily rubbed dry, so that evaporation is prevented. In the open air, however, especially if there be much wind, the evaporation is rapid, and the sensation of cold, thus produced, and superadded to that occasioned by the bath, is at times overpowering to the feeble and the delicate; but, in all cases, in which the bath agrees with the individual, a sensation of glow soon comes on, and there is an apparent, but not perhaps real, increase in the capillary action, and especially in that which is concerned in calorification. This has been termed "reaction," and has been likened to the excitement, that follows the cold stage of a febrile paroxysm. This reaction is not great, although it seems to be so to the bather, in consequence of his previous sensations of cold. Our sensations, indeed, with regard to heat and cold, are entirely relative. They enable us merely to judge of the comparative conditions of the present, and the past: hence it is, that deep cellars appear warm to us in winter, and cool in summer. At a certain distance below the surface, the temperature of the earth indicates the medium heat of the climate; yet, although this may be stationary, our sensations on descending to it in winter, and in summer, would be by no means identical.

On the whole, then, although the common opinion is, that the cold bath is in all cases tonic, it ought, with more propriety, to be esteemed sedative; and hence it is better adapted for the robust and the vigorous, than for the weakly and the delicate. With many, in the latter condition, the glow is long in being established, and the feeling of privation of heat, and of nervous and vascular depression, persists so long as to occasion apprehension, that permanent mischief has been produced. It would be obvious, therefore, from these effects of the cold bath, that it will be improper after the system has been much fatigued by immoderate exercise of any kind;—walking, running, dancing, &c.

The foregoing remarks apply yet more forcibly to water at a much lower temperature than the medium heat of the climate.

The observations, previously made on the impropriety of exposing children unnecessarily to the cold air, with the view of hardening them, are equally applicable to this form of applying cold. Strong children may withstand the test; but the feeble and the delicate will succumb.

An estimate of the effects of the cold bath will lead to the following deductions:—that being inadmissible wherever there is great debility and exhaustion, it is obviously less adapted for the periods of life, when the functions are more feebly executed, than when they are accomplished in full vigour; accordingly, it is less applicable in infancy and old age, than in youth, and in the age of virility:—that it is not well suited for such as are liable to sanguineous congestions, or determinations in internal organs;—and that great caution is requisite in employing it during the existence of cutaneous affections,—especially such as are apt, after a sudden disappearance, to be followed by internal mischief in the lining membrane of the bowels, or in other organs. For similar reasons, caution is requisite in recommending it during the existence of the catamenial discharge, when the system of the female is irritable, and peculiarly susceptible of modification by deranging influences. When a cold bath is taken for health simply, perhaps no greater range than between 50 and 75° should be indulged; and the precise point may be regulated by the feelings of the patient. If the "shock" on first immersion, be too severe, when the temperature is near the lower of these points, the water may be raised a few degrees higher; or, if the uneasy feelings during immersion should indicate too depressed a temperature.

The ordinary temperature of the *warm bath* is between 90° or 92°—that is, six or eight degrees below the heat of the body—and 96° or 98°. Even when it is as low as the former point, we find, on immersion, a pleasurable feeling of warmth, because the temperature of the air is generally below this point, and the body, therefore, is commonly parting with more caloric. Those of languid circulation will prefer the higher temperature; those of active circulation and hot skin the lower.

The warm bath is a well known luxurious enjoyment to the wayworn traveller, removing from his surface the accumulation of cutaneous secretion, united with the dust which impedes the exhalation from the parts of the body exposed to it, and imparting fresh vigour to the frame. Every one, who has had recourse to it under such circumstances, must have been struck with the rapidity with which his enfeebled powers have been renovated. With like effect it has been habitually and advantageously used by persons advanced in life.

The effect of the warm bath is to diminish the frequency of the pulse, especially where it has been higher than natural, and this effect is generally in proportion to the duration of the immersion. It also renders the respiration slower, and lessens the temperature of the body; these effects being greatly induced by the freedom with which the blood circulates in the capillary vessels, so that the force of propulsion in the heart need not be as energetically exerted, and less fluid is sent, in the same space of time, to the lungs, whilst the soothing influence of the warmth and moisture diminishes the action of the organs of calorification. The same influence, exerted upon the capillaries of the surface, is extended, by sympathy, to the great nervous centres, and a disposition to sleep is the consequence. It is by virtue of these properties, that the warm bath produces, indirectly, the good effects that result from its use after a long and fatiguing journey, when the circulation, and respiration have become hurried, and the sensorial system is inordinately excited. We can hence understand the beneficial effects of warm bathing in all diseases of nervous, or vascular excitement; and why the warm bath should be better adapted than the cold for the feeble and the delicate,—the nervous and those of a cold constitution.

The *hot bath* is one in which the temperature of the water exceeds 98° of Fahrenheit, or is higher than that of the body. It differs essentially in its effects upon the system from the warm bath. Whilst the latter is soothing and disposing to mental and corporeal quietude; the former is stimulating,—communicating heat to the frame, and exciting the vascular and nervous systems to a degree, which, in particular predispositions, and habits, and during the existence of certain diseases—those of vascular, or nervous excitability for example—is positively and markedly injurious. This becomes signally manifest, when we reflect upon the effects occasioned by immersing the healthy body in a bath of this kind. The bulk of the extremities is increased, so that rings become too small for the fingers; the fluids expand, and hence the supervention of all the symptoms of the most manifest plethora. The pulse becomes quick and full; the respiration accelerated and embarrassed; the veins are turgid, and the carotid and temporal arteries beat violently; the functions of sensibility are blunted; a feeling of anxiety and constriction is experienced in the præcordial region; and these symptoms are, at times, accompanied, or followed, by palpitations, fainting, vertigo, and occasionally by apoplexy. All these effects are the more marked, the hotter the bath, the longer the person remains in it, and the greater the degree of plethora. When he leaves the bath, copious perspiration generally succeeds; and a state of languor and exhaustion follows the previous excitement.

The phenomena, produced by the hot bath, will lead to a satisfactory appreciation of the cases to which it can be appropriated, as a hygenic agent. It ought obviously to be employed with caution by those of the apoplectic make—of large head, short neck, and florid complexion—and by such as are predisposed to hemorrhage, or violent internal inflammations. It is rarely or never used as a hygienic agent.

The *tepid bath*, or one from 75° to 90° Fahrenheit, is well adapted for those cases of nervous excitability, in which the shock of the cold bath is too great. It is also an excellent preparative for the cold bath, when the properties of the latter are indicated. Two or three immersions in tepid water—the temperature being slightly diminished at each successive immersion—will enable the system to reap every advantage from the cold bath: this, when first used, ought to be near the temperature of the lowest grade of the tepid, after which the temperature may be depressed as far as the physician considers advisable. It excites less inconvenience than any of the varieties, and may be advantageously used in those equivocal cases, where the indications are by no means decisive.

The division of baths according to temperature has differed, within slight limits, with different observers. The following has been proposed by a recent able writer (Forbes, Art. *Bathing*, in *Cyclopædia of Practical Medicine*) " as one founded on practical observations, and therefore likely to be useful"—leaving it always to be understood, as he properly remarks, that in fixing the precise boundaries by individual degrees, we are influenced more by motives of convenience than from any belief that these are the exact and true limits of the different classes of baths.

| | | |
|---|---|---|
| 1 The cold bath | from | 33° to 60° |
| 2 The cool bath | from | 60° to 75° |
| 3 The temperate bath | from | 75° to 85° |
| 4 The tepid bath | from | 85° to 92° |
| 5 The warm bath | from | 92° to 98° |
| 6 The hot bath | from | 98° to 112° |

*Sea bathing* differs from the fresh water bath in the saline impregnation, which modifies, in some respects, the effect upon the system. It may be used in the cold, warm, hot, or tepid form; but the main results are similar to those that follow the fresh water bath at the same temperature.

Dr. Bell has properly remarked (*On Baths*, &c. p. 167,) that, " if we merely had regard to the temperature of sea water we should consider immersion in it simply cold bathing, but there are circumstances, connected with the act, which modify materially its effects. Sea bathing is usually preceded by some exercise, a walk or a ride to the beach: it is accompanied by some muscular exertion, struggling against the waves, or, in the more robust, by attempts to swim: with others, again, the whole affair is attended by a dread of danger, which powerfully affects the nervous system, and causes hurried breathing, palpitation, and increased rapidity of the circulation. The immersion, also, is in a fluid largely impregnated with salts. Add to these, exposure to often a cool, and keen wind from the sea, which, on our coast, must of course be easterly, and we can readily conceive that sea bathing presents a more complex problem for solution than the mere use of a cold bath." Most of these circumstances, however, are applicable to bathing in a fresh water river, or lake. The main difference, after all, is dependent upon the one containing saline ingredients;—the other not. Owing to the saline impregnation the fluid does not evaporate as rapidly from the skin; and when the evaporation is accomplished, the saline residuum remains attached to the surface; and this, it is imagined, keeps up a mild degree of stimulation, which has been presumed sufficient to explain the well known fact, that persons are less liable to catch cold, after being drenched with salt water than with rain.

With respect to the manner of bathing, the most important point is to moderate the shock to the nervous, and the delicate. This, as a general rule, is best done by a sudden immersion of the whole body. The uneasy feelings are much augmented by the practice, adopted by the timid, of gradually permitting the water to ascend higher and higher until the whole body is immersed. A little fortitude is necessary to take the plunge, but after this little or no inconvenience is generally felt by repeating it; and, accordingly, this is the course recommended in all sea-bathing establishments.

The time best adapted for bathing demands also a passing comment. By general consent in many places early in the morning, before breakfast, is preferred, and it is considered to be improper whilst digestion is going on—or at least during the early stages. The process of digestion occasions a concentration of the vital activity on the stomach, and this is morbidly modified by any cause that acts powerfully on the nervous system, or interferes with the general vascular, and nervous action, as bathing certainly does.

But although before breakfast is the *best*, it is not the *only* time for bathing. Under similar circumstances it may be advantageously had recourse to, whenever digestion is completed, or considerably advanced. As regards sea-bathing, the time of day is generally regulated more or less, by the state of the tide. Dr. Forbes, however, is of opinion, that for the majority of persons for whom the cold bath is prescribed, either as a measure of hygiène, or as a remedy, the best time for using it will be about noon; that is, he says, " two or three hours after breakfast." " At this time we may presume that the system is sufficiently recruited by the assimilation of the morning's meal; and we may yet farther be enabled to ensure reaction by such previous exercise as may be deemed proper." In this country, where, at the bathing places, the time of breakfast is two or three hours earlier, the best time for bathing may be fixed between 10 A. M. and 1 P. M.; and it is that chiefly adopted at most of our watering places.

To prevent the injurious effects of the hot rays of the sun during summer from beaming upon the head, an oil-skin cap is generally worn by the delicate especially.

The best general rules for guidance, as to the use of the cold bath when performed at seasonable times, are—not to employ it when the individual is cool or chilly, or when the heat is undergoing resolution by the establishment of perspiration, which is a cooling process.

The length of time, that the bather should remain immersed, must depend upon circumstances. The feeble, and the delicate, who experience a considerable shock, especially in the cold bath—or whose nervous, and vascular systems are much depressed—should withdraw after the first immersion, and be well dried, and rubbed, until a cheerful glow is produced on the surface. This is more particularly necessary as the depression—the diminution of vascular action, and of the powers of calorification—is still farther lowered after the bather has come out of the water, and remained for a few minutes exposed to the air. They, who are more vigorous, may remain in for several minutes; but if uneasy feelings should supervene—as chilliness, faintness or vertigo—

they ought immediately to withdraw, and adopt every means to avoid the depression, subsequently excited by the evaporation of the water from the surface of the body. With this view, the bather should cover himself with a dry flannel garment, which will absorb the fluid and prevent the loss of heat; after which, the ordinary clothing must be resumed as soon as practicable, and moderate exercise be taken,—short of inducing fatigue.

At times, after bathing, the delicate remain chilly, and uncomfortable, so as to render the warmth of bed advisable, with frictions over the surface, or the application of heat to the pit of the stomach, by means of a bladder half filled with hot water, a bag of hot salt, or hot flannels.

In the warm bath a much longer sojourn may be indulged than in the cold;—from a quarter of an hour to half an hour, or longer, according to the feelings, and constitution of the individual. This is the length of time commonly adopted in this country; but on the continent of Europe the bather often remains in much longer. In Germany, an hour is a common period, and in the mineral baths of Switzerland, as in those of Leuk and Baden, often four or five hours,—the bath being not unfrequently repeated twice a-day. (Osann, Art. *Bad*, in *Encyclopäd. Wörterb. der medicinisch Wissensch.* iv. 555, Berlin, 1830.) The first effect of the warm bath, especially one of the highest temperature, is commonly somewhat exciting, and, therefore, like the hot bath, it is not adapted for such as are liable to determinations of blood towards the head, lungs, or other important organs; but after a sojourn in the bath of ten or fifteen minutes, a relaxant agency is exerted. In the artificial bath, however, it is difficult—if not impracticable—to keep the temperature at the same point; but this is easily accomplished in the natural warm bath, such as that of the Warm Springs of Virginia.

Of the *vapour baths* much need not be said in a work on hygiène. Their medicinal virtues are entensive, but the consideration of them belongs properly to materia medica. Of the impunity, with which we may pass from one of them to a medium of a much lower temperature, we have already spoken,—in referring to the Russian vapour baths, and to Dr. Traill's observations, and experience in one of them. The greater the temperature of the steam the greater will be the stimulation produced by it. The Russians, as we have seen, are extremely fond of it; and its effects, as described by them, are agreeable and refreshing; yet if pushed to too great an extent, it can scarcely fail to induce a degree of lassitude, and depression, corresponding to the amount of previous excitation.

The *shower bath* acts, in the main, like the ordinary bath, as far as respects temperature,—producing sedative effects when cold; stimulating when hot. The shock, however, or the impression made on the nervous system, is generally greater, and hence it is not suitable for those of great nervous susceptibility. For such as are predisposed to certain head affections, this form of bath is a valuable hygienic agent,—the shock, and the refrigeration being applied directly to the head, whilst derivatives may be applied at the same time to the lower extremities.

*Affusion* or the pouring of water over the naked body, is a form of the shower bath; and its effects are similar,—the impression made upon the nervous system being more irregular, and therefore more powerful, than when the water is applied over the whole surface, as in the ordinary bath.

*Ablution* is the application of water to the surface by the hands, a sponge, towel, &c. The shock is not as great in this form as in any of the others, and the reaction is consequently less. Independently of the advantage of ablution, as a means of cleanliness, it is a useful hygienic, and therapeutical agent. Accustoming the surface to being washed daily with tepid, or cold water, would seem to lessen the tendency, so marked in some individuals, to affections induced by atmospheric vicissitudes. Washing the throat or the chest with cold water has seemed to diminish the proclivity to inflammatory sore throat, and the different varieties of catarrh.

The effect, resulting from deranged capillary action of the feet, has been more than once referred to. It is one of the most common causes of catarrh, and hence the importance of keeping them removed, as far as possible, from the sources of irregular action —by appropriate clothing; or by accustoming them, as it were, to moderate vicissitudes, by bathing them every morning in tepid water, and gradually diminishing the temperature of the fluid, until cold water is employed. In this way, the tendency to catarrh, from irregular action of the capillaries of the feet, may often be obviated. It is owing to this extensive and intimate sympathy between every part of the capillary system, that the good effects of ablution, as a refrigerant in fever, are produced. If cold water be repeatedly applied to the arms, when the skin is hot and dry, the temperature of the surface, with which the fluid is made to come in contact, is reduced; the action of the vessels of the part diminished, and the sedative effect extended, by sympathy, to the rest of the capillary system, so that, in this way, cold ablution is one of the most valuable temperants of morbid heat that we possess.

The *douche, douse, dash*, or *spout bath* is the local application of water by means of a canal, or tube; but it is more used as a therapeutical, than as a hygienic agent. The effects are dependent both upon the shock, and the temperature of the fluid; but especially the former. It can be applied at any temperature, and its effects are of course modified according to the degree of heat, like the ordinary baths, and according to the size of the stream, and the force with which it is made to impinge upon the part. The cold douche is one of the most efficacious means ever devised for taming the furious maniac. For this purpose, the patient is placed beneath a reservoir situate above the ceiling of the apartment, from which a plug can be drawn, so that a column of water of the size of the aperture may fall from a height upon the naked head. The most violent paroxysm is in this way speedily brought to a close, and the impression, made upon the nervous system, is so overwhelming, that tranquillity generally succeeds rapidly to the state of cerebral excitement and turmoil.

Of the partial baths, the hip bath, *coxæluvium*, and the foot bath, *pediluvium*, are most used. The coxæluvium is generally employed therapeutically in affections of the uterus, or rectum; as well as for strengthening the functions of the pelvic viscera, when their action is not duly energetic.

The foot bath, or pediluvium, is employed both as a hygienic, and therapeutical agent. The daily use of the cold foot bath, as we have had occasion to mention, lessens the susceptibility to catarrh in those that are especially prone to it; and, indeed, to all affections that are produced by derangement of the capillary system. There is no better prevention against chilblains,—an affection produced directly by the vicissitudes of temperature, to which the feet are so much exposed, occasioning capillary derangement, in the mode previously explained. If the feet be regularly and daily bathed in a cold fluid, they become so adapted to atmospheric changes as to resist their morbific influence.

PRACTICES ACCESSORY TO BATHING.—*Flagellation* is used by the Russians for the purpose of exciting action on the surface of the body. It is employed especially after the cold bath, and particularly in the case of those in whom reaction is established with difficulty. It is administered by means of a rod of birchen twigs, used lightly so as to excite rubefaction, and a sense of heat.

*Frictions* act in a similar manner; and the stimulation they produce on the surface extends by contiguous sympathy to the muscles, which become adapted for energetic and ready contraction. For this reason, they were always had recourse to by the athletæ of old, prior to their trials of strength. Friction is employed, with us, after cold bathing, especially in the case of the feeble, the delicate, or the aged, who remain chilly, and uncomfortable after the bath; and it is a useful means for exciting reaction.

*Shampooing*, (French, *massage, massement*) consists of a number of accessory operations conducive to the same end. It is a Hindoo process, introduced into Europe of late years, and is thus described by Anquetil; (Deslandes, *Manuel d'Hygiène*, p. 222) " One of the attendants on the bath extends you upon a bench; sprinkles you with warm water; and presses the whole body in an admirable manner. He cracks the joints of the fingers, and of all the extremities. He then places you upon the stomach; pinches you over the kidneys; seizes you by the shoulders, and cracks the spine, by agitating all the vertebræ; strikes some powerful blows over the most fleshy and muscular parts; then rubs the body with a hair glove until he sweats; grinds down the thick and hard skin of the feet with pumice stone; anoints you with soap, and lastly shaves you, and plucks out the superfluous hairs. This process continues for three quarters of an hour; after which a man scarcely knows himself; he feels like a new being."

*Kneading* has been used in affections of the limbs and joints; as well as in cases of spinal distortion, dependent upon debility of the muscles of the back—the great cause, indeed, of many of these affections. It was, at one time, conceived to be the height of impropriety to add to the weight pressing upon the spinal column, and complex instruments were invented for taking off the weight of the head, which was regarded as having much agency in the production of these affections. A great improvement has, however, taken place in the mode of viewing these unfortunate cases; and instead of keeping the muscles of the head, neck, and back in a state of inaction, every effort is made to arouse them to energetic contraction; for this purpose, a weight is placed on the head, and the individual is made to walk about daily for some time: by which means the muscles, that extend the spine, are excited to action to prevent the disposition to flexion of the vertebral column, which the weight on the head occasions; and thus the deformity is at times, altogether removed, when the treatment is duly persevered in.

Of late years, the operation of kneading has been more used with us in cases of dyspepsia, dependent upon torpor or debility of the muscular coat of the stomach and intestines. It has been affirmed, that owing to this pathological cause the food may be detained so long in the stomach, or small intestines, as to undergo fermentation, followed by distention, and other symptoms of indigestion, and that the best plan for obviating this condition is—to excite the muscular fibres of the stomach and intestines, by pressure employed in the manner mentioned. That good effects have resulted from this practice is certain; and it may be beneficially employed in cases of dyspepsia of the kind described, but it is manifestly inapplicable to the variety, which is dependent upon inflammatory irritation of the mucous membrane, and in which the mechanical violence, constituting the process of kneading, could not be tolerated. When had recourse to in dyspeptic cases, the operation consists in pressing on the abdomen so as to force the intestines up towards the stomach, and the latter organ against the diaphragm; thus occasioning a degree of succussion of those organs, and exciting the muscular structures concerned to a more vigorous effort; but it is probable, that a part of the effect is produced by the influence of the *moral* on the *physique*. The long continued operation keeps the mind, and nervous system, actively engaged, and directed towards the seat of the process, and a salutary agency is thus exerted on the torpid organs, which materially aids the direct stimulation, induced by the pressure and succussion. As a remedy, therefore, in those varieties of dyspepsia, that are dependent upon torpor, kneading is not to be despised, and it ought not to be subjected to the fate, that has befallen many useful agents, which, in consequence of their having been introduced, and fostered by quackery and selfishness,—although unquestionably efficacious under proper administration,—have fallen into total, and unmerited neglect, as soon as they were revealed to the world. A wise discrimination can select from every passing system and observance something capable of being retained, and of being philosophically and usefully employed for the relief of suffering humanity.

*Anointing* was followed by all the nations of antiquity. The Romans were in the habit of smearing the skin, either with oil or butter,—not only after, but often before, taking a bath; and the Russians, East Indians, and Egyptians still adopt a like practice.

The effect of the application of oleaginous substances to the skin is to render it less susceptible of impression from external temperature—oil being an imperfect conductor of caloric. Hence the practice of anointing, when the bather passed from a warm to a cold bath, or into the cooler temperature of the air of the apartment.

---

MINERAL SPRINGS.—In another work (*General Therapeutics and Materia Medica*, ii. 430) the Author has animadverted on the evil, that must necessarily result in various diseases, from the indiscriminate mode in which different mineral waters are drunk at their sources; and to a less degree, the evil is experienced, when they are employed by those in health. He has there remarked, that every intelligent physician, at fashionable watering places, has deplored the ignorance of invalids and their medical advisers, which has doomed many a hopeless case to a most inconvenient pilgrimage; for although the accomodations of such places ought to be adapted expressly for the comfort of the sick, attention appears to be paid rather to the sound, who are able to enjoy the pleasures of the table, and to administer, therefore, in a greater degree to the interest or cupidity of the proprietors. It is, however, of the latter class, that we shall have to treat more especially here;

—referring to the work cited, for the applications of the subject to the diseased.

Allusion has already been made to the eminent advantages to health from simple change of air. To this, indeed, and to a change of diet and regimen, much of that benefit which results from a journey to the sites of our mineral springs must, doubtless, be ascribed. (See p. 127.) Hence it is, that neither the waters drunk at a distance, nor any artificial waters, can be taken with the same advantage, as those fresh from the spring: and if the artificial mineral waters were sent from Philadelphia and taken at the spring whose waters they are designed to imitate, they would, in most, if not in all, cases produce the same effects as the latter, especially if the individual were not aware, that he was taking an artificial preparation.

When an inquiry is made into the character of the diseases, that are most benefited by a visit to watering places, it is found that the large mass of them are really such as are removable by simple change of air. That a change of air and of habits is, indeed, capable of accomplishing all that can be effected by our mineral waters is sufficiently demonstrated by the W a s s e r c u r or Hydropathy, in which no article of the materia medica, and nothing but the pure element, is used; and it is found, that the cures are mainly effected upon such patients as are wont to be sent to watering places. The founder of the plan—Priessnitz—proposes to cure all diseases, that are not in such a stage as to be absolutely incurable, by cold water used externally and internally, along with constant exposure to mountain air; active exercise; total abstinence from all distilled and fermented liquors; plain coarse food; hard straw mattresses; and in Priessnitz's own establishment, we are told, the sojourner inhales an atmosphere not of the purest,—being contaminated by a smell, in part arising from the cows that are kept in stables beneath the house; in part from *cabinets d'aisance* upon the staircase, and from the kitchen beneath the common room, which opens into it by a trap door, through which the cooked food as well as the various odours, find entrance. Priessnitz lives in the mountains of Silesia, and when we take into consideration the entire change that must be experienced by his patients in their journey thither, and, in the case of the better classes more especially, in their mode of life when they get there, we need hardly be surprised, that all those affections, which are capable of being removed by such revellents should yield to his efforts.

From the temperature and prominent ingredients of mineral waters, we can readily pronounce as to their general medicinal virtues. Some of them are cathartic; others tonic: almost all, in appropriate quantities, are diuretic; and capable of modifying the condition of the circulating fluid, and thus of changing the whole system of nutrition, so as to break in upon various morbid conditions of a chronic nature. Still, as regards all these actions, the same results would probably ensue upon the employment of an artificial water of a similar kind, if it had the same extrinsic circumstances associated with it. Nothing is more preposterous than the practice almost universally inculcated, and followed at different mineral springs, of directing immense quantities of the water to be taken early before breakfast: ten tumblerfuls is not an uncommon quantity at Saratoga; and, accordingly, we ought not to be astonished, that so many persons visit these and other mineral springs of the country in the possession of health, and leave them in a state of disease; when, if they had taken the waters in moderation, the tone of their systems might have been materially improved. It is absurd to prescribe the same formula for all cases, and to load the stomach so much in any case; yet such is the popular custom at most of the watering places.

If the sojourner at the springs be in good health, let him avoid the waters altogether, or take them sparingly; leaving the other hygienic influences to be fully exerted upon him; but should he be a valetudinarian, the waters must be had recourse to under appropriate rules, suggested by the nature of the case, and the peculiar mineral impregnation. Few, however, of the searchers after health will believe that the least important hygienic agent is the water; and were they convinced of this, they might perhaps be less disposed to visit, and pass their time at, the springs, and to reap the other extrinsic advantages to which allusion has been made. The drinking of the waters is an object for undertaking a journey; and if the journey be undertaken, it may happen, that the use of the waters will be found unnecessary, if not injurious.

# CHAPTER V.

### EXERCISE.

Effect of posture on certain of the functions—shock produced by exercise—active exercises—their effects on the functions—exercise should be accompanied with mental amusement—travelling exercise—walking—leaping—running—dancing—the chase—fencing—boxing—wrestling—singing—declaiming—reading aloud, &c.—passive exercise, or gestation—riding in a carriage, litter, palanquin, sedan chair, &c.—sailing, &c.—exercises of the infant—tossing—rocking, &c.—indolence, and its evils.

There is no hygienic agency of more importance than the due exercise of the body; and there is none that could be employed more injuriously, in certain cases of diseased action. Even the erect attitude, as well as the sitting posture, in which there is no concussion communicated to the frame, or to any of its organs, and where the muscular effort demanded is in the extensors of the head, neck and back chiefly, may be injurious in certain diseases, and morbid tendencies, from the mere effect of gravity. The physician is compelled to attend to this circumstance in the management of disease, or of morbid predisposition. With this view, he directs one labouring under encephalic inflammation, or predisposed to apoplexy, to keep his head higher than his body—to diminish the flow of blood along the arteries distributed to the head, whilst its return by the veins is facilitated by gravity. In like manner, the erect attitude is improper for one having varices in the veins of his legs, or any affection of the lower extremities, which is capable of aggravation by too great an afflux of blood to it.

When the erect attitude is accompanied by exercise, which communicates a *shock*, its effect upon the diseased conditions of depending organs is yet more powerful, and in this way pelvic and abdominal affections are often aggravated.

Exercise may either be *active* or *passive:*—in other words, it may be accomplished by the individual himself, by calling into action the various muscles of locomotion; or he may be entirely inactive, and resign himself to the action of bodies extraneous to him.

ACTIVE EXERCISE is attended by *local* and *general* effects;—the former being exhibited in the muscles exerted; and the latter being produced by the succussion, and excitement occasioned by the exercise. It gives firmness and elasticity to the muscles, and they experience such increase in their nutrition, that the muscles of the arm of the prize-fighter and fencer become, under its influence, models for the statuary. The fat is absorbed from between the muscles and their fasciculi, and their outlines become well marked. On the other hand, if a limb be suffered to remain at rest, the nutrition of the muscles is less active; the muscular fasciculi lose their prominence, and the limb ultimately appears shrunken.

Another effect of active exercise is—to increase the action of the heart; the blood, consequently, more readily reaches the capillaries, and a free circulation takes place in them, so that obstructions are prevented; but it will be readily seen, that if any such obstructions should already exist, exertion may be prejudicial, by propelling the blood too strongly into the obstructed capillaries, and thus exciting disease in the minute vessels.

Again, active exercise—and especially travelling exercise—improves the digestive function. The desire for food recurs more regularly and energetically; and hence the indolent, and sedentary residents of the city—shut up in their confined habitations—have much less appetite, than the rural labourer, whose toilsome calling leads him altogether into the fresh air. These, however, are the results of moderate exercise only. If it be pushed too far, so as to produce fatigue, the effect is very different; and the stomach speedily exhibits its participation in the state of exhausted muscular action.

When the stomach is distended by a full meal, active exercise is not advisable, but when it has begun to dispose of its contents, it may be employed in moderation, not only with impunity, but with advantage.

The invigorating influence of travelling exercise on the digestive function has been observed by all, and has been already referred to.

The function of respiration is so intimately connected with that of circulation, that if the latter be excited inordinately, the former becomes so likewise. Accordingly, when, after violent exercise— running, dancing, wrestling, &c.—the heart beats violently, and the pulse is accelerated, and stronger, the respiratory movements participate in the turmoil so as at times to threaten suffocation; whilst the necessary aeration of the blood is interfered with,—the experiments of Allen and Pepys, and of Jurine showing, that the expired air contains less oxygen, and more carbonic acid, than during a state of tranquillity.

As the capillary action is augmented by exercise, it will be understood, that the functions, referred to the capillary arteries, will be augmented likewise; and hence that secretion, and nutrition may be accelerated. In this manner, we account for the greater development, acquired by parts that are constantly exercised; and as a nice balance exists between the exhalants and absorbents in a state of health, it is probable, that the function of absorption is likewise rendered more energetic, but not to so great a degree as that of exhalation;—the body, consequently, acquires bulk, and vigour, provided the exercise be not pushed too far. Should it be so, however, and a due supply of nutriment not be derived from the food, the fat of the body becomes absorbed, and the weight is speedily reduced. This is the method adopted for reducing jockeys to the proper point. They are loaded with heavy clothes, and made to run until they sweat immoderately, whilst their diet is restricted.

Over-exertion of the whole body is a cause of early decease in many occupations, in consequence of its wearing out, as it were, the excitability of the frame, and giving occasion to irregular action of capillaries, which lays the foundation for organic mischief. Such is especially the case with coal-heavers; those engaged in canal making, mining, &c.

On the sensations and intellectual faculties moderate exercise acts as a salutary excitant; but, again, if it be carried too far, the contrary is the case: the fatigued condition of the muscles is responded to by a similar state of the brain, and nervous system, and the feeling of lassitude renders the individual unfit for all intellectual meditation. The frequent repetition of muscular efforts communicates, as we have seen, to the muscles a predominance of development; and this, it has been conceived, is unfavourable to the development of the function of sensibility; whilst, on the other hand, indolence is apt to induce irritability or impressibility of the nervous system; the sensations become acute; the perceptions exaggerated; and hence the various nervous affections to which the sedentary are liable.

Dr. James Johnson refers to an effect of travelling, which, he conceives, has not been noticed by any other writer. He affirms, that the exercise of the body, taken on the road, or while wandering about seeing objects of curiosity, is not favourable to intellectual operations, and he thinks it probable, " that a high range of health is incompatible with the most vigorous exertion of the mind, and that this last both requires, and induces a standard of health somewhat below par." "It would not be difficult," he says, " to show, that the majority of those, who have left behind them imperishable monuments of their intellectual powers and exertions, were people of weak bodily health: Virgil, Horace, Voltaire, Pope, and a thousand others might be quoted in illustration;—and he adds,—" be this as it may, it is certain, that travelling exercise while it so much improves all the bodily functions, unhinges and unfits the mind *pro tempore* for the vigorous exercise of its higher faculties. I much doubt, whether the immortal effusions of Byron were penned immediately after the impressions were made on his mind by the Rhine, the Alps, the lakes of Helvetia, the ruins of Italy and Greece, with all their classical, and historical associations. But the first excitement being over, the memory of scenes and circumstances, together with the reflections, and recollections attendant thereon, furnish an ardent mind with rich materials and trains of thought, that may, by gifted individuals, be converted into language; and thus conveyed to thousands."

It is probable, however, that this effect of travelling exercise, in unhinging and unfitting the mind for the vigorous exertion of its higher faculties, is but little connected with its improving " all the bodily functions." It may be accounted for by the fact, that whilst, in a rapid journey, the sensations are kept vividly engaged, the mind is altogether occupied in the reception of ideas, and no time is permitted for the exertion of the " higher faculties." But every one, who has lived in a romantic region, will admit, that a residence in such a situation adapts the mind for loftier flights of the intellect, than one which furnishes no food for contemplation, or for mental elevation. All this, however, is probably independent of any corporeal effect of travelling.

When moderate exercise is taken, the effect of the succussion or shock, given to the body, can scarcely be separated from that of the muscular contraction. This, at least, is the case with those who are in health: but when labouring under disease, the slight succussion of ordinary walking may excite considerable uneasiness,— as in cases of stone in the bladder,—or it may occasion abortion, or uterine hemorrhage in such as are strongly predisposed to it;— excessive uneasiness if some of the viscera be inflamed;—aggravation of headach, &c. If such be the effect of moderate succussion, it may readily be conceived what must be the result of more violent shocks, in rapid succession. Hernia may be induced, or, if already existent, a farther protrusion may occur, followed by all the symptoms of strangulation: abortion may suddenly supervene; an aneurism may be ruptured; or concussion of the brain, or spinal marrow might be occasioned.

As regards, then, the effect of active exercise on the different functions we may infer, that moderate exercise has a beneficial or tonic influence; whilst, if it exceeds the bounds of moderation, it may have an opposite result, and may be attended or succeeded by irritations of one kind or other;—and that when the more violent exercises are taken, succussions or shocks are given to organs, which, if not too severe, may augment the action of some of them, when torpid; but if pushed beyond the due limits, may give rise, in others, to more or less serious dislocations or other mischief;— as hernia, aneurisms of the large vessels; dilatation of the cavities of the heart; hemorrhages from the lungs or nose; sprains and lacerations of muscles, &c. Of all these, hernia is the most frequent lesion, and it is accordingly often met with amongst those artisans, who are compelled to use much violent muscular exertion —as porters, draymen, &c.

But, in order that exercise shall produce the full benefit on the functions, of which it is capable, it ought to be combined with mental amusement. Much may depend upon the mere exercise of the muscles, and much upon the change of air, that attends many of the varieties of exercise; but a combination of mental occupation, and amusement with these is of high importance to the invalid. It is on this combination, that the beneficial results of travelling exercise are dependent. "The mere *act of travelling* over a considerable extent of country," says an intelligent writer, whom we have more than once cited, " is itself a remedy of great value, and when judiciously conducted, will materially assist the beneficial effects of climate. A journey may, indeed, be regarded as a continuous and rapid change of climate, as well as of scene; and constitutes a remedy of unequalled power in some of those morbid states of the system, in which the mind suffers as well as the body. The continued change of air seems to do that for the corporeal part, which the constant succession of new scenes, and objects does for the mind. In chronic irritation of the mucous surfaces of the pulmonary, and digestive organs, especially when complicated with a morbidly sensitive state of the nervous system, in hypochondriasis, &c., travelling will often effect more than any other remedy with which I am acquainted." (Sir James Clark, *Sanative Influence of Climate*.)

The constant succession of new or of interesting objects in travelling arrests the attention so powerfully as to absorb or detract from all other sensations, and prevents the mind from dwelling on the gloom and depression, which ill health so naturally induces. Hence its salutary agency on the hypochondriac, and the monomaniac, distracting the former from his thoughts of self-torment, and the latter from the corroding idea that engrosses him. "A sportsman habituated to ease and luxury," says Dr. Kitchener, " will rise with the sun, undergo the most laborious exercise in hunting a stag, hare or fox, for the space of half a day, not only without fatigue but with benefit to health, owing to the amusement and hilarity, which the mind enjoys; but were the same gentleman compelled to go through half as much exercise, which afforded no amusement, his fatigue and disgust would be insupportable. This is every day the miserable experience of men, who were once engaged in the habits of industrious trade, and bustle, and whose success, and wealth have encouraged, and enabled them to retire from business: they find life a burden, and not having a pleasing object to encourage exercise, they acquire a painful *ennui;* and find they have exchanged the *otia* for the *tædia vitæ.* It is here that various exercises have been suggested as succedanea; but, alas! they all fail because they want the pleasurable zest. The dumb bell is tugged, the feet and legs are dragged along the walks, and avenues of a garden, but alike uselessly." Exercise, in short, to convey its full benefit, should always be combined with mental amusement. It is in this way, that dancing is not only not improper, but salutary, when the same amount of exercise of the limbs, uncombined with the hilarity, which the music and society engender, might, in particular cases, be positively injurious. " Troops who march in silence are more easily fatigued than when their step is regulated by the drum and fife. In some gymnastic schools of the continent, the young athletes are made to perform their exercises to the sound of music, to diminish their fatigue. The rope dancer mainly depends on it—the Canadian boatmen, and the gondolier, seek instinctively to increase their energy, as well as lighten their labours, by their native melodies." (Belinaye, " *Sources of Health and Disease in Communities,*" p. 21 ;—See, also, Combe, *Op. cit.* p. 113.)

The object of gymnastics and of calisthenics is to subject the locomotive apparatus to regulated action, for the purpose of communicating precision to the movements, augmenting the action of organs, rectifying deformities, and contributing to the preservation, and restoration of health ; and the wise gymnast endeavours to throw in as much amusement as possible, and to take away from his pupil every idea of forced exercise. When this idea prevails, more than half the benefit, that would otherwise accrue, is lost. Fortunately, with the varied food offered to it, in a well arranged, and well attended gymnasium, the mind of the youth is kept in a state of constant occupation and cheerfulness, which largely aids the good effects of muscular exertion, as well as of the succussion attendant on several of the exercises ; and many instances have presented themselves in which a due adaptation of these influences has infused vigour into the youthful frame, when every other kind of agency had been fruitlessly invoked. It was, indeed, the opinion of an experienced American physician—Dr. Parrish— that " vigorous exercise, and free exposure to the air" are by far the most efficient remedies, even when pulmonary consumption is present. " It is not, however," he remarks, " that kind of exercise usually prescribed for invalids,—an occasional walk or ride in pleasant weather, with strict confinement in the intervals,—from which much good is to be expected. Daily and long continued riding on horseback, or in carriages over rough roads, is, perhaps, the best mode of exercise; but when this cannot be commanded, unremitted exertion of almost any kind in the open air, amounting even to labour, will be found highly beneficial. (See page 144; and, also, *North American Medical and Surgical Journal*, for 1829 and 1830.)

Keeping the general effects of exercise in mind, we shall have but little difficulty in understanding the phenomena that result from the different kinds of active exercises.

*Walking* is one of the gentlest of these, when on a plain, and in moderation. The muscles of the abdomen, trunk, neck, and extremities are exerted, but without exciting in them any feeling of fatigue. Not so when we ascend or descend, an inclined plane. In the former case the muscles of the anterior part of the thigh of the limb carried forward are powerfully exerted to draw the body upwards, and fatigue is experienced in them. The effort required, too, hurries the circulation, and respiration,—producing anhelation or panting in the most vigorous, if the ascent be long, and steep, —and developing it, almost instantaneously, in such as labour under asthma, or serious heart disease: indeed, one of the earliest evidences of the existence of the latter may be the panting, and sense of impending suffocation, when the individual ascends even a moderate flight of stairs. In descending, there is a tendency of the body to fall forwards, which is counteracted by the vigorous contraction of the extensors of the back, and neck; and hence these muscles become first fatigued.

The shock or succussion in walking is inconsiderable, unless a false step is made; and on this account it is better adapted for such as require caution in their locomotive exertions than any of the varieties of voluntary locomotion, which we have to mention.

In *leaping*, the shock is greatly dependent upon the height to which the body is raised from the ground. It is adapted only for the period of youth, when the cartilages are elastic, and the viscera can more readily endure the jar to which they are subjected.

In old age, the cartilages become shrivelled, and possessed of less elasticity; and accordingly the shock from a leap or fall is not deadened as in youth, but is communicated in considerable intensity to the brain, and other viscera.

*Running* is between a walk and a leap, or rather it is a succession of leaps. In this exercise, every muscle of the body is more or less concerned, and hence its fatiguing character. It hurries also the respiratory, and circulatory movements, and is consequently inappropriate for such as are liable to affections of the lungs, heart or great vessels.

*Dancing* is likewise a union of stepping, and leaping. When used in moderation, so as not to induce too much fatigue, and when the motion of gyration is not too long continued—as it is apt to be in the waltz—this cadenced movement constitutes a wholesome exercise, besides communicating a degree of grace, and freedom to the motions, which they might not otherwise acquire. To the sedentary individual, and therefore to the civic resident, who is generally accustomed to a life of more or less corporeal inactivity, it is peculiarly appropriate. If, however, it be indulged too long or too violently, inconvenience may be sustained from the succussion being communicated to different organs; and dislocations or displacements of parts may occur, as in other varieties of powerful exercise. For obvious reasons, it is but little adapted for the pregnant female, or for one who is menstruating, although in both conditions it is not unfrequently practised. One of the causes of its injurious tendency in the latter condition is—the irritability of the system at the menstrual periods, and the great liability to irregular actions, which are apt to be developed, partly in consequence of the exertion, and partly in consequence of the too frequent concomitant,—exposure to cold after having been inordinately heated.

The injurious consequences, indeed, from dancing are usually more referable to the latter circumstance than to the severity of the exercise.

The *chase* is a combination of walking, running, leaping, and indeed, of every variety of muscular exertion. It is, in moderation, healthful, and the constant mental amusement prevents fatigue from being experienced to the extent that it would be—provided the mind were uninterested.

*Fencing* developes the muscles more immediately concerned—the biceps and pectoral muscles, for example; but its action is not confined to these muscles: it is requisite that the body should be kept in the due attitude, and hence the muscles of the lower extremities, and of the abdomen are greatly exerted; and the concussion is occasionally so considerable as to produce visceral displacements. When the cut and thrust exercise was introduced, some years ago, into the British army, the number of cases of hernia was found to be largely augmented. It has been said, too, that the exercise of the tread wheel, which consists in a similar action of the muscles of the lower extremities, and a similar concussion, has caused the same affection, or aggravated it greatly when already existent.

Fencing has the advantage of keeping the mind actively engaged to guard against the *coups* of the adversary, and hence it can be indulged longer without fatigue than many other varieties of active exercise.

Similar remarks are applicable to the exercise of *boxing*.

*Wrestling* is a violent muscular exertion, in which the different muscles of the body are powerfully contracted in turn, not only to preserve equilibrium, under the exertions of the antagonist, but to overcome them. Under its employment, the body acquires great vigour, and the muscles become developed so as to exhibit the prominences, which we observe in the representations of the ancient athletæ. The constant efforts, however, necessarily interfere with both circulation and respiration. The chest is made a fixed point for the efforts: the breath is consequently retained, and the blood is sent more forcibly to the head: the consequence is, that congestions are apt to take place there, and occasionally a vessel is ruptured in that cavity, or in the lungs; or transudation of blood takes place through the coats of the vessel.

From what has been said, the effect, produced by different gymnastic exercises, can be readily appreciated. This is dependent upon the particular muscles, that are thrown into action; the succussion, communicated to the frame, and the degree of mental amusement associated with them.

*Singing, declaiming, reading aloud,* &c., influence but a small portion of the body directly. Their effects are limited chiefly to the throat, larynx, parietes of the chest, and to the different thoracic and abdominal viscera: in moderation, they are not prejudicial, but the contrary. The voice acquires more extent, firmness, and suppleness, and the development of the thorax, and of its viscera is favoured. More exertion is required in singing, than in ordinary speaking, and hence it is more fatiguing. Declaiming, too, for any considerable period, is very distressing. When carried to too great a length, especially if accompanied with much mental excitement, the circulation is interfered with; the blood is sent from the heart with augmented force, whilst the impeded respiratory functions retard its return from the head; and hence, as we have the misfortune to hear frequently, a vessel gives way in the brain, or effusion of blood takes place by diapedesis, inducing apoplexy. Frequently, too, the action of the heart ceases under the influence of the excitation, and death is immediate. Some of our distinguished public speakers have had their career of usefulness cut short in this manner. In the same way, we can account for the supervention of hæmoptysis, and of serious thoracic disease, especially in such as are predisposed to them. But even where the lungs are delicate, proper exercise of them may have the effect of strengthening their tissue. Cuvier was in the habit of ascribing his own exemption from consumption to the invigorating effects of this kind of exercise. When he was appointed to a professorship, it was believed that he would fall a sacrifice to that disease; but the exercise of lecturing gradually strengthened the pulmonary organs, and his health improved so much, that he was never afterwards threatened with any serious disease of the lungs.

In a still more delicate condition of the lungs, the same exercise might, however, have proved fatal. In all such cases, consequently, the greatest caution must be observed: the kind of pulmonary exertion must be adapted to the particular exigency; and in all, the use of instruments, which interfere with the due play of the respiratory functions, must be sedulously avoided.

The effects of PASSIVE EXERCISE, or *gestation*, are dependent upon the muscular efforts, required to preserve the necessary attitudes, and upon the shock, communicated by the extraneous body, which is the vehicle.

Of the passive exercises,—*riding on horseback* requires the greatest muscular effort to preserve equilibrium, in consequence of the numerous impulses communicated by the varied motions of the animal. When the animal walks, the preservation of equilibrium is easy, and requires but little effort; but in riding rapidly, and especially if the animal be spirited, violent exercise is necessarily taken, and such as is but little adapted to the feeble, and the delicate. Equilibrium in such case is maintained with difficulty, and strong muscular contraction becomes necessary to fix the rider firmly in his seat: the shock is, at times, sudden and overpowering. This effect varies largely with the pace. Walking and ambling are attended with less succussion than galloping; and galloping with much less than trotting. The last is consequently the worst pace of all, for such as require this form of gestation at as little expense of muscular exertion as possible.

Horseback exercise, in moderation, where there is torpor, and inactivity of function—especially of the gastric and hepatic—is better than any other variety of passive exercise. It can be borne by those who are unable to take exercise on foot, and it admits of a more agreeable alternation of air, and scenery, than any of the active exercises;—keeping the mind constantly occupied, and allowing a modification of the physical influences of the atmosphere, so as to be serviceable in many diseases, and morbid tendencies. When the shock, however, is violent and long continued, it is improper in all those affections, that have already been referred to, as aggravated by the shock of the severer active exercises. It can thus be readily understood, why hernial displacements are more common amongst the cavalry than the infantry of an army. Different inconveniences, too, arise from the pressure of the saddle—as hemorrhoids and abscesses in the neighbourhood of the anus, followed by fistula,—and swelling of the testes is apt to be produced by the projection of the body against the pommel.

*Riding in a carriage* must differ in its effects according as the carriage is well hung, or the contrary. In the first case, it demands but little effort, and is therefore well adapted for the convalescent, the feeble, and the aged; but in the latter case—especially if the roads be rough—the whole economy may be disturbed, and much muscular exertion may be required to maintain equilibrium. This kind of gestation is comparatively inactive, and does not suit those who have been accustomed to foot exercise. The changes, indeed, from the one to the other—as in those who have amassed wealth, after having been accustomed to laborious exercise on foot—has often been prejudicial,—the action of the various organs, which went on satisfactorily under the constant succussion of active exercise, becoming diminished in energy, when the excitation has been withdrawn, or lessened by the adoption of passive exercise.

In the *litter, palanquin,* and *sedan chair,* we have but little of the beneficial results of riding exercise; hence they are generally used only as means of transport for the body. They may be employed in the case of those, who are so feeble, that any other variety of gestation is fatiguing or inconvenient, and where fresh air is still indicated.

The good effects of *sailing* are greatly dependent upon the constant mutation of atmospheric influences, and on the mental entertainment, which the change affords. When the water is still, there is but little muscular effort, and no shock. When, however, it is agitated, considerable exertion is required to preserve equilibrium; and the constant agitation, with many, brings on vertigo, nausea, and all the symptoms of sea sickness. This is not usually the case, however, on fresh water—not because the water contains no saline impregnation, but owing to the difference in the swell, and to the character of the motion impressed on the vessel in salt water. It is the impression, made upon the brain by the motion of the waves and of the vessel, that appears to be the first link in the chain of phenomena attending sea sickness; and the sensation of nausea, and the actual vomiting are produced consecutively, through the influence of that organ on the stomach. The precise manner, however, in which this is effected, is beyond our cognizance—like every other phenomenon, indeed, of the nervous system. We know, that the sight of a disgusting object, an offensive smell, or a nauseous taste, will, at times, as certainly cause sickness, as any of the more direct medicinal agents that are exhibited for the purpose of exciting it. In such cases, the impression must manifestly be conveyed to the brain by the organs of sense, and from this organ the sensation must emanate. It is probable, that when emetics produce their effects after being injected into the veins, the first effect takes place on the brain, and the stomach is impressed secondarily. To get rid of the affection, therefore, requires, that the brain shall be accustomed to the impressions made upon it through the motion of the vessel, and this occasionally requires a long period. The late Lord Nelson, it is said, was subject to sea sickness on every fresh embarkation, and whenever the sea was much agitated, and this has happened to many other eminent naval officers. Under this view of the subject it can be understood, that if any vivid impression be made upon the mind of the voyager, the nausea may be postponed, or prevented, as the force of the impression, made by the motion of the sea on the different senses, is thus detracted from; and accordingly most of the agents, that have been considered serviceable against sea sickness, have exerted their beneficial effects in this manner. Under feelings of confidence in the virtue of the prophylactic employed, the brain cannot be as vividly impressed;—the first link in the chain of phenomena is defective; and time, the great remover of the disposition to the malady, is afforded for the nervous system to become accustomed to the novel impression.

A similar kind of sickness is induced in many persons, by swinging, riding in a carriage with the back to the horses, &c.

Easy as is the exercise taken in a sea voyage, when the weather is propitious, and great as may be the mutation of atmospheric influences, it is not in this manner alone, that a sea voyage acts in the restoration of invalids—those predisposed to consumption especially. The situation on board ship greatly resembles that on the smaller islands. The air—as we have elsewhere shown, (page 180,)—before it reaches the vessel, when it is at any distance from land, becomes shorn of its heat, if it proceed from the equatorial regions, and tempered if from the arctic climes, so that the range of the thermometer is much less at sea than on land.

To the monomaniac, or to one predisposed to the dread calamity, a sea voyage is one of the most efficacious hygienic, or therapeutical agents that could be suggested. The sea sickness, in the first place, acts as a powerful revellent, distracting the mind from the corroding idea that engrosses it; and, added to this, the new objects which present themselves to one, who has never been on ship-board—and when the voyage is not tediously long, and unvaried—keep the mind from brooding over the product of morbid imagination, by continually attracting the attention to the scene before it. "These effects," says M. Londe, "will be still more marked, if the calm of navigation should be broken by storms. The commotions, which then strike the brain, force the most deeply affected monomaniac to tear himself from the object that constantly possesses him, to give his attention to the terrible spectacle, which surrounds him." (Art. *Gymnastique,* in *Dict. de Méd. et de Chirurgie Pratiques.*)

Such are the chief passive exercises, which we are accustomed to employ. The young infant is subjected to another—*tossing in the arms of the nurse*—an exercise which ought not to be

33*

dispensed with. It has been already remarked, that at one time the free use of the limbs was never permitted, and that the infant was swathed from head to foot, under the notion that the force of cohesion between its parts was insufficient—without such precaution—to prevent serious injury from accruing,—as dislocations of the vertebræ, &c. Nothing is now better established, than that the health of the child is signally improved by permitting the muscles to be freely exercised, and that there is no such risk as was at one time idly apprehended. Accordingly, at the *Hospice de Maternité* of Paris, and other similar institutions, in which the practice of swathing was once universal, the infants are placed upon the floor of a large, well-aired saloon, as soon as they are able to move their extremities freely, and nothing perhaps is more gratifying to the visiters of these establishments, than the sight of so much marked enjoyment, associated with so much innocence.

The exercise of the *cradle* is another variety of the passive kind. It is of much the same nature as swinging—occasionally practised, as a source of amusement, by the youth of both sexes. It is rarely, however, employed as an exercise, but rather as a means of quieting the child, and more readily inducing sleep. In the long run, the balance is probably against the nurse, in the article of trouble; for the child, once accustomed to be soothed to sleep by the motion of the cradle, will not afterwards go to rest without it; whilst, if habituated to sleep, without any such adventitious aid, from the commencement of existence, it does not subsequently become necessary.

Thus much, as regards the effects of exercise.—The evils, arising from a neglect of it, are sufficiently intelligible, and have been understood at all times and by all nations. Indolence was regarded as criminal by the nations of antiquity; and it has always been looked upon with detestation by the uncivilized, and without favour by the more cultivated.

Thus, Shakspeare:—

> " What is a man,
> If his chief good, and market of his time,
> Be but to sleep, and feed; a beast, no more.
> Sure, he, that made us with such large discourse,
> Looking before, and after, gave us not
> That capability, and godlike reason,
> To fust in us unused."

And Burton.—"Idleness is the badge of gentry, the bane of body, and mind, the nurse of naughtiness, the step-mother of discipline, the chief author of all mischief, one of the seven deadly sins, the cushion upon which the devil chiefly reposes, and a great cause not only of melancholy, but of many other diseases; for the mind is naturally active, and if it be not occupied about some honest business, it rushes into mischief, or sinks into melancholy."

All the functions of the individual, who resigns himself to inglorious inactivity, suffer; the nervous system acquires excessive impressibility, whilst the muscular system loses its strength, and the different vital functions are executed sluggishly, and with so much irregularity, that obstructions are apt to occur in the capillary system of vessels, followed by organic disease, of more or less serious character. All the secretions and excretions, with the exception of the secretion of fat, languish: the powers of nutrition are enfeebled, so that although the bulk of the body may be augmented, the texture of the organs is less firm and healthy; and thus the foundation is laid for hypochondriasis, hysteria, and the whole train of nervous diseases, and for many grave bodily ailments;—whilst

> "The languid eye, the cheek
> Deserted of its bloom, the flaccid, shrunk,
> And wither'd muscle, and the vapid soul,
> Reproach their owner with his love of rest. Cowper.

In this way sedentary habits are injurious; and hence literary men, clerks, and many artisans—as tailors, shoemakers, jewellers, &c.—suffer, although particular parts of the body may be well exercised in some of these occupations. Other parts may, however, be subjected to injurious pressure. The tailors are said to be so liable to fistula ani—from the pressure, occasioned by the position they are compelled to assume in their labours—that in London they have a "fistula club."

# CHAPTER VI.

### SLEEP.

Objects of sleep—evils from protracted watchfulness, and from too much sleep—temperature of the room—state of the bed—position, &c.—proper time for retiring to rest—time to be consumed in sleep—early rising—siesta.

The consideration of sleep, in its hygienic relations, is a proper sequent to the chapter on Exercise.

The different animal functions cannot be exerted for any length of time, without fatigue resulting, and a necessity arising for the reparation of the nervous energy or excitability, which has been more or less expended during their action. After a time—the length of which is somewhat influenced by habit—the muscles have no longer power to contract, nor the external senses to receive impressions; the brain ceases to appreciate; mental and moral manifestations are no longer elicited; the whole of the functions of relation become torpid, and remain in this condition, until the nervous system is renovated, and adapted for the repetition of those functions, which, during the previous waking condition, had been exhausted. This state constitutes sleep, which may consequently be defined,—the periodical suspension of all, or of most of those functions, that connect us with the universe. The suspension occurs in these functions, and in these only; the nutritive functions —digestion, absorption, respiration, circulation, nutrition, calorification, and secretion continuing in action, although in intermittent action, from the earliest period of embryonic life to the cessation of existence.

Sleep being thus "man's rich restorative," it cannot be long postponed, without certain phenomena resulting, which may be themselves morbid, or the causes of disease.

When watchfulness is long protracted—either in consequence of corroding care, intense anxiety or application, or the use of excitants—irregularity of action is induced in the great nervous centres, from which the effect is extended to every part of the nervous system; and, owing to this irregular—and indeed debilitating—condition, the various functions of the body, and markedly those of the capillary system—which are largely under the influence of the nervous system—become enfeebled; emaciation, and symptoms of anæmia, or of deficiency or of impoverishment of the blood, supervene, as indicated by paleness—etiolation—and incapacity for muscular exertion; the digestion is impaired; and, indeed, there is not a function that does not suffer. These are a part of the inconveniences attendant upon literary habits—the evils dependent upon such habits arising mainly from collateral circumstances, of which privation of rest, or irregularity in this respect, is one of the most injurious.

But the mischiefs, resulting from too great indulgence in sleep, are not less signal than those arising from its privation. The whole nervous system becomes blunted, so that the muscular energy is enfeebled, and the sensations, and moral and intellectual manifestations are obtunded. All the bad effects of inaction become developed; the functions are exerted with less energy; the digestion is torpid; the excretions are diminished, whilst the secretion of fat accumulates to an inordinate extent. The memory is impaired; the powers of the imagination are dormant, and the mind falls into a kind of hebetude, chiefly because the functions of the intellect are not sufficiently exerted, when sleep is too prolonged or too often repeated. Magendie, indeed, (*Précis de Physiologie*, 2de. édition, vol. ii. p. 574,) asserts, that protracted indulgence in sleep sometimes occasions serious diseases,—as idiocy and lunacy.

The physical circumstances, that modify the healthful exercise of this function—for so it must be regarded—of the nervous system, are numerous. The advantages of having the sleeping apartment so spacious, that the air cannot readily become greatly deteriorated, and with facilities for adequate ventilation, are now universally admitted; and in public institutions, where a number of beds is indispensable, the wards are always so constructed as to prevent stagnation of the air, polluted by the exhalations, and excretions from so many inmates. In many of our seminaries of learning, it is the custom for the student to sleep in the room in which he studies through the day. To this there are objections, not easily removeable however. In cold and wet weather, a fire becomes necessary; due ventilation cannot be effected; or if it can, the occupant is exposed to vicissitudes which cannot be regarded as wholly devoid of danger; and in the measures of cleanliness, that are demanded in the apartment, he is compelled frequently to expose himself to the inclemency of the weather without, or to the dampness necessarily existing within. Such being the facts, it is surprising, that we do not observe more sickness occasioned by the system than actually results from it. This, however, is a good deal dependent upon the degree of salubrity of the locality; and in situations that are liable to malarious disease, it is apt to develope much indisposition.

The soundness of repose, and the extent of renovation from it, are more or less interfered with by the character of the couch; and in this, custom—" the tyrant custom"—which

> "Can make the flinty, and steel couch of war
> A thrice-driven bed of down"

has much to do. Every one must have experienced the restlessness that attends any change of bed, especially if the texture, number of clothes, pillows, &c. have differed much from what he has been habituated to. The bed, or mattress should be of medium consistence;—neither too hard to be disagreeable, nor too soft to envelope the sides of the body, so as to allow it to be overheated. On the whole, perhaps the ordinary hair mattress is best adapted for both winter and summer. (Kitchener, *Op. cit.* p. 76.)

Of late, air beds have been much recommended. Of these we have had no personal experience, but a modern writer (Macnish, '*Philosophy of Sleep,*' Amer. edit. 1834, p. 268,) who has used them, affirms, that they are the worst, that can possibly be employed, as they become very soon heated to such an unpleasant degree as to render it impossible to repose upon them with any comfort; and this objection, he considers, applies with equal force to air pillows, which he several times attempted to use, but was compelled to abandon, owing to the disagreeable heat that was generated in a few minutes.

We shall not follow the various writers on hygiène, by descending to minutiæ, respecting the propriety of having furniture to the bed, or of using blankets, which Dr. Macnish regards as doubtless wholesome than sheets. All these points, we think, should be regulated by the feelings of the individual; and we should conceive it as injudicious to reject the use of warm bed clothing in winter, as that of warm body garments. The same feelings have induced Dr. Macnish to lay down the rule,—that when a person is in health, the atmosphere of his apartment should be cool, and that, on this account, "fires are exceedingly hurtful, and should never be had recourse to except when the individual is delicate, or the weather intolerably severe;" but this does not look like philosophy. Why should the body be surrounded by a temperature nearly equal to its own, whilst the face is in contact with air —perhaps near the freezing point, and often loaded with humidity? There is certainly more wisdom in the opinion of Dr. Kitchener, (*Op. cit.* p. 78,) that a fire in the bed room is sometimes indispensable—and, that during half of the year, those who can afford it would do wisely to have one at least once in every week. " The fire should be lighted about three or four hours before, and so managed that it may burn entirely out half an hour before you go to bed,—then the air of the room will be comfortably warm, and certainly more fit to receive an invalid, who has been sitting all day in a parlour as hot as an oven, than a damp chamber that is as cold as a well."

A recent intelligent writer, Sir George Lefevre, to whom we have had occasion to refer more than once, who spent many years in Russia, and who cautions the unattacked, but predisposed, to pulmonary consumption " to *beware of cold*, and to *cherish* warmth," strongly animadverts upon the system of warming houses, which prevails in England, and is almost, if not quite, as objectionable in this country. After stating, that in Russia the inner rooms of the houses, and those that surround them,—the halls, the corridors, the staircases, are heated by stoves, he adds—" The bed-room offers this striking contrast to the English dormitory, that it is warmer in winter than in summer. Not chilled with cold, slipping off his clothes with all possible speed, does the inhabitant of St. Petersburg jump into his bed, and bury himself under an enormous weight of blankets, to get out of the cold stage. He undresses himself leisurely, and is warm enough under a common quilt and a single blanket. He does not dread that most awful of all moments, when he must leave a warm bed, with his teeth chattering in his head as he emerges into a frost-chilled room from out of his close-drawn curtains. No warming-pan, lackered and shining, is seen suspended near his kitchen fire-place. He is not troubled with a species of barking, which may be denominated the *bed-room cough* characteristic of an English house, so audible when the transit is made from the face-scorching fireplace to the cold freezing dormitory." And he subsequently observes. "The Russian rooms are provided with stoves, but these are not necessary. A well-built fireplace, which throws the heat into the room, and allows only the smoke to go up the chimney,—not one of the old-fashioned sort, which takes in half of one side of a drawing room,—but a well-constructed, well-fitted grate, is quite sufficient to keep the apartment warm, provided that the doors and windows be air-tight; but there must be no rattling of casements, no gust of wind from under the doors, to make the carpet dance,—or adieu to COMFORT. This English word, so little understood by foreigners, is not even so by ourselves, as regards either the construction of our houses, or the mode of heating them. In cold weather, fires should be kept up day and night. The secret consists in *keeping the enemy out of the house.* If he enter, it is difficult to turn him back. By well regulated fires, Russian stoves may be dispensed with. The air is more pure, too, in rooms where there are grates; and if the doors and windows be tight, there will be no draft of consequence. The room which requires the most attention, and which is always the most neglected, is the *ante-room,* or *hall,* or *long passage,* or that place into which the *street door* opens. Hence a warm stove is imperative.— Who is not acquainted with the sound of the instantaneous, spasmodic, choaking cough, which seizes the invalid in his transit from the warm parlour through the cold hall, and up the chilly staircase. This is a cruel experiment for tender lungs,—an antidote to all the good, which medicine can effect. Here is the comfort of a day destroyed in a few seconds, and a night of cough and uneasiness ensues, which might be avoided. It is in this respect, that Russian houses are so preferable. The hall is the warmest of all the apartments, for it is the most heated, in order to defy the admission of the greatest cold. How is this to be accomplished in English houses? It is not easy to alter their construction. A stove will, however, warm the ante-room, and it might be so constructed as to allow of a long chimney, which could be carried along the wall and up the staircase. The wealthy only can accomplish these comforts, but, by so doing, they may remain more securely at home than by seeking warmth under Italian skies. No houses are so ill constructed for invalids as the English. The Scotch flats are infinitely preferable, and will allow more easily of all these improvements; but the inhabitant of an English house has to descend from the drawing-room to the parlour; whence, again, to the former; thence, perhaps, mounting two flights of cold stairs to the bed-room. Health may brook the varieties of temperature, to which these operations expose us; but very delicate beings cannot, and the patient may fall a sacrifice. In traversing from a warm apartment through cold corridors, or mounting a staircase, the invalid should be provided with a large shawl, with which to envelope the head and neck. Thus protected, the bed-room may be reached without danger. If this be not so warm as is desirable, let it at least be made as warm as circumstances will admit. A warm quilted dressing gown is an essential part of the bed-room apparel. It should be close at hand, and lie upon the foot of the bed, so as to be slipped on before the patient has totally emerged from the couch. It should be worn during the toilet operations. The feet should be shod in slippers lined with fur or wool. This clothing, than which nothing can be warmer, guarantees the invalid against bed-room cold so far as clothing is capable of doing it. The same should be worn at night, previously to going to bed whilst undressing. As to the cold ague fit, which is produced by getting between clean mangled sheets;—how is that to be avoided? The warming-pan presents the only remedy, and the use of that should never be omitted. By a strict attention to all these matters—by warming the house throughout as effectually as possible—by avoiding all currents of air—by exposing the body, as little as possible, to impressions of cold, which may be effected by the use of proper clothing—and by ever bearing in mind, that all affections of the lungs are aggravated by the neglect of these precautions, some good may be promised to the community." (*Thermal Comfort*, p. 28.)

The plan adopted, of late years, in many of the better houses of this country, of warming by means of heated air, ensures equability of temperature in every part of the establishment provided due attention be paid. Care is likewise necessary, that proper ventilation be effected.

The habit of keeping the chamber as warm as is the practice with many—in some of the southern states more especially—whilst the passages are almost as cold as the external air, cannot certainly be conducive to health, and is particularly objectionable in the nursery, where proper ventilation is not easy; and it has appeared to us, that those persons have enjoyed the greatest share of health, who have only had recourse to fires, when coldness or humidity has suggested them—so as to change the thermometric, and hygrometric conditions of the room before they retired to rest. In malarious districts, the use of a fire in the sleeping apartment is often a valuable hygienic resource, by promoting ventilation, and obviating humidity, which is a great predisponent to malarious disease. Sir James Clark, indeed, expresses his belief, that a person might sleep with perfect safety in the centre of the Pontine marshes, by having his room kept well heated by a fire during the night. In such localities, the entrance of the external air during the night should be avoided, by keeping the doors and windows fast; but in healthy situations the windows may be thrown open during the night, when the thermometer is very elevated, with complete impunity. In many of the southern portions of the Union, young and old sleep with the doors and windows open, and with a current of air blowing over them; but the air is so warm, that no mischief results from it; and, in many parts of the torrid regions of the globe, windows are not in use. For upwards of eight years, the Author was in the habit, in Virginia, of sleeping in a draught of air, during the hottest nights of summer, and he does not recollect any bad consequences to have been produced by it, when the air was dry. Some delicate persons are, however, extremely susceptible of the morbific action of the night air, and have consequently to be careful in admitting it to circulate freely through the chamber, even during the hottest nights. There are others, again, who have habituated themselves to admit fresh air into the chamber, even in the depths of winter. Such is said to have been the practice of the late Dr. James Gregory of Edinburgh—long, one of the most distinguished ornaments of the celebrated university of that city.

Humidity of the air of the chamber is, however, by no means as pregnant with danger as the same condition of the bed clothing. In large hotels, where the ingress and egress of travellers is incessant, it is often extremely difficult to have this important point attended to; and unless the traveller is careful, he is apt to be put into a damp bed, and—in consequence of the irregular action of capillaries, thus induced—to be attacked with catarrhal, rheumatic, or other inflammations of a dangerous character. Some of the worst cases of rheumatism, that the Author has ever met with, have been ascribed—and perhaps with justice—to this cause.

To the individual, who is in perfect health, and free from any predisposition to disease, the position he assumes in bed is a matter of small moment, and too trivial to merit notice, but where the make is apoplectic—as characterized by full habit, short neck, florid complexion, &c.—and especially where apoplexy has occurred in the family, position is of some consequence; and the head should be elevated, so as to throw some impediment in the way of the flow of blood to the brain, whilst its return is facilitated. In such, too, as are liable to disturbed dreams, nightmare, or somnambulism, position has to be attended to. These are more apt to be produced, when the person is upon his back, owing perhaps to the viscera pressing upon the great vessels, which course along the spinal column;—for whatever interferes with the due course of the circulation, or with respiration, gives occasion to uneasy sensations, which are appreciated by the brain, and, in consequence of the irregularity there excited, it is roused into action, so as to induce the phenomena we are considering. It can thus be understood, why a hearty supper, in one unaccustomed to it—especially if it have consisted of materials difficult of digestion—may occasion disturbed rest, frightful dreams; and, in those that are predisposed to it, somnambulism. Sir Charles Bell remarks, that the incontinence of urine, to which children are liable, frequently arises from lying on the back, and that it may be prevented by accustoming them to lie on the side.

Although the condition of the bed, the position, and the presence or absence of noise, light, &c., may interfere somewhat with sleep, it is more frequently broken by internal, than by external irritants; so far, at least, as regards the phenomena we have been considering. During sleep, both external and internal irritants excite the greater effect, owing to the nervous system being no longer stimulated by the ordinary impressions made on the external senses; and if such impressions be insufficient to prevent sleep, they may still excite dreams. It is on this account, that impressions, made on the sense of touch, for example, will excite the most exaggerated representations in the brain, in the shape of dreams. The bite of a flea appeared to Descartes the puncture of a sword; an uneasy position of the neck may excite the idea of strangulation; a loaded stomach, that of a house or a castle, or of some powerful monster pressing on the stomach. (See the Author's *Human Physiology*, 5th edit. ii. 545, and Macnish, *Op. cit.* p. 54 for many such cases.) But, although a full supper is frequently attended with the consequences described, there are some who, from habit, are unable to sleep without this meal, and in Great Britain, amongst the middle ranks of society, it was formerly the most comfortable repast; yet they appeared to enjoy as large a share of health as any portion of the population. As a general rule, however, we should consider it more wholesome to avoid repletion with solid food at this meal, and to complete it two or three hours, or more, before retiring to rest.

As to the oft disputed questions,—the hour at which we ought to retire to rest; and the length of time that should be passed in sleep,—it is difficult to say any thing precise. Of the bad effects, resulting from the conversion of the night into day, we have already spoken. Night is the proper period for rest, for obvious reasons; and the day for exertion. Yet it is too much the habit, in civic life especially, to disregard this; and, what is worse, to make the period of retiring to rest, as well as that indulged in sleep, extremely irregular. Such is apt to be the case also with the student, especially if his social habits lead him, in the day and the early part of the evening, to participate in the pleasures of society, and of the table. Dr. Macnish affirms, that it may be laid down as a rule, that to make a custom of remaining up for a later period than eleven is prejudicial. " Those, therefore, who habitually delay going to bed till twelve, or one or two, are acting in direct opposition to the laws of health, in so far as they are compelled to pass in sleep a portion of the ensuing day, which ought to be appropriated to wakefulness and exertion : (*Op. citat.* p. 278 :) and Dr. Kitchener observes :—" whether rising early lengthens life we know not, but are sure, that sitting up late shortens it,—and recommend you to rise by eight, and to retire to rest by eleven; your feelings will bear out the adage, that "one hour's rest before midnight is worth two after." (*Op. citat.* p. 62.) These views are doubtless just, but much depends upon habit; and if the individual were regularly to retire to rest at twelve, and consume the necessary time in rest no injury from this course ought to be anticipated:— so much depends upon the habit which may have been formed. It is irregularity in these respects, as before observed, that is the main cause of mischief, provided the hour of retiring to rest does not encroach too much upon the morning.

What ought to be the time consumed in sleep depends upon so many circumstances, that, no positive rule can be established. From six to eight hours is the period assigned by many physiological and hygienic writers. Dr. Macnish asserts, that no person, who passes only eight hours in bed, can be said to waste his time in sleep; whilst Dr. Kitchener considers, that the time requisite for restoring the waste, occasioned by the action of the day, depends on the activity of the habits, and on the health of the individual; but that it cannot in general be less than seven, and need not be more than nine, hours.

Where attempts have been made by literary characters to assign a proper period for sleep, they have either been guided by their known capabilities; or by what they have esteemed themselves capable of effecting; or they have been led—in their ignorance of physiology—into Utopian considerations, regarding the time *wasted* —as they conceive—in rest. How else can we account for the idea of Jeremy Taylor, that three hours only, in the twenty-four, should be devoted to sleep? In an equally arbitrary manner, Baxter fixes on four hours, Wesley on six, and Lord Coke on seven. So much depends upon the constitution, and habit of individuals, that if some were restricted to the period, allotted by Baxter, or Taylor especially, their lives could not fail to pay the forfeit. Men of active minds, whose attention is engaged in a series of interesting employments, sleep much less than the lazy, and the listless. In them, the excitability is soon expended, but it is readily restored. It is probable, that in those cases the sleep is more intense, and that such of the animal functions, as indispensably require rest, are completely suspended, or asleep, during the whole period allotted to it. How otherwise can we explain the perfect renovation, experienced by those, who accustom themselves to two or three hours' rest only ? It is a common observation with the sailor, that he can sleep as much in four hours—the period of his watch—as the landsman can in ten. General Pichegru informed Sir Gilbert Blane, that in the course of his active campaigns he had, for a whole year, not more than one hour of sleep, on an average, the twenty-four hours; and the great Frederick, and yet greater Napoleon are said to have passed a surprisingly short time in sleep, during the active periods of their career. This may be partly accounted for by the fact, that the earliest part of our sleep—as every one must have observed—is the soundest. It rarely happens, that this is the period of dreams, which come on later in the night, or towards morning. The sleep, therefore, is at this time most restorative ; and every medical practitioner must have been surprised to find, when he has been disturbed after one or two hours' rest, how greatly the excitability of the nervous system has been restored. The powers of the sensorium, as Sir Gilbert Blane, suggests, seem to be wound up, as it were, at the most rapid rate, in the first period of sleep; and great part of the refreshment, in the later hours, seems more imputable to the simple repose of the motive organs than to the recuperative power of sleep.

In infancy, and youth, when the functions of the nervous system are unusually active, the necessity for sleep is greatest ; in mature age, when time is more valued, and cares are more numerous, it is less indulged in ; whilst the aged may be affected in two opposite modes—they may be either in a state of almost constant somnolency, or their sleep may be short and light.

It has been a common remark, that women require more sleep than men; and M. Georget assigns them a couple of hours more,—allotting to men six, or seven hours, and to women eight, or nine; but Dr. Macnish judiciously doubts, whether the female constitution properly speaking, requires more sleep than the male ; at least he says " it is certain that women endure protracted wakefulness better than men, but whether this may result from custom is a question worthy to be considered." The fact is, however, too general to permit us to invoke custom, and it would seem, that the female frame, although far more excitable than that of the male, is longer in having that excitability exhausted, and that the recuperative powers are greater, so that the excitability, when exhausted, is more readily restored. The notion, that the female requires more rest than the male, appears, indeed, to be traditionary, and, like most traditions, to have been handed down from one individual to another without due examination: the degree of muscular, and mental exertion, to which the male is accustomed, would seem indeed, to indicate, that a longer period of rest, to admit of the necessary restoration of excitability, ought to be required by him.

It has been an old fashion to inculcate, somewhat too abstractedly, the pre-eminent advantages of early rising; and a very recent writer has asserted, that " almost all men, who have distinguished themselves in science, literature, and the arts, have been early risers ;" (Macnish, *Op. cit.* p. 282;) but the exceptions, we are satisfied, are more numerous than the rule itself. By far the majority of the studious spend so much of the night in study, that early rising would not only be prejudicial, but impracticable. Far safer is the maxim,—

> " Early to bed, and early to rise
> Will make a man healthy, wealthy, and wise:"

because, in this case, repose is indulged at the period best adapted for it, whilst a due quantity of rest can be taken so as to admit of early rising. If an individual, whose frame seems to demand a repose of eight hours, be in the habit of retiring to rest at midnight, it would be idle for us to expect, that he should rise at the same hour as if he retired to rest at nine or ten. The time of rising will, therefore, have to be regulated somewhat by the time of going to bed. Where this is not attended to, and where the individual rises before he has had his due allowance of sleep, he is apt to be drowsy and indolent during the whole day, and totally unfit for any great intellectual, or corporeal exertion.

As respects the *siesta*, or the " nap" after dinner, it has been questioned, whether it can be indulged with impunity. It is certain, that after a full meal both man and animals feel a propensity to sleep, but it is not so certain, that digestion is facilitated by it: on the contrary, it has been maintained, that it is more tardy than in the waking condition. The difference in this last respect is so great, that, as Broussais remarks, the appetite recurs many hours before the usual time when long watching is indulged, and an additional meal becomes necessary,—proving the truth of the old French proverb,—"*qui dort dine :*"—"he who sleeps, dines." Dr. Kitchener has collected a number of opinions in favour of remaining quiet after dinner; but all the respectable individuals cited would not have regarded sleep with equal favour. Absence from all active exercise doubtless aids digestion, and we are not prepared to say, that, even admitting a short siesta to somewhat retard digestion, we have ever known evil to result from it. In hot climates, indeed, it is a universal practice, and its impunity has led to the universality of its adoption: yet it has been described by a writer, whom we have more than once quoted, as "pernicious." "On awaking," he remarks, " from such indulgence, there is generally some degree of febrile excitement in consequence of the latter stages of digestion being hurried on; it is only useful in old people, and in some cases of disease:" (Macnish, *Op. citat.* p. 274:) but if "pernicious" in the abstract, it is not easy to see how it can be useful under the circumstances specified.

If, therefore, the desire for sleep after dinner—or indeed at any period of the day—be urgent, it ought to be indulged for a short time; for as Dr. Kitchener asks, (*Op. citat.* p. 58,) " is it not better economy of time to go to sleep for half an hour, than to go on noodling all day, in a nerveless, and semi-superannuated state,—if not asleep, certainly not effectively awake for any purpose requiring the energy of either the body or the mind? 'A forty winks' nap,' in a horizontal posture, is the best preparative for any extraordinary exertion of either."

# CHAPTER VII.

#### CORPOREAL AND MENTAL OCCUPATIONS.

Influence of professions limited to a few circumstances; exposure to vicissitudes; variations of temperature; mineral and other exhalations, &c.—literary pursuits not often the cause of disease—head affections ascribed to them—imagination said to act injuriously on the body—duration of life amongst authors—bad effects of too early application—necessity of health for the full exercise of the intellect—intense mental excitement injurious—effects of emotions, when inordinate.

The varied occupations of mankind have a manifest agency upon health, and many of them become the source of serious disease. The mischief is not, however, so extensive as might be presumed, even in the most insalubrious callings—owing to the power possessed by the living economy of habituating itself, in some measure, even to the most malign influences. Sooner or later, however, if these influences be prolonged, inroads are made on the healthy function, and organic and fatal mischief results.

If we cast our regards on the different trades and occupations, we find that their influence on the human body is caused by a few circumstances; and of these—the degree of exertion, of elevation or depression of temperature, of greater or less exposure to vicissitudes, the sedentary or other character of the calling, and the presence or absence of noxious exhalations, are the most prominent.

During the early periods of life, the organs of the body are accustomed to constant succussion in the different exercises adapted to the age; and if a sedentary employment be chosen in the period of adolescence or virility, the organs—no longer experiencing the succussion to which they had previously been habituated—execute their office languidly, and hence the frequency of torpor of the digestive function in such cases, and the occurrence of dyspepsia among the sedentary and inactive. On the other hand, severe exercise, accompanied by exposure to atmospheric vicissitudes, is apt to lay the foundation for obstructions in the capillary tissues of different organs, and to consequent disease and disorganization, in parts whose integrity is necessary for the continuance of health, and even of life. Hence it is, that, in such, the diseases are apt to be of a highly inflammatory character, or very acute; whilst the diseases of the sedentary, and of those less subjected to sudden variations in the atmospheric influences, are of a more chronic kind.

It was estimated by Sydenham, that two-fifths of mankind die of acute diseases, and that of the remaining one-third, two-thirds—or one-ninth of the whole—die of pulmonary consumption. But pulmonary consumption is developed by the same atmospheric irregularities, which give occasion to acute diseases in general; so that we can readily understand, that those occupations which expose their followers to such morbific agencies, must be most fatal to man. Under another head, reference was made to the harmlessness of exposure to cold, provided ordinary precautions be taken; and it was at the same time remarked, that constant exposure to great heat is not as innocuous; but that it occasions considerable erethism in the dermoid tissue—both skin and mucous membranes—which erethism is extended from the part of the latter, lining the upper portion of the intestinal canal, to the liver; so that super-excitation may occur in that organ leading to morbid effusion, tumefaction and induration; and, accordingly, those occupations, which are carried on in an elevated temperature, are apt to lead to visceral and other engorgements of dangerous tendency.

On the whole, we may infer—that, *cæteris paribus*, such occupations as are conducted in the open air, and in which the amount of exercise is not excessive, are most conducive to health. We say *cæteris paribus*, for much will depend upon diet and regimen. The butcher, for example, is apt to indulge in animal food, whilst his avocation does not require him to take much exercise—he therefore becomes plethoric, and the diseases that assail him are mostly of this character. The coal-heavers, the brewers' draymen, and the ballasters of London, are allowed large quantities of strong beer:—the first and last being accustomed to severe exertion, do not experience as much injurious influence from the plethora, and over-stimulation, occasioned by this article of diet; but the draymen, not exerting themselves to the same degree, become plethoric, bloated, and over excited ; so that if inflammation attacks any of their tissues, such inflammation is apt to be of the more unhealthy or erysipelatous, rather than of the phlegmonous, character; and so much tendency to increased action of capillary vessels is induced, that the slightest wound, or bruise, is usually succeeded by that variety of inflammation.

It has already been remarked, (page 75,) that occupations, in which putrid miasmata are exhaled, are not so productive of disease, as might be imagined, but that on the contrary, the knackers and the catgut-spinners—who are pre-eminently exposed to such miasmata—are healthy—surprisingly healthy—and many of them long-lived. We can hence understand, that glue and size boilers, who live in the most disagreeable stench, may be fresh-looking and robust ; and that tallow chandlers—also exposed to offensive animal odours—may attain considerable age.

Again, it is manifest, that those employments which give occasion to the exhalation of impalpable powders, or gaseous substances, may exert a positively detrimental influence on the organism, by being received into the lungs, and producing mischiefs directly in those organs, or indirectly in other parts of the frame.

Millers, who breathe an atmosphere loaded with an impalpable powder, which enters the lungs with the air of inspiration, are liable to irritation and inflammation of those organs, and therefore to phthisis pulmonalis, asthma, &c. Hence they are pale and sickly; and, according to Mr. Thackrah, very rarely attain old age. Tea-sorting, coffee-roasting, paper-making, machine-making, iron-filing, &c. may be, in this way, injurious.

In like manner, substances may be volatilized in different processes—as in brass founding, and in the arts of the coppersmith, plumber, house painter, operative chemist, and potter—and may exert their ordinary deleterious agency on the frame ;—the latter occupations, in consequence of the lead employed in them. It is not always, however, by the lungs that the lead enters in these cases. Since proper precautions have been taken, in some of the large smelting establishments of Great Britain, it has been found, that much fewer cases of lead paralysis and lead colic have occurred than formerly. These precautions consist in compelling the workmen, before going to their meals, to change their clothes, and to carefully wash their hands with the aid of a nail brush, so as to remove every particle of the metal, and thus prevent it from entering the digestive organs along with the food. The result has shown most satisfactorily, that the cause, in such cases, is generally applied through these passages, rather than through the skin or lungs.

Occupations, again, in which the gases are exhaled, are wholesome or injurious, according to the nature of the gases. Grooms and hostlers—for example—inspire ammoniacal gas, but this—being devoid of noxious properties—of course exerts no insalubrious agency. They appear, indeed, to be generally robust, healthy, and long-lived. On the other hand, the gold-finders are exposed to a most deleterious gas—the sulphuretted hydrogen—which, if sufficiently concentrated, kills, and in lesser doses is productive of disease.

Thus much we know regarding the general circumstances, which may render particular occupations insalubrious; but when we descend to greater minuteness, our deductions are any thing but satisfactory; and, accordingly, the different statements which have been published on this subject, have not led to any definite conclusions, as regards the comparative salubrity of different avocations. As respects classes of congenerous occupations, compared with others that are dissimilar, we may pronounce somewhat positively; but when we descend to genera and species, our inferences are by no means as satisfactory. (See the article *Artisans, Diseases of the,* in *Cyclop. of Pract. Medicine.* Amer. edit. Philad. 1844.)

Great attention has been paid, of late years, to the influence of occupation and customs on human health, and more especially of the factory system on the health of operatives; and valuable information has been elicited. Much light has been thrown on these matters by the *Sanitary Reports* presented to the British Parliament, and by the inquiries of Messrs. Ure, Villermé, Noble, and others,—to some of the results of which reference has been made in an early part of this work. All these investigations would seem to show, that the evils, which have been presumed to appertain to manufactoring pursuits in Europe, have been greatly exaggerated; and the same, doubtless, applies to this country. It is positively asserted by Dr. E. Bartlett (*A Vindication of the Character and*

*Condition of the Females employed in the Lowell Mills,* p. 13. Lowell, 1841,) that "the manufacturing population of Lowell is the healthiest portion of the population;" "and there is no reason," he adds, "why this should not be the case. They are but little exposed to many of the strongest and most prolific causes of disease, and very many of the circumstances, which surround and act upon them, are of the most favourable hygienic character. They are regular in all their habits. They are early up in the morning, and early to bed at night. Their fare is plain, substantial and good, and their labour is sufficiently light to avoid the evils arising from the two extremes of indolence and over exertion. They are but little exposed to the sudden vicissitudes, and to the excessive heats or colds of the seasons; and they are very generally free from anxious and depressing cares." In a former chapter (p. 110,) a table of the average age of death among the different classes of people in Manchester and Rutlandshire, England, was given, with the view of showing, in a striking manner, the difference between the amount of civic and rural mortality; but the table exhibits no less signally another important fact,—that whilst in Manchester the average age of death among professional persons and gentry and their families was 38; that of tradesmen and their families was 20; and that of mechanics, labourers and their families 17. A like difference is shown in the country districts of Rutlandshire; and, so far as investigations have been made in this country, the results would seem to be analogous. In an address to the members of the Massachusetts Medical Society, presented to the counsellors of that body, by Drs. John D. Fisher, Edward Jarvis and O. W. Holmes, in February 1844, it is stated, that the Committee had obtained an analysis of the ages, and also of the domestic and social condition, of 1767 persons, who had died in Dorchester, Massachusetts, within the last 27 years; by which it appeared, that the average duration of life in the families (including father, mother and children,) of labourers, fishermen, journeymen mechanics and factory operatives was - - 27 years 5mo.
Mechanics who carry on business on their own account - - - - - - 29 " 6
Merchants, capitalists, professional and salaried men, amateur farmers - - - - 33 " 2
Farmers who own and cultivate their lands 45 " 8

and, that the difference is not ascribable to occupation merely was shown by the fact, that it was found to be greatest among the little children at their homes. "This great difference of mortality between the children of the poor and of the comfortable farmer"—the Committee add—" cannot be caused by the employment of the head of the family. There must be a cause or causes connected with the domestic condition, or management, to produce this discrepancy. But it is yet a question to be solved by farther and wider observation, whether this, although a general fact in England and Wales, is here more than a particular fact in regard to Dorchester."

Dr. Guy, in the *Journal of the Statistical Society* of London, (cited in the *Provincial Med. and Surg. Journal* for Dec. 16, 1843; and in the *Philadelphia Medical Examiner* for March 9, 1844,) has inquired at some length into the influence of employments upon health. He confirms the results arrived at by other observers, in showing the great advantage, which the better classes enjoy over other members of society. They appear to live longer, and probably enjoy better health. This is doubtless owing to better ventilation and food, and the greater attention bestowed on the places which they inhabit. It is partly also due, as Dr. Guy has suggested, to the facilities which they enjoy for exercise in the open air. The great difference between the gentry and other members of society is not more worthy of notice than the slight advantage which the tradesman in Great Britain enjoys over the class of working men: according to Dr. Guy, if we limit the comparison to the average age, we find that the tradesman lives about three quarters of a year longer than the entire class of workingmen— little more than a year and a half longer than the class employed solely within doors—two years longer than the men following the more sedentary occupations, and about three years longer than the class which consists chiefly of domestic servants. On the other hand, the life of the tradesman is shorter by about a quarter of a year than that of the entire class of out-door labourers. The little advantage possessed by the tradesman over the mass of workingmen, Dr. Guy thinks, probably results from the sedentary life he leads, his want of proper exercise, and the small space which the necessities of business allow him to appropriate to the accommodation of himself and family. Taking one tradesman with another, it is, perhaps, not unreasonable to suppose that he habitually breathes an air as impure, and follows an occupation nearly as unwholesome, as the class beneath him. The labour, which the workingman has to undergo, provided it is not carried to excess, is more favourable to health than the confinement to which the tradesman is subject; and this confinement raises him in the scale of mortality but little above men following the more sedentary occupations. Both classes of men, the tradesman and the workingman, are doubtless exposed to unwholesome influences, which might be wholly removed or greatly mitigated by the interference of others, or by their own precautions.

A simple inspection of the comparative average of death in Manchester and in Rutlandshire might readily lead the superficial to the belief, that manufactures are the cause of the increased mortality in the former situation: yet a reference to the table of the mean annual mortality of females in twelve metropolitan districts, at page 122 of this work, will show, that the difference of mortality is dependent rather upon locality, inasmuch as the greatest mortality is at times found to prevail where no factories exist. (Mr. Chadwick's *Sanitary Report*, p. 159. Lond. 1842.) On the whole, in the existing state of knowledge, we are justified in concluding, with a recent writer, (*British and Foreign Medical Review*, April, 1843, p. 313,) that no peculiar evils to health and life attach necessarily to manufacturing pursuits;—that the position of the labouring classes, as a whole, is comparatively prejudicial in these respects; and more particularly of those who inhabit the ill-conditioned localities of large towns; and that in so far as factories, and other corresponding places of labour, interfere with the right conditions of health, they of course lead to the production of disease, and to the shortening of life; but that these evils appertain rather to their *domestic* than to their *industrial* relations."

It has been imagined by many, that literary occupations are positively injurious to health; and that this may occasionally be the case can scarcely be doubted. They are probably, however, less frequently the cause of disease than is imagined. Few are injured by study, unless the frame is unusually excitable, or the mental application unusually protracted; but it is more consolatory to the relatives to have this cause assigned, although, in too many of the cases, study has had but little agency in the result. More than once, indeed, we have known diseases, brought on by juvenile indiscretion, referred to excessive application at the desk, or in the study. There is something soothing in the idea, that even self-immolation has been voluntarily incurred by habits, which have been esteemed so creditable in all ages, but especially in youth; and the suffused eye of the mourning relative gleams with melancholy pleasure when she reflects on the honourable path which the unfortunate *victim* was pursuing.

The diseases, that have been usually ascribed to hard study, are such as implicate the great organ of the intellect more especially; as mania, epilepsy, and palsy. Such affections would appear to have been occasionally, though rarely, produced by the cause assigned. The diseases, with which the literary are especially afflicted, are those to which the sedentary are liable, even when the intellect is suffered to lie dormant; and accordingly dyspepsia, and its gloomy concomitant—hypochondriasis—with general torpor of the digestive apparatus, owing to corporeal inaction, are the common results; but these diseases are of a chronic nature, and by no means liable to destroy, although most distressing to the sufferer; and, therefore, it may, we think, be unhesitatingly affirmed, that literary men, as a body, attain as high a degree of longevity as those of any other avocation. This has been the case in all ages. In antiquity, it was most remarkable; and all our associations of ancient wisdom are attached to the hair whitened by time, and to those venerable busts, which exhibit the characteristics of the accumulated wisdom of ages. Germany affords us an example of a class of men, who devote themselves from an early age to literary pursuits exclusively; and their longevity has been every where a subject of comment. It has, indeed, been maintained—and with much evidence in its favour—that the pursuit of letters in Germany, as every where else, is eminently favourable to longevity. The distinguished physician and naturalist, Blumenbach, asserts, that for the half century and more of his connexion with one of the most celebrated universities in Europe, he has not known a solitary example of any youth falling a victim to his ardour in the pursuit of intellectual distinction; and Eichhorn, one of the most voluminous writers of the day—the eminent philologist and historian—is said to affirm boldly "that no one ever died of hard study. The idea is preposterous. A man may fret himself to death over his books, or any where else, but literary application would tend to diffuse cheerfulness, and rather prolong than shorten the life of an infirm man." (*American Quarterly Review*, No. xi. p. 203:—also, an article, by the Author, in the same Journal, No. xxix, p. 214.) Our experience is completely in accordance with theirs. We cannot, indeed, recollect a solitary case of serious mischief, induced by too great intellectual exercise, although, as has been remarked, the cause has not unfrequently been assigned.

A modern writer (Dr. R. R. Madden, *Infirmities of Genius*, &c. chap. vi.) is disposed to infer, from tables drawn up by himself, but which are far from unobjectionable, that there is more wear and tear from literary pursuits in which the imagination is vigorously exerted, than where any other faculty of the mind is as energetically called into action; and farther, he thinks, the earlier the mental powers are developed; the sooner do the bodily powers begin to fail. "For the purpose," he remarks, "of ascertaining the influence of different studies on the longevity of authors, the tables, which follow, have been constructed; in which the names and ages of the most celebrated authors, in the various departments of literature and science, are set down, each list containing twenty names of those individuals, who have devoted their lives to a particular pursuit, and excelled in it. No other attention has been given to the selection than that which eminence suggested, without any regard to the ages of those, who presented themselves to notice. The object was to give a fair view of the subject, whether it told for, or against the opinions, that have been expressed in the preceding pages. It must, however, be taken into account, that as we have only given the names of the most celebrated authors, and, in the last table, those of artists in their different departments, a greater longevity in each pursuit might be inferred, from the aggregate of the ages, than properly may belong to the general range of life in each pursuit. For example, in moral or natural philosophy, a long life of labour is necessary to enable posterity to judge of the merits of an author, and these are ascertained not only by the value, but also by the amount of his compositions. It is by a series of researches, and recasts of opinion, that profound truths are arrived at, and by numerous publications, that such truths are forced on the public attention. For this a long life is necessary, and it certainly appears, from the list that is subjoined, that the vigour of a great intellect is favourable to longevity in every literary pursuit, wherein imagination is seldom called on."

From tables, formed on this plan, Dr. Madden deduces the following order of longevity, and the average duration of life of the most eminent in each pursuit.

|  | Average years. | Average years. |
|---|---|---|
| Natural Philosophers, | 1494 | 75 |
| Moral Philosophers, | 1417 | 70 |
| Sculptors and Painters, | 1412 | 70 |
| Authors on Law and Jurisprudence, | 1394 | 69 |
| Medical Authors, | 1368 | 68 |
| Authors on Revealed Religion, | 1350 | 67 |
| Philologists, | 1323 | 66 |
| Musical Composers, | 1284 | 64 |
| Novelists and Miscellaneous Authors, | 1257 | 62½ |
| Dramatists, | 1244 | 62 |
| Authors on Natural Religion, | 1245 | 62 |
| Poets, | 1141 | 57 |

It is manifest, however, that in the formation of all such tables, much room is allowed for the intrusion of error. Different individuals may have different views, as regards those who are the most eminent, and the greatest discrepancy may be exhibited in the results, although the investigators may have been equally disposed to discard intentional error. In illustration of this, we shall take one of the lists—as selected by Dr. Madden—of individuals, with whose acquirements, and titles to distinction he may, from his profession, be presumed to be most familiar, and place alongside it one chosen by ourselves, with the view of exhibiting the difference that may readily, and honestly arise in such estimates. But although we are disposed to award honesty to the selection of Dr. Madden, there is some slight reason for believing, that the maxim he was desirous of inculcating—" that the vigour of a great intellect is favourable to longevity in every literary pursuit, wherein imagination is seldom called on"—may have unconsciously biassed him ; otherwise, how can we account for his omission of the name of Bichat— distinguished above his contemporaries for the light, which his observant and penetrating mind diffused over the different departments of medical science ; and of some of which he may, indeed, be regarded as almost the founder ;—Bichat, of whom Corvisart so feelingly, and justly remarked—in his letter to the first Consul, announcing his death :—" Bichat vient de mourir sur un champ de bataille, qui compte aussi plus d'une victime : personne en si peu de temps n'a fait tant de choses et aussi bien ;"—yet this illustrious man has been passed over, whilst Corvisart—far his inferior—is there, with Tissot, Jenner, and Fordyce, who, whatever services they may have rendered to medical science, were certainly not pre-eminent as medical authors. Darwin, too, might with much more propriety be classed with the poets, for there is more of poetry than of history in his few medical publications; and Paracelsus is elevated to a rank, of which so notorious a charlatan is unworthy.

| Name. | Age. | Name. | Age. |
|---|---|---|---|
| 1. Brown, John | 54 | 1. Béclard | 40 |
| 2. Corvisart | 66 | 2. Bichat | 31 |
| 3. Cullen | 78 | 3. Boerhaave | 70 |
| 4. Darwin | 72 | 4. Chaussier | 82 |
| 5. Fordyce | 67 | 5. Cullen | 78 |
| 6. Fothergill | 69 | 6. Fothergill, J. | 68 |
| 7. Gall | 71 | 7. Frank, J. P. | 76 |
| 8. Gregory, (John) | 48 | 8. Gall | 70 |
| 9. Harvey, (W.) | 81 | 9. Georget | 33 |
| 10. Heberden | 92 | 10. Godman | 36 |
| 11. Hoffman | 83 | 11. Good, J. M. | 62 |
| 12. Hunter, J. | 65 | 12. Gregory, James | 68 |
| 13. Hunter, W. | 66 | 13. Haller | 69 |
| 14. Jenner | 75 | 14. Hunter, J. | 65 |
| 15. Good, J. M. | 64 | 15. Laennec | 45 |
| 16. Paracelsus | 43 | 16. Mead | 81 |
| 17. Pinel | 84 | 17. Pinel | 81 |
| 18. Sydenham | 66 | 18. Reil, J. C. | 54 |
| 19. Tissot | 70 | 19. Soemmering, S. T. | 75 |
| 20. Willis, T. | 54 | 20. Sydenham | 65 |
| Total | 1,368 | Total | 1,249 |

In our list, the names of Béclard, Bichat, Georget, and Godman have been added, amongst others, none of whose ages exceeded forty, and but one attained it. The first of these distinguished men was professor of anatomy in one of the most celebrated medical schools of the age. His talents were of a high order ; his views profound, and his mode of communicating them lucid. His publications were not numerous, but they were most creditable. The *" Elements of General Anatomy"* have been translated both in this country and in England; and they signally exhibit the author's acquaintance with the complicated organism of man. His additions, too, to the *Anatomie Genérale* of Bichat, have tended to illustrate and develop the views of his distinguished master. Of that master we have already spoken, and although we are almost irresistibly impelled to dwell on the deeds of one, whose fame must endure as long as the memory of the worthies of by-gone days can be preserved, we must restrain our feelings.

Of M. Georget's claims to respectful notice—had we not possessed the pleasure of personal knowledge—his Essay on "*Insanity*," and his "*Physiology of the Nervous System*," and especially of the Brain, would have been amply sufficient to convince us. He was one of the original projectors of, and contributors to, the *Dictionnaire de Médecine*, and he enriched that useful publication with many valuable monographs. One of these was the basis of his Essay on Insanity. A pupil of the celebrated Esquirol, and a constant attendant at La Salpêtrière,—the great Parisian hospital for those of unsound mind,—his attention had been particularly directed to the physiology and diseases of the brain; and the results of his observations, and reflections—as contained in his various publications—have stamped him as a deep, and original thinker, and as an accurate discriminator of those singular cases of mental aberration, which so frequently present themselves, and are appreciated with so much difficulty.

The propriety of introducing into the list the name of Godman, who—in spite of the disadvantages of fortune, and a brief existence, spent in sickness, and in suffering—succeeded in elevating himself to a high rank amongst physicians, and naturalists, no one will dispute. Nor from such a list could the name of Laënnec have well been excluded. Although his pen was by no means prolific, he has the merit of having proposed a most valuable mode of investigating diseases of the chest, now adopted in every quarter of the globe.

Such are the characters of those in the list we have selected, who died young in years, but old in honour.

If we refer to the list cited, from Dr. Madden, we find the average duration of the lives of medical authors to be sixty-eight; so that their longevity is, in his table, next below that of the authors on law and jurisprudence, and immediately above that of the authors on revealed religion. The corresponding table, formed by the Author, gives the average at less than $62\frac{1}{2}$; and if he had inserted—in the place of names perhaps not more distinguished—those of Miquel of Paris, Gordon of Edinburgh, and Dorsey of Philadelphia—none of whose ages perhaps exceeded thirty-five—the average would have been as low as in some of the tables, where imagination is presumed to have exerted such disastrous effects upon the frame.

It is a common observation, that physicians are more short lived than the members of many other professions and callings;—and the irregularities in diet, and sleep—with the exposure attendant upon the active exercise of their profession—cannot but have an injurious influence on the health of many:—" aliis inserviendo consumuntur, aliis medendo moriuntur." Researches, undertaken by Casper, of Berlin, (*Wochenschrift* u. s. w. Jan. 1834; and *Annales d'Hygiène*, April, 1834) have led him to deduce the following comparative longevity of different callings:

Of 100 theologians, there have attained the age
of 70 and upwards . . . . . . 42
Agriculturists and Foresters . . . . . 40
Superintendents . . . . . . . 35
Commercial and industrious men . . . . . 35
Military men . . . . . . . 33
Subalterns . . . . . . . 32
Advocates . . . . . . . 29
Artists . . . . . . . . 28
Teachers, Professors . . . . . . 27
Physicians . . . . . . . 24

M. Quetelet (*A Treatise on Man*, p. 40. Edinb. edit. 1842) properly remarks, that it would seem to follow from this table, that mental labour is more injurious to man than bodily; but that the most injurious state of all is when fatigue of body is joined to that of the mind. Observations have been too few to enable us to deduce any accurate comparison; but the results of Casper certainly confirm the common observation alluded to above; and it would seem, that the statistical inquiries of Mr. Chadwick (*Report on the Sanitary Condition of the Labouring Population of Great Britain.—Supplementary Report on the Results of a Special Inquiry into the Practice of Interments in Towns*, p. 13. Lond. 1843) have led him to a similar inference. The mortuary registration for the year 1839 gives the following as the average age of death of persons in the three professions in England—Clergymen 59; Lawyers 50;

and medical men 45. Still, as we have seen, amongst the medical authors, many of whom were in extensive practice, we have numerous instances of the attainment of a good old age.

It is somewhat singular, that in Dr. Madden's list we should not find the name of any individual under forty-three years of age, and but one so young—the notorious Paracelsus. The next youngest is Dr. John Gregory, who died at the age of forty-eight. Dr. Madden must, consequently, have had some reason for rejecting those whose deaths were so untimely. If we inquire into the nature and number of the contributions made to science by many of those on his list, we find, that but few of them had distinguished themselves, at the same age, to any thing like the extent of Bichat, Béclard, Georget, or Godman, and if we suppose for a moment what might have been produced by these individuals, if they had been permitted to live as long as Corvisart, Hoffman, or Tissot, it cannot but be believed, that their title to distinction would have been yet more signal. They, who are cut off early in their career, and have left imperishable memorials of their existence, are, indeed, the most fitting subjects for such lists.

It must be obvious, however, that all such tables are liable to the objection, that no correct approximation can be attained by them. So much is left to the whims and caprices of compilers, and so much depends upon their pre-conceived notions, that no two estimates will be found to agree, and, consequently, no such general rule, as that deduced by Dr. Madden—and believed by him to be canonical—can be embraced. Every thing in his tables goes to satisfy him, that imagination, over exerted, is a fell destroyer of mankind. But let us inquire, whether it be true, that poets are shorter lived than other writers; or, in other words, whether the play of the imagination in poetical composition have the effect of curtailing the duration of existence. So far as such individuals are frequently persons of acute sensibility—natural or acquired—the remark may be just, within proper limits. The signal influence exerted by the *moral* on the *physique*—and conversely—is a topic of interesting investigation with the physiologist; and nothing is better established than that there is a wide difference amongst mankind in these respects; and that the nervous, the delicate, the easily impressible—they whose nervous systems are so tenderly organized as to feel the slightest shocks—are more liable to morbid derangements—mental as well as corporeal—than such as are —to use the language of Meiners—more inflexible. This, however, does not apply to the poet solely; but to many who are not alive to the beauties of poetry in any of its subdivisions;—to many of the fairer part of the creation, who are proverbially nervous and hysterical; acutely sensible to impressions;—and to all those, perhaps, who are regarded, and with propriety, to possess genius, —whether this genius may exhibit itself in poetry simply, or brilliantly illumine those departments of science, or art, in which the more staid faculties of the mind are exerted, and which are regarded by Dr. Madden as markedly longevous. The possessor of the attributes, which are looked upon as the characteristics of genius, is apt to be led into irregularities less likely to befall those who are not as highly gifted; and these irregularities—acting upon a frame unusually susceptible and easily thrown off the track by deranging influences—have probably a larger share in the causation of diseases to which such individuals are liable.

In the table of Dr. Madden, in which he contrasts the natural philosophers with the poets, there is certainly a great disparity in the average amount of years attained by the twenty persons on each list;—the former amounting to 1494 years, the latter to 1144; or being to each other in the ratio of 1000 to 763.

| NATURAL PHILOSOPHERS. | | POETS. | |
|---|---|---|---|
| Name. | Age. | Name. | Age. |
| 1. Bacon, | 78 | 1. Ariosto, | 59 |
| 2. Buffon, | 81 | 2. Burns, | 38 |
| 3. Copernicus, | 70 | 3. Byron, | 37 |
| 4. Cuvier, | 64 | 4. Camoens, | 55 |
| 5. Davy, | 51 | 5. Collins, | 56 |
| 6. Euler, | 76 | 6. Cowley, | 49 |
| 7. Franklin, | 85 | 7. Cowper, | 69 |
| 8. Galileo, | 78 | 8. Dante. | 56 |
| 9. Halley, (Dr.) | 86 | 9. Dryden, | 70 |
| 10. Herschel, | 84 | 10. Goldsmith, | 44 |
| 11. Kepler, | 60 | 11. Gray, | 57 |
| 12. La Lande, | 75 | 12. Metastasio, | 84 |
| 13. La Place, | 77 | 13. Milton. | 66 |
| 14. Leeuenhoek, | 91 | 14. Petrarch, | 68 |
| 15. Leibnitz, | 70 | 15. Pope, | 56 |
| 16. Linnæus, | 72 | 16. Shenstone, | 50 |
| 17. Newton, | 84 | 17. Spencer, | 46 |
| 18. Tycho Brahe, | 55 | 18. Tasso, | 52 |
| 19. Whiston, | 95 | 19. Thomson, | 48 |
| 20. Wollaston, | 62 | 20 Young, | 84 |
| Total | 1494 | Total, | 1144 |

A simple inspection of the list of poets will show, however, that some distinguished names might have been substituted for those selected, which would have raised the total amount much above what it is in the table. Chaucer, for example, whose title to distinction none can dispute, died at the age of 72: Göthe, the poet of philosophy—the universal poet—as he has been termed, died at the age of 83;—Klopstock—the German Milton—lived to the age of 79; and Wieland, distinguished for his rich and boundless imagination, attained the same age. Similar examples could be adduced from the history of any of the modern nations of Europe, and if we go to ancient times, we are struck with surprise at the advanced age, which their poets, as well as their literary men of all classes, attained.

If we inquire, however, into the habits of life of many of the poets, in the list of Dr. Madden, we may discover abundant cause for their early decease. Burns, for example, was notoriously addicted to the use of spirituous liquors, until he completely ruined his constitution, and brought on the disease that destroyed him. His is, consequently, by no means a fair case for elucidating the effects of poetical pursuits on health. His productions, too, were not the offspring of application. His poetry was produced fitfully, and whenever his imagination suggested; but he was not the poet of application. Yet Dr. Madden has chosen him for lengthened disquisition, and for the elucidation of a position, which his case is well calculated to overthrow. The following extract from his work offers a satisfactory explanation for the premature deaths of others on the list.

" In Burns's time intemperance was much more common in his walk of life than it now is. In Pope's day we find not a few of his most celebrated contemporaries and immediate predecessors addicted to drunkenness. ' Cowley's death,' (Pope says,) ' was occasioned by a mere accident, while his great friend Dean Pratt was on a visit with him at Chertsey. They had been together to see a neighbour of Cowley's who (according to the fashion of the times,) made them too welcome. They did not set out on their walk home till it was too late, and had drunk so deep, that they lay out in the fields all night. This gave Cowley the fever that carried him off. " Dryden, like Burns, was remarkable for sobriety in early life, ' but for the last ten years of his life (says Dennis,) he was much acquainted with Addison, and drank with him even more than he was used to do, probably so far as to hasten his end.' Yet in his case, as Byron's, wine seems to have had no exhilarating influence; speaking of his melancholy, he says,—' nor wine nor love could make me gay.' And Byron speaks of wine making him savage, instead of mirthful. Parnell, also, (on Pope's authority,) ' was a great follower of drams, and strangely open and scandalous in his debaucheries, (his excesses, however, only commenced after the death of his wife, whom he tenderly loved,) and those helps, (he adds,) that sorrow first called in for assistance, habit soon rendered necessary, and he died in his thirty-sixth year, in some measure a martyr to conjugal fidelity, somewhat we presume in the way

'Of Lord Mount Coffeehouse, the British peer,
Who died of love with wine last year.'

" But another account describes Parnell's taking to drunkenness on account of his prospect declining as a preacher at the queen's death, ' and so he became a sot, and finished his existence.' Churchill was found drunk on a dunghill. Prior, according to Spencer, used to bury himself for whole days and nights together with a poor mean creature, his celebrated Chloe, who, unlike Ronsard's Cassandra, was the barmaid of the house he frequented. And even Pope, we are told by Dr. King, hastened his end by drinking spirits."

So that, according to Dr. Madden's own admission, four of the poets on his list, were addicted to habits more tangible and destructive than the simple pursuits of the imagination; and three of these—Burns, Dryden, and Pope—are considered to have hastened their end, if not to have actually destroyed themselves, by drinking.

But let us inquire dispassionately—so far as relates to our subject—into the circumstances connected with the lives of some of the others on Dr. Madden's list. Of the history of the " divine Ariosto" we know but little. We mean of his private history. His age, at the time of his death, was respectable. Byron, whose habits were none of the best, died of fever, brought on by exposure in a most unhealthy locality, united with epilepsy, to which he had been subject, and which is one of the diseases presumed by Dr.

Madden to be "literary." The age of Camoens—the most celebrated of the Portuguese poets—is given by Dr. Madden at 55. He died in his 62d year, notwithstanding he had spent a great part of his life in the unhealthy regions of India, and on his return to Portugal was in such penury, that a slave, whom he carried with him from India, begged in the streets to support the life of his master. Collins, the poet of the passions, in every sense of the word—as possessor and depicter—was of the most irregular habits; so little control, indeed, did he exert over his unfortunate propensities, that it was thought best to confine him in a lunatic asylum. He died at the early age of 36;—not 56, as Dr. Madden has it. Cowper in spite of his insanity, lived to the goodly age of 69,—almost the "three score years and ten;" and died ultimately of dropsy. The life of Goldsmith—eventful as it was in misery—was terminated by a low fever, which appears to have been in no respect induced by the play of the imagination. Beautiful as are the outpourings of his muse, they are few in number, and could not have occupied so much of his time and attention, as those of his productions in which the imagination is less invoked. It is, indeed, difficult to know how to class an individual, who, as Dr. Samuel Johnson observed, left no species of writing untouched, and adorned all to which he applied himself. He was certainly as worthy of being ranged amongst the dramatists as some that Dr. Madden has placed there. Gray died of gout in the stomach, in his fifty-fifth year, a complaint not likely to have been induced by the cause to which Dr. Madden is desirous of ascribing it. Tasso—the victim of multifarious misfortune—subject also to insanity, died of a violent fever, in his fifty-second year; and Thomson—who was remarkably indolent, and too much disposed to sensual indulgences—of a cold, caught on the Thames, in his 48th year.

It is painful to drag the frailties of eminent individuals from their "dread abode," but it is indispensable to do so in order to arrive at correct conclusions. They are, besides, matters of record, and sufficiently testify, that the views, maintained by Dr. Madden, are untenable; and that other causes than mere imagination were connected with their early fate. Nor ought we to be surprised, that the productions of the imagination should be more largely furnished by those under forty years of age, than the more severe efforts of the judgment, which often require a life of application. Youth is proverbially the period of the imagination, and some of the best efforts of the poet have been made at a time of life, when others are about to commence the prosecution of the transcendental studies of a physical nature,—and after the age of forty, we generally find, that the ardour of the poet, and his productive powers begin to fail, so that the efforts of his muse are few, and far between, and perhaps generally less dazzling than those elicited at an earlier age.

We think, then, it may be established as a general axiom, that literary pursuits are directly favourable to long life, whether they require the exercise of the memory, the judgment, or the imagination; and that where the health is apparently injured by them, the evil is dependent rather on collateral circumstances,—on irregularity of habits, as regards eating, drinking or sleeping,—often acting upon a frame unusually susceptible of impressions, for such is the common accompaniment, of genius; and that these views are just, is strongly corroborated by examining the history of female authors, most of whom have been extremely long lived; doubtless, in a great degree, because they were exempt from that irregularity of life, which we have seen to be so destructive to the poets, whose productions have appeared in youth, and the celebrity arising from which has led them into society, and into habits, that have too frequently been destructive. In a late number of the *London Quarterly Review*, there is the following list of some of the most celebrated female authors of Great Britain. Their united ages amount to 1429 years, and the average to $71\frac{1}{2}$;—placing them next below the class of natural philosophers, as given by Dr. Madden.

| Names. | Age. | Names. | Age. |
|---|---|---|---|
| 1. Lady Russel | 87 | 12. Mrs. Lennox | 84 |
| 2. Mrs. Rowe | 63 | 13. Mrs. Trimmer | 69 |
| 3. Lady M. W. Montagu | 73 | 14. Mrs. Hamilton | 65 |
| 4. Mrs. Centlivre | 44 | 15. Mrs. Radcliffe | 60 |
| 5. Lady Hervey | 70 | 16. Mrs. Barbauld | 83 |
| 6. Lady Suffolk | 79 | 17. Mrs. Delany | 93 |
| 7. Mrs. Sheridan | 47 | 18. Mrs. Inchbald | 68 |
| 8. Mrs. Cowley | 66 | 19. Mrs. Piozzi | 81 |
| 9. Mrs. Macaulay | 53 | 20. Mrs. Hannah Moore | 88 |
| 10. Mrs. Montague | 81 | | |
| 11. Mrs. Chapone | 75 | | 1429 |

Such, we think, are the correct general deductions from an examination of the evidence we possess on this subject. We might even go farther, and affirm, that the pursuit of letters—whatever may be the intellectual faculties mainly exerted—does not necessarily induce infirmities of body or mind, except in the young, and in frames unusually impressible—as those of some men of genius, as well as of men of no genius at all, are at times found to be;—and that the exercise of no one faculty of the mind appears to produce more wear and tear of the economy than another.

We have said, that literary occupations cannot be closely pursued with the same impunity in the young as in the adult, and this for reasons, that are sufficiently intelligible. When study is indulged to excess in early life, it may have a tendency to induce a predominance in the nutrition of certain organs at the expense of others. It is well known, that if any organ be energetically exercised, its vital activity is exalted, and a larger afflux of blood takes place towards it, so that it attains a greater degree of development than where it is less used. Hence we can conceive, that a constant overstraining of the intellectual powers, especially when conjoined with irregularity in exercise, diet, sleep, &c. may occasion augmented flow of blood to the brain, and consequent disease in that viscus, even in the adult. Still more likely is this to ensue, if the same application be made before the organs have undergone their full evolution; and hence we may conceive, that early and intense study may lay the foundation to faulty development in other parts of the frame, and to great energy of nutrition in the brain. But whilst we admit, that this *may* be the case, we are satisfied it happens but rarely—far less frequently than is apprehended—the impaired health of the studious being generally referable, as before observed, to collateral circumstances rather than to cerebral disorder thus directly induced; yet the idea of the morbific agency of great intellectual application prevails universally, and has been adopted by many writers on the physiology, and pathology of the nervous system. "Men of exalted intellect," says a modern writer on insanity, (Scipion Pinel, *Physiologie de l'homme aliéné*, p. 177,) " perish by their brains, and such is the noble end of those, whose genius procures for them that immortality, which so many ardently desire." The same idea, by the way, is conveyed by Pliny. "Morbus est etiam aliquis per sapientiam mori." Dr. Madden, too—after having entered into a lengthened description of the character of the incomparable genius, Sir Walter Scott, and after having mentioned, that he died of palsy—asserts, that this disease is the too frequent termination of literary life; and he enumerates, amongst the "martyrs to literary glory," Copernicus, Petrarch, Linnæus, Lord Clarendon, Rousseau, Marmontel, Richardson, Steele, Phillips, Harvey, Reid, Johnson, Porson, Wollaston and Scott—" a few of the many eminent names of those, who have fallen victims to excessive mental application, by paralysis, or apoplexy." Yet many of these persons were not distinguished as severe students; several are classed by Dr. Madden in the tables of literary occupations, not characterized by the higher flights of the imagination; some did not die of apoplexy, or palsy; and most of them attained a good old age, although the hibits of one in particular were such as would destroy any person, who did not possess a constitution of iron. Copernicus, and Wollaston, and Linnæus belong to the table of natural philosophers—"the first on the list of studies conducive to longevity"—the first of whom died in his 71st year; the second at the age of 62; and the last at the age of 72. Petrarch is in his list of poets—he attained the age of 68, and probably died of heart disease, for he was found dead early in the morning with his head resting on a book. Clarendon, and Rousseau died at the age of 66; Marmontel, in his 77th year; Richardson at 71; Steele at 58; Harvey, the illustrious discoverer of the circulation of the blood—who is said to have shortened his life by a dose of opium—at 81; Reid—the metaphysician—in his 86th year; Johnson in his 75th : and Porson, whose grossly intemperate habits were well calculated to shorten existence, at the age of 49.

This list is sufficient to show the longevous effects of literary pursuits, although these worthies are considered by Dr. Madden to have fallen " victims" to " excessive mental application." We suspect that there are but few corporeal avocations, which could exhibit greater longevity; and few in which the same number of cases of apoplexy or palsy might not be readily selected.

Dr. James Johnson (*'Change of Air,'* or the *Philosophy of Travelling,*) has hazarded the opinion, that a high range of health is probably " incompatible with the most vigorous exertion of the mind, and that this last both requires and induces a standard of health somewhat below par." "It would not be difficult," he adds, " to show that the majority of those, who have left behind them imperishable monuments of their intellectual powers, and exertions, were people of weak bodily health. Virgil, Horace, Voltaire, Pope, and a thousand others might be quoted in illustration."

Such impaired condition of the functions was doubtless present in the cases referred to, and it has existed, and does exist, in numerous others. But these are only coincidences, affording examples of high intellectual attainments and productions, in spite of the bodily infirmities under which those distinguished individuals laboured, but by no means showing that they were the consequence of such infirmities. Nothing, indeed, would seem to be clearer than that full intellectual development requires, that the different corporeal functions should be faithfully and regularly executed. It is impossible for the mind to aspire to lofty conceptions, or for the various intellectual faculties to be fully accomplished, unless the body is devoid of suffering. Whatever distracts the mind from its own operations enfeebles the results, and nothing does this more effectually, and unpropitiously, than suffering of any kind. Every one must have felt the difficulty of bending the intellectual powers on any important topic, when the stomach has been deranged simply by over distention; and still more, when food, difficult of digestion, has been taken; and how much more must this be the case under the continued pressure of functional, or organic disease! It can be easily conceived, however, that although sickness may interfere with the vigorous exercise of the " higher faculties," it may yet be the occasion of greater production than a state of health. Disease, or infirm health necessarily confines the invalid, and hence incites to intellectual exercise, for the purpose of dispelling the *ennui*, which such a condition induces, and thus the *production* may be greater, although the *capabilities* may be less.

But although to an overwhelming proportion of those, who devote themselves to quiet and regular intellectual persuits, and who attend properly to collateral circumstances, the excitement of the brain may be salutary rather than prejudicial, there may be a few—a very few—who experience mischief from close mental application. Such are they, as we have said, of frames unusually impressible, and in whom, when any organ is thrown into unwonted exercise, a sudden afflux to it of vital energy ensues, which, in the case of the brain, might give rise to headach, confusion of thought, with the whole train of nervous symptoms. The individuals, thus circumstanced, we say are few, although it is a common excuse, urged by such as are indisposed to intellectual application, and is generally received as valid. The evil, too, may be greatly obviated by habit—by never forcing the intellectual powers, but bending them daily on their object, until they become accustomed to the exercise; and being especially careful not to permit them to interfere with those collateral agencies, the regularity of whose application is essential to health. When the mind is well disciplined, it is surprising what may be accomplished by a proper use of time. No one, in modern times, has surpassed, in productive capabilities, Sir Walter Scott: yet, by proper economy of time, he was enabled to avail himself, as fully as the most unoccupied, of the pleasures of social and domestic intercourse. When asked by Captain Hall, how many hours a day he could write for the press with effect, he replied. "I reckon five hours and a half a day is very good work for the mind, when it is engaged in original composition. I can very seldom reach six hours, and I suspect that what is written after five or six hours' hard mental labour is not worth much." On being asked how he divided those hours, he said: "I try to get two or three of them before breakfast, the remainder as soon after as may be, so as to leave the afternoon free to walk, or ride, or read, or be idle." (*Fragments of Voyages and Travels*, 2d and 3d series, chap. i.)

Very different is the intense mental excitement, produced in those who have the cares of empires reposing upon them; or of the merchant engaged in deep and involving speculations. The effects, here, resemble rather those of the passions, or emotions than of the tranquil—comparatively tranquil—mental exertions of the closet. To the former the most towering intellect may succumb: we have offered sufficient reason to show, that the latter need entail no such evils. It may be said, indeed, that if mental application occasions increased flow of blood to the head, it must necessarily be followed by morbid phenomena; but, when such augmented afflux is within due bounds, it no more follows, that cerebral disease should result, than gastric derangement, whenever an increased flow of blood takes place to the stomach; as always happens, in truth, when it is performing its healthy functions.

In cases where a portion of the scull has been removed, opportunities have occurred for witnessing the state of the brain during mental emotion; and an injection of its tissue appears to have been all that was especially noticed. In the case of a young gentleman taken to Sir Astley Cooper, who had lost a portion of the scull just above the eyebrows—" On examining the head " says Sir Astley, (*Lectures on Surgery*, vol. i.) " I distinctly saw the pulsation of the brain was regular, and slow; but at this time he was agitated by some opposition to his wishes, and directly the blood was sent with increased force to the brain, and the pulsation became frequent and violent ;"—and he properly infers, that if, in the treatment of injuries of the brain, we omit to keep the mind free from agitation, our other means may be unavailing. Although, therefore, we admit the dangers, that are presumed to result from violent mental emotions, owing to the consequent augmented vital action in the encephalon, we may yet deny, that a slighter degree of the same exaltation will be attended with equally—or with any —unfavourable consequences. Indeed, the mischiefs, that occasionally result from violent mental contentions, are more frequently exerted upon the nervous function itself than upon the vessels distributed to the nervous centres: the heart beats irregularly—convulsively as it were—and at times ceases at once to act, so that the individual dies suddenly of fatal syncope. Although the action of the heart is but indirectly under the nervous influence, we know it is powerfully acted upon by the emotions, so that in sudden paroxysms of joy, or grief, or fear, its irritability is, at times, irretrievably exhausted. The individual does not in such cases die of apoplexy, which begins in the brain; but of syncope beginning in the heart. This last organ, in other words, is the first to die.

In this way, the *moral* may act most injuriously on the *physique*. We have already seen how largely the former is influenced by the latter. Fortunately for us, it happens, that fatal consequences rarely result except from the sudden influence of overpowering emotions. The same mental excitation—when of a somewhat less degree—may be experienced for a long time, and yet the system may and does ultimately rally. Corvisart observes, that diseases of the heart were extremely common in the times of the French revolution, when the minds of all classes were kept in a state of constant agitation and alarm. Where mischief is done by such causes, the organ that suffers will generally be the heart; although the functions of the brain are occasionally perverted, and mental aberration, in the form of mania, succeeds to the violence done to the brain and nervous system, when the emotion is overwhelming; or, melancholy—" thick ey'd, musing, and curs'd melancholy," is the product of its more lengthened and corroding application. Happily, however, notwithstanding the affecting tales we hear of broken hearts, such cases are not frequent either literally or metaphorically. We say literally, for it is asserted, that Philip the Fifth of Spain died suddenly on learning the disastrous rout of his army near Plaisance, and Zimmermann states, that on opening his body the heart was found burst. Where the heart breaks metaphorically, the main morbid impression is made on the nervous system—and especially on the great nervous centres: owing to the concentrated action on these, watchfulness is induced, and the different functions carried on under the presidency of this system —especially the functions of nutrition—become impaired, so that the health declines; the organs are insufficiently nourished, and atrophy gradually dries up the fountains of life. But such calamitous cases—as already observed—are passing rare. In referring to " the class of mental emotions, denominated *fear, grief, sorrow*, and *anxiety*, which make the greatest depredations on the functions, and structure of the central organ of the circulation," and to some " curious allusions" in certain of the ancient writers to this subject, Dr. James Johnson (*Treatise on Derangement of the Liver*, &c. p. 221,) adduces the following remarks of Melanchthon, which he designates as " the most remarkable passage of *antiquity*," and as one " that would not dishonour the first pathologist of the present day."—" Mœstitia cor quasi percussum constringitur, tremit, et languescit, cum acri sensû doloris. In tristitiâ, cor fugiens attrahit ex splene lentum humorem malancholicum qui effusis sub costis in sinistro lateri hypochondriacos flatus facit ; quod sæpe accidit iis qui diuturnâ curâ et mœstitiâ conflictantur." That is, to adopt the unsatisfactory translation cited by Dr. Johnson,—" Sorrow strikes the *heart*, makes it flutter and pine away with *great pain ;* and the black blood drawn from the spleen, and diffused under the ribs on the left side, makes those perilous hypochondriacal flatulencies, which happen to those that are troubled with sorrow." This, Dr.

Johnson says is " a true picture of cardiac disorder from the nervous irritation of grief or sorrow and ought to be kept in mind, both by patient and physician;" but it strikes us as mere verbiage, conveyed in a learned language it is true, but not on that account the less unmeaning; and we think, we are justified in adding, not only unworthy of, but unintelligible to, *any* pathologist of the present day.

Yet, although the violent passions, when often indulged—or the deeper, but less manifest emotions, when long protracted—may be injurious, the regulated indulgence of the emotions, especially those of an exciting character, is not only innocuous but salutary : under their play, the action of the different organs goes on with more vigour, and there is a greater resistance to morbific impressions than where the functions are executed with a languid sameness. In childhood, indeed, and in youth, which are the ages of active and boisterous enjoyment, the full play of the passions, and of the organs on which their effects are exhibited, appears to be almost indispensable to health ; and evil has been found to result from any plan, which has prevented the accustomed juvenile enjoyments. " The crying and sobbing of children," says Dr. Combe, (*Op. citat.* p. 188 ; and his book on *Infancy*, edited by Dr. Bell, Philad. 1840) "contribute much to their future health, unless they are caused by disease, and carried to a very unusual extent. The loud laugh, and noisy exclamations attending the sports of the young have an evident relation to the same beneficial end, and ought therefore to be encouraged instead of being repressed, as they are often sought to be, by those who, having forgotten that they themselves were once young, seek in childhood the gravity and decorum of more advanced age. I have already noticed an instance on a large scale, where the inmates of an institution were, for the purpose of preserving their health, shut up within the limits of their hall for six months, and not allowed to indulge in any noisy and romping sports. The aim of the directors was undoubtedly the purest benevolence, but from their want of knowledge, their object was defeated, and the arrangement itself became the instrument of evil."

Dr. Combe's views are perhaps carried somewhat too far, but there is much truth in the advantage, which he ascribes to the proper indulgence of the different emotions.

# APPENDIX.

Deposition, involving questions regarding the effect of draining a malarious soil—table of the mean temperature, &c. of the seasons, in different places in America, Europe, &c.—tables of the temperature of St. Augustine, &c. during certain months—mean temperature, &c. of corresponding months in certain winter retreats—temperature, &c. of Campeche, and of Santa Cruz— table of the comparative digestibility of different alimentary substances.

AFTER the observations on malaria, in the first edition, were written, the author was requested to give in a written deposition, before a court of justice, on questions of hygiène, involving some of the theoretical, and practical points comprised in the consideration of that subject; and as this deposition sets forth the notions, which he entertains regarding this "fitful pest," as briefly expressed as the nature of the case would admit, he thinks it well to add them in a supplementary chapter.

Many years ago, one of the most eminent agriculturists of Virginia attempted to drain a marsh or "creek"—as it is termed by one of the contending parties—situate on one of the large rivers of that state; and below tide water. This he endeavoured to effect by making two dams,— an upper, and a lower; the former of which is alone referred to in the deposition. To a certain extent he succeeded, and a part of the marsh was put into cultivation; but, in the year after the draining, much sickness was experienced, especially in ——, a village in the neighbourhood. It is asserted, however, by the one party, that this sickness was not confined to the vicinity of the marsh, but was marked throughout the whole extent of the river valley. After this, the land remained long unreclaimed; but very recently the present proprietor determined upon repeating the attempts made by his ancestor. An injunction was, however, obtained against him, and it was in consequence of such injunction, that the author was called upon for a written answer to various queries, proposed by the counsel for plaintiff, and defendant,—the parties having mutually agreed, that the answers should be read as evidence, without being put in a legal form.

It may be well to remark, that the "upper dam," to which reference is frequently made, was thrown across the marsh, to exclude the tide water from about seventy-five acres of wet, boggy, or marshy land above it; and that the water from rains and springs had been intercepted, and conducted to the river, by ditches, and canals, cut along the margin of the dry land, and around the whole circumference of the meadow. Before these operations were undertaken, the tide water, and that from rains and springs, flowed into, and spread over, the whole seventy-five acres. Subsequently, and at various times, about sixty acres had been cultivated, and produced variable crops of Indian corn, according to the seasons, and other casualties. About ten acres, which might have been cultivated, have never been; and about five have at all times been too wet for grain. The meadow is surrounded by high banks, and the bank on the side of the village is covered with a growth of trees, and thick underwood, varying in width from thirty to forty yards. The nearest part of the meadow to the first house in the village is about three-fourths of a mile, and the farthest about a mile and a-half: the whole marsh lying north of west from the village. The meadow above the upper dam is the subject of contention; the lower dam having been cut so as to admit the tide water as usual; and the whole undertaking, so far as relates to the reclamation of the land between the two dams, has been abandoned.

QUESTIONS SENT BY THE PARTIES.

*By the Defendant.*—Dr. Dunglison is requested to state, whether he ever examined the marsh on the estate belonging to —— ——, in the county of ——, called ——; if so, he is requested to give his opinion on the following points.

1. The tendency of the marsh, in its present unreclaimed condition, to affect the health of those residing in its immediate vicinity?

2. Whether it is probable, that the health of ——, (the village,) is affected by miasma emitted from that part of the marsh, which is located above the upper dam?

3. Whether the reclamation of that portion of the marsh lying above the upper dam will have any, and if any, what effect upon the health of ——, (the village,) and what is likely to be the effect upon the health of that place, of the means resorted to, to effect such reclamation, whilst the work is in progress?

*By the Plaintiffs.*—1. What opportunities have you had of ascertaining the effect of the operations of draining this meadow or creek of Mr. ——'s, on the health of ——, (the village?)

2. Do you know any thing from experience of the effects of stagnant water, or illy drained land in eastern Virginia, on the health of the per-

sons living in the vicinity of such land or water; and if so, what are the effects?

3. Are the remittent and intermittent fevers, so common in autumn in eastern Virginia, occasioned by local causes—if so, what are those local causes?

*Answers to the Defendant's questions.*

In answer to the Defendant's inquiry, whether the undersigned has ever seen the marsh in question? he replies, that he had an opportunity of personally inspecting it in the latter end of June, 1833; and in reply to the first query,—as regards "*the tendency of the marsh, in its present unreclaimed condition, to affect the health of those residing in its immediate vicinity?*"—he has no hesitation in expressing his opinion, that it is more likely to produce malarious disease, in its present condition, than if it were thoroughly reclaimed.

In its existing state, indeed, it appears to be most favourable for the generation of malaria. It is alternately submerged, and exposed to the solar rays with the flowing and ebbing of the tides; and, during the neap tides especially, a large surface is necessarily exposed to the sun's heat. This is, in the undersigned's opinion, and experience has proved the truth of it, a most favourable condition for the evolution of febrific miasmata: indeed, Dr. Ferguson—a writer who had extensive experience in tropical regions on this matter—asserts, that there seems to be one only condition indispensable to the production of the "marsh poison," as he terms it,— the *paucity* of water, where it has previously and recently *abounded*. "To this," he says, "there is no exception in climates of high temperature," and thence, he thinks, we may justly infer, that the poison is produced at a highly advanced stage of the drying process. The observation of the undersigned leads to opinions somewhat analogous to those of Dr. Ferguson; and these, he thinks, are applicable to the marsh in its present condition; for during the heats of summer and autumn, considerable portions must be undergoing alternate overflow and desiccation, and thus be in a condition eminently adapted for the copious evolution of malaria.

The undersigned doubts not, therefore, that there are constantly exhaled from the surface of the marsh, during the heats of summer and autumn, febrific miasmata, capable of injuriously affecting the health of persons living "in its immediate vicinity."

QUESTION 2d.—"*Whether it is probable, that the health of ——, (the village,) is affected by miasma emitted from that part of the marsh, which is located above the upper dam.*"

*Answer.*—Although the undersigned considers, that miasmata are exhaled in sufficient abundance from the part of the marsh above the upper dam, to affect injuriously those living "in its immediate vicinity," he does not consider that this can apply to the inhabitants of ——, (the village,) which is on the same level with the marsh, and the nearest house of which, if he recollects right, is at least three quarters of a mile distant; whilst the malarious ground is surrounded by high banks, and the bank on the side of the village is protected by an intervening growth of trees and thick underwood, varying in width from twenty to fifty yards, more or less. Nor, unless he is mistaken in the direction in which the village lies from the land in question, can the malaria be often driven towards the village. The marsh lies to the north of west, and during the seasons of summer and autumn, the prevalent winds are not from that quarter. For all these reasons, the undersigned does not conceive it probable, that the health of —— is much affected by miasma emitted from that part of the marsh, "which is located above the upper dam."

QUESTION 3d.—"*Whether the reclamation of that portion of the marsh, lying above the upper dam, will have any, and if any, what effect upon the health of ——, and what is likely to be the effect upon the health of that place, of the means resorted to, to effect such reclamation, whilst the work is in progress.*"

*Answer.*—A part of the answer to this question is comprised in the one just given. If, in its present state, it does not, for the reasons assigned, materially affect the health of the inhabitants of ——; it probably would not, under any process, that might be undertaken for reclaiming the marsh, even were such process to give rise to a greater evolution of malaria. If, however, the desiccation be properly performed, the admixture of the tide-water with that from rains and springs will be altogether precluded, and the surface will be put into a condition less adapted for the exhalation of the miasm in question.

From what the undersigned has already remarked, it will appear to be his belief, that whenever the solar rays can evaporate the water covering a malarious soil, so as to thoroughly desiccate that soil, malaria will be given off; but this disengagement does not take place to any amount, except soon after the first draining, and if the access of water be entirely prevented, the evil will be corrected as far as the circumstances will admit. Under this view, it may be said, that if the whole marsh be drained, the surface exhaling the miasm will be, for a time, greater than it is now; and that, as is proved by experience, the first warm seasons after the draining of land will be liable to malarious affections. Such might, and probably would be the case with the land in question, if the desiccation were attempted at an improper period, as during the seasons of spring, summer, or early in the fall; but if it be undertaken towards the close of autumn, in winter, or early spring, and be effectually done, so as to exclude the overflowing of the tide-water, and that of the rains and springs, and to prevent the stagnation of water on the surface, the ground would be cultivated and put into a favourable condition before the accession of the summer and autumnal heats; and this course cannot fail, in the undersigned's opinion, to detract largely from the amount of mischief which now exists, under circumstances extremely favourable for its generation, and which will continue to exist unless such reclamation be effected.

The undersigned does not, therefore, conceive, that the reclamation—that is, the effectual reclamation—done at a proper season, of the marsh lying above the upper dam, will have any effect upon the health of ——; nor does he think, that the means resorted to for effecting such reclamation can have any influence on the health of that place, whilst the work is in progress. In stating this opinion, he has used the expression "effectual reclamation," because he regards this as the great end to be accomplished; but even if imperfectly performed, he cannot imagine that the surface can be left in a state much better adapted for the disengagement of miasmata than it is in at present.

### ANSWERS TO THE PLAINTIFF'S QUESTIONS.

QUESTION 1.—"*What opportunities have you had of ascertaining the effects of the operations of draining this meadow or creek of Mr. ——'s on the health of ——?*"

*Answer.*—Personally, the undersigned has had none. He knows nothing except what has been stated to him, and these statements have been most discordant, although all were referred to *experience*. The undersigned need hardly say, that, in every such case, *reputed experience* should be received with caution, and that the evidence should be narrowly sifted. Whenever the rights and feelings of individuals are arrayed against each other,—especially if such feelings involve the health of families and of districts,—*coincidents* are apt to be regarded as *consequents*, and, with the greatest disposition to be just, injustice is often committed. The undersigned esteems it proper to make this remark, in connexion with the opinions he has expressed touching the propriety of draining this marsh—the great mode of accomplishing what the French term the *assainissement* of marshes. With them *assainissement*, or the "act of rendering salubrious," as applied to marshes, is almost synonymous with *draining*. There are, indeed, but two ways in which this desirable object can be accomplished—the one is destruction by submerging; the other reclamation by *desiccation* or *draining*. Now it is possible, that after the desiccation of the marsh more malarious disease may prevail, although, as the undersigned has remarked in one of his answers to a query from the defendant, if done in the manner advised, this is not likely to result from the process; but he trusts, if such should be the case, it may not be hastily ascribed to the desiccation, but that dispassionate inquiry may be made, whether other situations on the river are not at the time more than usually insalubrious.

QUESTION 2.—" *Do you know any thing from experience of the effects of stagnant water, or illy drained land, in eastern Virginia, on the health of persons living in the vicinity of such land or water; and if so, what are the effects?*"

*Answer.*—On this subject, the undersigned has necessarily had much experience in different regions of the globe. The history and effects of malaria have, indeed, been with him, for years, an interesting topic of inquiry. So long ago as the summer of 1823, he had occasion to publish an article on the subject, in the *London Quarterly Review*—which was one of the earliest *ex professo* essays on malaria that had appeared. In that essay, the opinions he has expressed in this communication are contained,—but slight modification having been produced in them by subsequent experience.

His opportunities in eastern Virginia—and the remark does not apply solely to it—have shown, that in certain districts, the inhabitants, in the vicinity of stagnant water, and of imperfectly drained land, have been subject to malarious disease; whilst in other districts, and apparently under the same circumstances, there has not been a solitary case of intermittent, and no greater number of remittent fevers than in localities of a different description. In other words, the soil itself must be malarious, in order that miasmata shall be exhaled. The undersigned does not recollect, that during the eight or nine years in which he resided at the University of Virginia, he had one marked case of intermittent under his management produced by the locality; although there is a meadow not far from the buildings, not more, perhaps, than two hundred yards, which is annually submerged during the winter, and at times till late in the spring. Within the circuit, too, of some miles, and along the south-western range of mountains, although there are many collections of stagnant water, millponds, &c., intermittents scarcely exist, and remittents are by no means rife; whilst in other localities, and in some not far distant from those mentioned, and, indeed, through perhaps the whole of eastern Virginia below tide water, such local conditions could not fail to be the *foyers* of much endemic disease. The steeping of hemp is proverbially a most unhealthy process, where the soil is malarious, but on the mountain chain, to which the undersigned has referred, the herb is cultivated, and the process of making hemp accomplished, without the induction of any thing like miasmatic disease.

If, therefore, the question of the plaintiff be restricted to eastern Virginia, the answer of the undersigned will have to vary according to the precise district. Indeed, the question might equally have included western Virginia, for, along the Shenandoah and in other situations, malarious soils exist, causing disease to as great an extent as in many of the unhealthy localities of eastern Virginia.

In such malarious districts, then, as those lying on the —— river, which experience shows to be malarious, stagnant water, or illy drained land does produce injurious effects " on the health of persons living in the vicinity of such land or water:" the diseases, thus induced, are chiefly intermittent and remittent fevers; and the great mode of permanent *assainissement*, in all such cases, as the undersigned has already remarked, is to thoroughly desiccate the faulty locality at a proper season.

QUESTION 3.—" *Are the remittent and intermittent fevers, so common in autumn in eastern Virginia, occasioned by local causes—if so, what are these local causes?"*

*Answer.*—On this question a volume might be written. It involves indeed "a bone of contention," which has been gnawed for ages, and yet the marks of the teeth are scarcely perceptible. Whilst it has been maintained by some, that *all fevers* are produced by malaria; others, and distinguished members of the profession, have held, that malaria is not necessary for the production of any, and that it merely adds to their malignancy when once induced. Others, again, have gone farther, and have ascribed every malady characterized by periodicity, or that recurs at intervals, to the agency of this emanation. The first opinion is unworthy of comment: the second is true within certain limits only; and the last is too sweeping in its character.

The view of the undersigned is, that malaria is an essential agent in the production of the diseases referred to in the question; and that this malaria is a " local cause," but of what nature he knows not. It has hitherto escaped the researches of the chemical analyst. It is an emanation from soils, that are marshy, in particular situations, but not in all. In this country, there are many marshy districts, which are not marked by any predominance of the exhalation; whilst in others, not marshy, malarious fevers occasionally prevail with fearful malignity. At times, also, a situation previously free from malarious disease becomes extremely subject to it; and conversely. The banks of many of the large rivers of the United States were at one time healthy, where they are now almost uninhabitable. Two or three years ago, on the shore of Long Island, at the Narrows, malarious fevers prevailed with great virulence, yet, for forty years previously, they were almost unknown there. The whole of the Maremma district of Italy—stretching from Leghorn to Terracina —is a prey to these affections, yet in many parts of it there are no marshes within several miles. The inference, therefore, is, that although in marshy lands, and in the oozy shores of our streams, localities exist favourable to the evolution of malaria, this morbific effluvium may yet be evolved from soils in no respect paludal. The bilious remittent is a common disease in every part of Virginia, although more prevalent in the lower than in the upper country. In the latter, it presents itself in localities where we may seek in vain for marshes, or for any thing resembling them.

The reply, then, of the undersigned to this query of the plaintiff, is;—that he considers the remittent and intermittent fevers, common in autumn in eastern Virginia, to be mainly occasioned by local causes; but with regard to the nature of those local causes he is consummately ignorant; all he can say is, that experience has proved certain localities to be malarious, but what the precise nature of the soil exhaling the malaria, or of the malaria itself, is, the chemical pathologist has yet to learn.

From all, then, that has been said it will appear,—that the undersigned is of opinion, that to permanently remove or diminish the evolution of malaria from the meadow in question,—and the remark might be extended to malarious marshes in general—it is important, that a thorough reclamation should be effected at a proper season; that it should be put into cultivation, so as to prevent the solar rays from beaming upon the reclaimed soil during the heats of the subsequent summer, and that if this be accomplished, the undersigned does not conceive, that the health of —— could be in anywise injuriously affected, but that,˙on the contrary, if any effect were induced, it would probably be one of amelioration.—All of which the undersigned humbly, and respectfully submits, as his deliberate and conscientious belief.

ROBLEY DUNGLISON.

*Baltimore, June,* 1834.

# TABLE OF MEAN TEMPERATURES.

Table, showing the Mean Temperature of the year, and of the different seasons—with the Mean Temperature of the warmest and coldest months—of different places in America, &c., as deduced from the Paper of Von Humboldt on Isothermal Lines, the Meteorological Registers kept by the Surgeons of the United States' Army, the work of Sir James Clark on Climate, &c., &c.

| PLACES. | Latitude. | Mean temperature of several years. | Mean temperature of different seasons. | | | | Mean temperature of | |
|---|---|---|---|---|---|---|---|---|
| | | | Winter. | Spring. | Summer. | Autumn. | warmest month. | coldest month. |
| Nain, Labrador,........ | 57.°08' | 26.°42 | 0.°60 | 23.°90 | 48.°38 | 33.°44 | 51.°80 | 11.°20 |
| Fort Brady, Mich...... | 46.39 | 41.37 | 14.09 | 37.69 | 61.83 | 43.94 | 62.87 | 12.65 |
| Quebec, L. C.......... | 46.47 | 41.74 | 14.18 | 38.84 | 68.00 | 46.04 | 73.40 | 13.81 |
| Eastport, Me,......... | 44.54 | 42.44 | 23.44 | 38.58 | 60.54 | 45.43 | 63.52 | 20.91 |
| Fort Howard, Mich..... | 44.40 | 44.50 | 20.82 | 41.40 | 68.70 | 45.18 | 73.67 | 17.95 |
| Fort Crawford, Miss... | 43.03 | 45.52 | 23.76 | 43.09 | 69.78 | 46.74 | 71.34 | 20.14 |
| Cambridge, Mass...... | 42.21 | 50.36 | 33.98 | 47.66 | 70.70 | 49.82 | 72.86 | 29.84 |
| Conncil Bluffs, Missouri. | 41.25 | 50.82 | 27.38 | 46.38 | 72.84 | 48.60 | 75.92 | 27.19 |
| Newport, R. I......... | 41.30 | 51.02 | 33.82 | 46.87 | 68.70 | 53.83 | 71.46 | 32.14 |
| Philadelphia,.......... | 39.56 | 53.42 | 32.18 | 51.44 | 73.94 | 56.48 | 77.00 | 32.72 |
| New York,............ | 40.40 | 53.78 | 29.84 | 51.26 | 79.16 | 54.50 | 80.78 | 25.34 |
| Cincinnati,............ | 39.06 | 53.78 | 32.90 | 54.14 | 72.86 | 54.86 | 74.30 | 30.20 |
| Monticello, Va......... | 37.58 | 55.40 | 37.67 | 54.67 | 73.33 | 56.50 | 75.00 | 36.00 |
| Washington, D. C...... | 38.53 | 55.56* | 36.80 | 53.83 | 75.90 | 56.59 | 79.13 | 34.66 |
| Smithville, N. C....... | 34.00 | 58.88 | 53.44 | 64.76 | 80.46 | 68.15 | 82.93 | 50.69 |
| Charleston, S. C....... | 32.47 | 60.18 | 51.09 | 66.73 | 80.89 | 67.55 | 82.81 | 49.43 |
| Natchez, Miss......... | 31.34 | 64.76 | 48.56 | 65.48 | 79.16 | 66.02 | 79.70 | 46.94 |
| Pensacola, Florida,.... | 30.28 | 68.77† | 55.13 | 69.67 | 82.57 | 69.05 | 83.55 | 53.80 |
| St. Augustine, do...... | 29.48 | 72.23 | 59.29 | 71.47 | 82.73 | 75.15 | 83.94 | 56.60 |
| Tampa Bay, do........ | 27.57 | 72.37 | 61.24 | 72.93 | 80.14 | 75.28 | 80.72 | 58.70 |
| Vera Cruz,............ | 19.11 | 77.72 | 71.96 | 77.90 | 81.50 | 78.62 | 81.86 | 71.06 |
| Havanna,............. | 23.10 | 78.08 | 71.24 | 78.98 | 83.30 | 78.98 | 83.84 | 69.98 |
| Bahamas,............. | 26.40 to 27.5 | 78.3 | 71. | 77. | 83. | 80. | 90. | 64. |
| Barbadoes,........... | 13.10 | 79.3‡ | 76.7 | 79. | 81. | 80. | | |
| Cumana,.............. | 10.27 | 81.86 | 80.24 | 83.66 | 82.04 | 80.24 | 84.38 | 79.16 |

\* St. Louis, Missouri, Lat. 38.°46'. Mean temperature 55.°86. New Harmony, Lat. 38.°11' Mean temperature 56.°74.

† New Orleans, Lat. 30.° Mean temperature 69.°01. Baton Rouge, Lat. 30.°26'. Mean temperature 68.°07.

‡ Jamaica, coast, Mean temperature, 80.°6.

TABLE of the Temperature, &c. of St. Augustine, during the months of December, 1833, and of January, February, March, and April, 1834,—as indicated by a self-registering thermometer—from a register kept by Dr. Peter Porcher, now of Charleston, S. C.

The temperature of Germantown, during the same months, is taken from the meteorological register, published in the "Journal of the Franklin Institute." The observations were taken at sunrise and at two o'clock, P. M.; they consequently give the temperature of the *day* only; whilst those of Dr. Porcher indicate the maximum and minimum during the 24 hours.

The medium temperature of the corresponding months in Baltimore is given on the authority of Professor Hall—whose observations were taken at 8 A. M., at 2 P. M., and at 11 P. M.

## DECEMBER, 1833.

|    | TEMP. |      | WIND.       | WEATHER.                                  |
|----|-------|------|-------------|-------------------------------------------|
|    | Max.  | Min. |             |                                           |
| 1  | 63    | 35   | N.E.        | Rain.                                     |
| 2  | 70    | 45   | N.          | Fair.                                     |
| 3  | 62    | 52   | "           | "                                         |
| 4  | 64    | 52   | "           | "                                         |
| 5  | 63    | 57   | N.E.        | Cloudy.—Windy.                            |
| 6  | 62    | 55   | "           | Rain.                                     |
| 7  | 63    | 52   | "           | "                                         |
| 8  | 59    | 48   | "           | "                                         |
| 9  | 58    | 49   | "           | Cloudy.                                   |
| 10 | 59    | 42   | "           | Rain.                                     |
| 11 | 56    | 42   | "           | "                                         |
| 12 | 60    | 52   | "           | "                                         |
| 13 | 55    | 52   | "           | "                                         |
| 14 | 55    | 39   | W.          | Fair. Windy and uncomfortable.            |
| 15 | 63    | 46   | N.W.        | "                                         |
| 16 | 58    | 38   | S.W.        | Rain.                                     |
| 17 | 50    | 34   | W.          | Fair. Cold and windy.                     |
| 18 | 50    | 32   | "           | "                                         |
| 19 | 51    | 42   | "           | "                                         |
| 20 | 55    | 53   | N.E.        | Rain.                                     |
| 21 | 63    | 46   | S.W.        | "                                         |
| 22 | 53    | 46   | N.E.        | Cloudy. Raw and disagreeable.             |
| 23 | 60    | 56   | S.E. & N.W. | Clear morning. Rain, thunder and lightning, in the evening. |
| 24 | 63    | 50   | N.E.        | Cloudy. Evening,—thick fog.               |
| 25 | 57    | 33   | N.W.        | Fair.                                     |
| 26 | 50    | 45   | N.E.        | "                                         |
| 27 | 52    | 46   | "           | "                                         |
| 28 | 50    | 45   | "           | Cloudy.                                   |
| 29 | 53    | 53   | "           | "    Some rain.                           |
| 30 | 69    | 62   | S.W.        | "                                         |
| 31 | 74    | 59   | "           | Fair.                                     |

Mean temperature of the month 52°.85; maximum 74°; minimum 32°; range 42°. Mean daily range 11°. Greatest daily range 28°.

GERMANTOWN.—Mean temperature of the month, taken in the *day* only, 34°.16. Maximum height, 44°—on the 1st, 8th and 30th. Minimum, during the *day*, 21° on the 13th.

## TEMPERATURE OF ST. AUGUSTINE. 443

### JANUARY, 1834.

|    | TEMP. |     | WIND.     | WEATHER. |
|----|-------|-----|-----------|----------|
|    | Max.  | Min.|           |          |
| 1  | 74 | 60 | S.W.      | Foggy morning. Clear afternoon. |
| 2  | 74 | 44 | S.W. morn.| Changed to N.E., with lightning, thunder and rain,—evening. |
| 3  | 44 | 43 | N.E.      | Rain. |
| 4  | 44 | 39 | "         | "    stormy. |
| 5  | 44 | 35 | "         | " |
| 6  | 42 | 26 | "         | " |
| 7  | 42 | 35 | "         | Fair. |
| 8  | 49 | 40 | N.W.      | " |
| 9  | 59 | 49 | "         | " |
| 10 | 72 | 55 | S.W.      | "    foggy morning. |
| 11 | 72 | 58 | "         | "    morning, thick fog. |
| 12 | 79 | 51 | "         | " |
| 13 | 56 | 46 | N.E.      | Cloudy, with slight rain. |
| 14 | 50 | 46 | "         | "    " |
| 15 | 50 | 47 | "         | Rain. |
| 16 | 58 | 53 | N.       | " |
| 17 | 66 | 55 | S.E.      | Fair. |
| 18 | 67 | 54 | "         | " |
| 19 | 69 | 59 | "         | " |
| 20 | 69 | 57 | "         | " |
| 21 | 73 | 49 | S.W.      | Changed to N.E. at sunset. Fair. |
| 22 | 49 | 42 | N.E.      | Cloudy. |
| 23 | 50 | 37 | N.E.      | Rain. |
| 24 | 50 | 44 | N.        | Fair. |
| 25 | 58 | 49 | N.E.      | " |
| 26 | 66 | 45 | S.W.      | " |
| 27 | 53 | 48 | N.E.      | Cloudy. |
| 28 | 56 | 44 | "         | " |
| 29 | 53 | 46 | "         | Rain. |
| 30 | 52 | 47 | "         | " |
| 31 | 55 | 49 | "         | " |

Mean temperature of the month 52°.93; maximum 79°; minimum 26°; range 53°. Mean daily range 10°.9. Greatest daily range 30°.

GERMANTOWN.—Mean temperature of the month, taken in the *day* only, 28°.22. Maximum height, 59° on the 18th. Minimum during the *day*, 10° on the 7th.

BALTIMORE.—Mean temperature of the month, 33°.4.

## FEBRUARY, 1834.

| | TEMP. | | WIND. | WEATHER. |
|---|---|---|---|---|
| | Max. | Min. | | |
| 1 | 55 | 38 | N.W. | Fair. |
| 2 | 55 | 45 | N.E. | " |
| 3 | 57 | 45 | " | " |
| 4 | 64 | 49 | W. | " |
| 5 | 65 | 49 | S.W. | " |
| 6 | 69 | 50 | " | " |
| 7 | 70 | 53 | " | " |
| 8 | 63 | 50 | N.E. | " |
| 9 | 67 | 55 | W. | Cloudy. |
| 10 | 67 | 50 | N. | Fair. |
| 11 | 65 | 45 | " | " |
| 12 | 67 | 53 | S.E. | " |
| 13 | 68 | 55 | S.W. | " |
| 14 | 76 | 59 | " | " |
| 15 | 79 | 66 | " | " |
| 16 | 83 | 63 | " | " |
| 17 | 75 | 55 | S.W. to N.E. | with rain, lightning and thunder. |
| 18 | 58 | 53 | N. | " thick weather. |
| 19 | 63 | 59 | " | Cloudy morning. Fair evening. |
| 20 | 65 | 58 | N.E. | Fair. |
| 21 | | | | Omitted on account of absence. |
| 22 | | | | Weather fair, and mild. |
| 23 | | | | |
| 24 | | | | |
| 25 | 84 | 60 | N.E. | Fair. |
| 26 | 60 | 52 | " | " |
| 27 | 64 | 55 | " | Cloudy. |
| 28 | 56 | 45 | " | Rain. |

Mean temperature of the month 59°.52; maximum 84°; minimum 38°. Monthly range, 46°. Greatest daily range, 24°. Mean daily range, 13°.83.

GERMANTOWN.—Mean temperature of the month, taken in the *day* only, 39°.34. Maximum height, 65° on the 15th. Minimum, during the *day*, 20° on the 8th.

BALTIMORE.—Mean temperature of the month, 47°.4.

TEMPERATURE OF ST. AUGUSTINE.

MARCH, 1834.

|    | TEMP. |      | WIND. | WEATHER.                    |
|----|-------|------|-------|-----------------------------|
|    | Max.  | Min. |       |                             |
| 1  | 50    | 43   | N.W.  | Fair. Cold.                 |
| 2  | 63    | 34   | W.    | "                           |
| 3  | 50    | 40   | N.E.  | "                           |
| 4  | 60    | 50   | "     | "                           |
| 5  | 70    | 60   | S.E.  | windy.                      |
| 6  | 73    | 62   | S.W.  | Cloudy.                     |
| 7  | 75    | 60   | S.E.  | Foggy morning. Clear day.   |
| 8  | 75    | 64   | "     | Fair.                       |
| 9  | 64    | 58   | N.E.  | Cloudy. Gusty day.          |
| 10 | 62    | 56   | E.    | Rain.                       |
| 11 | 66    | 54   | N.E.  | "                           |
| 12 | 60    | 48   | "     | Cloudy.                     |
| 13 | 66    | 59   | "     | Fair.                       |
| 14 | 66    | 55   | S.W.  | Rain.                       |
| 15 | 66    | 53   | N.E.  | Cloudy.                     |
| 16 | 65    | 54   | "     | Rain.                       |
| 17 | 65    | 59   | "     | Cloudy.                     |
| 18 | 69    | 59   | "     | Overcast.                   |
| 19 | 69    | 60   | "     | Fair.                       |
| 20 | 73    | 62   | S.E.  | Rain.                       |
| 21 | 71    | 46   | N.W.  | Fair.                       |
| 22 | 55    | 44   | N.E.  | "                           |
| 23 | 66    | 54   | E.    | "                           |
| 24 | 76    | 59   | S.E.  | "                           |
| 25 | 81    | 65   | S.W.  | "                           |
| 26 | 80    | 59   | "     | Rain. Lightning.            |
| 27 | 70    | 59   | N.E.  | " Heavy thunder.            |
| 28 | 67    | 58   | "     | Cloudy.                     |
| 29 | 73    | 58   | "     | Rain.                       |
| 30 | 80    | 60   | S.E.  | Fair.                       |
| 31 | 75    | 61   | "     | "                           |

Mean temperature of the month 61°.76; maximum 81°; minimum 34°. Monthly range 47°. Greatest daily range 29. Mean daily range 12°.5.

GERMANTOWN.—Mean temperature of the month, taken during the *day* only, 41°. 64. Maximum height 70° on the 20th. Minimum, during the *day*, 21°. on the 22d.

BALTIMORE.—Mean temperature of the month, 49.°

APPENDIX.

APRIL, 1834.

| | TEMP. | | WIND. | WEATHER. |
|---|---|---|---|---|
| | Max. | Min. | | |
| 1 | 74 | 59 | S.E. | Fair. |
| 2 | 74 | 59 | " | " |
| 3 | 76 | 62 | " | " |
| 4 | 64 | 50 | N.E. | Gale with rain. |
| 5 | 50 | 40 | " | " " |
| 6 | 52 | 40 | N.W. | Cloudy. |
| 7 | 70 | 46 | W. | Fair. |
| 8 | 70 | 49 | S.E. | Overcast. |
| 9 | 70 | 50 | S.E. | Fair. |
| 10 | 73 | 61 | S.W. & N.E. | " |
| 11 | 70 | 55 | E. | " |
| 12 | 70 | 54 | S.W. | " |
| 13 | 73 | 55 | E. | " |
| 14 | 79 | 55 | S.E. | " |
| 15 | 75 | 56 | N.W. | " |
| 16 | 79 | 59 | W. | " |
| 17 | 79 | 60 | S.E. | " |
| 18 | 79 | 59 | " | " |
| 19 | 76 | 58 | variable. | Rain. |
| 20 | 78 | 58 | E. | Fair. |
| 21 | 81 | 62 | S.E. | " |
| 22 | 76 | 60 | " | " |
| 23 | 83 | 60 | S.W. | " |
| 24 | 80 | 62 | N.W. | " |
| 25 | 83 | 62 | W. | " |
| 26 | 70 | 58 | N.E. | Cloudy. |
| 27 | 70 | 53 | " | Fair. |
| 28 | 72 | 56 | " | " |
| 29 | 80 | 56 | S.W. | " |
| 30 | 84 | 64 | " | " |

Mean temperature of the month 64°.63; maximum 84°; minimum 40°. Monthly range 44°. Greatest daily range 24°. Mean daily range 17°.63.

BALTIMORE.—Mean temperature of the month, 59°.

# TABLES OF TEMPERATURE.

Although the preceding tables embrace but one year, they enable us to form some approximation to the character of the climate of St. Augustine, compared with that of other places of this country and of Europe. To exhibit this more clearly, the following tabular views are appended, which show the mean monthly temperature, maximum, minimum, and range, as well as the greatest daily, and mean daily range, during the corresponding months—but of different years—at some of the prominent retreats for the valetudinarian, in Great Britain, on the continent of Europe, and in the African islands. It is proper, however, to remark, that in no situations, except in those to which an asterisk is affixed, was the register thermometer used. In the others, the observations were made during the *day* only, and consequently the numbers given are far below the real range throughout the twenty-four hours.

The places are arranged in the order of their mean temperature.

### TABLE OF MEAN TEMPERATURE.

| PLACES. | December. | January. | February. | March. | April. |
|---|---|---|---|---|---|
| Sidmouth, - - | 43.00 | 36.30 | 42.00 | 45.00 | 51.00 |
| Penzance, - - | 46.50 | 43.00 | 44.50 | 46.50 | 48.50 |
| Pau, - - - - | 41.53 | 38.89 | 44.96 | 46.80 | 55.79 |
| Montpellier, - | 46.00 | 42.00 | 45.00 | 47.00 | 53.00 |
| Nice, - - - - | 48.60 | 45.85 | 49.00 | 51.45 | 57.00 |
| Rome, - - - | 49.62 | 47.65 | 49.45 | 52.05 | 56.40 |
| Naples, - - - | 50.50 | 46.50 | 48.50 | 52.00 | 57.00 |
| Madeira, - - | 60.50 | 59.50 | 58.50 | 61.06 | 62.50 |

### TABLE OF MAXIMUM, MINIMUM AND RANGE OF TEMPERATURE.

| PLACES. | December. | | | January. | | | February. | | | March. | | | April. | | |
|---|---|---|---|---|---|---|---|---|---|---|---|---|---|---|---|
| | max. | min. | range. | max. | min. | range. | max. | min. | range. | max. | min. | range. | max. | min. | range. |
| Sidmouth,* - - | 54 | 25 | 29 | 47 | 21 | 26 | 52 | 27 | 25 | 56 | 26 | 30 | 60 | 31 | 29 |
| Penzance,* - - - | 56 | 34 | 22 | 54 | 28 | 26 | 55 | 33 | 22 | 59 | 34 | 25 | 62 | 36 | 26 |
| Pau, - - - | 56 | 25 | 31 | 56 | 21 | 35 | 60 | 35 | 25 | 65 | 35 | 30 | 71 | 43 | 28 |
| Montpellier, - - | 57 | 32 | 25 | 53 | 27 | 26 | 55 | 30 | 25 | 58 | 35 | 23 | 64 | 41 | 23 |
| Nice, - - - | 59 | 40 | 19 | 58 | 27 | 31 | 58 | 37 | 21 | 65 | 41 | 24 | 69 | 46 | 23 |
| Rome, - - - | 60 | 31 | 29 | 58 | 29 | 29 | 60 | 33 | 27 | 65 | 37 | 28 | 74 | 44 | 30 |
| Naples, - - - | 61 | 34 | 27 | 58 | 29 | 29 | 60 | 31 | 29 | 69 | 38 | 31 | 78 | 43 | 35 |
| Madeira,* - - - | 68 | 52 | 16 | 69 | 50 | 19 | 68 | 51 | 17 | 69 | 51 | 18 | 72 | 55 | 17 |

TABLE OF DAILY RANGE OF TEMPERATURE.

| PLACES. | DECEMBER. | | JANUARY. | | FEBRUARY. | | MARCH. | | APRIL. | |
|---|---|---|---|---|---|---|---|---|---|---|
| | mean daily range. | greatest daily range. | mean daily range. | greatest daily range. | mean daily range. | greatest daily range. | mean daily range. | greatest daily range. | mean daily range. | greatest daily range. |
| Sidmouth, - - | | 13 | | 13 | | 12 | | 12 | | 13 |
| Penzance, - | 3 | | 4 | | 6 | | 8 | | 9 | |
| Pau, - - - - | 7 | 13 | 7 | 16 | 9 | 16 | 9 | 17 | 8 | 18 |
| Montpellier, - | 9 | | 8 | | 9 | | 14 | | 14 | |
| Nice, - - - - | 6 | 14 | 8 | 16 | 9 | 18 | 9 | 17 | 11 | 18 |
| Rome, - - - | 9 | 15 | 11 | 16 | 10 | 18 | 12 | 19 | 10 | 20 |
| Naples, - - - | 9 | 13 | 9 | 14 | 11 | 19 | 11 | 18 | 14 | 20 |
| Madeira,* - - | 11 | 14 | 11 | 17 | 9 | 13 | 10 | 14 | 9 | 13 |

# TEMPERATURE OF CAMPECHE.

TABLE of the Temperature in CAMPECHE, latitude 19°.51' N. during the month of February, 1834, as indicated by a self-registering thermometer, from a register kept in the consulate of the United States, by Dr. Henry Perrine.

|   | TEMP. Max. | TEMP. Min. | WIND. | WEATHER. |
|---|---|---|---|---|
| 1 | 75 | 74 | N. | Morning drizzly—day cloudy—afternoon drizzly. |
| 2 | 76 | 74 |  | Morning cloudy—afternoon clear. |
| 3 | 76 | 74 |  | Clear. |
| 4 | 77 | 74 | N.E. | " |
| 5 | 77 | 74 |  | " |
| 6 | 77 | 74 | S.E. & N.W. | " |
| 7 | 77 | 74 | " |  |
| 8 | 77 | 74 | " |  |
| 9 | 78 | 75 | " |  |
| 10 | 77 | 75 |  | Sky occasionally slightly obscur'd. |
| 11 | 77 | 75 | " |  |
| 12 | 77 | 75 | " |  |
| 13 | 77 | 75 | " |  |
| 14 | 83 | 75 | " |  |
| 15 | 83 | 76 | " |  |
| 16 | 82 | 76 | " |  |
| 17 | 82 | 76 | " |  |
| 18 | 83 | 77 | " & S. & W. |  |
| 19 | 84 | 78 | S.E. & N.W. |  |
| 20 | 84 | 78 |  | Sky slightly overcast in afternoon. |
| 21 | 84 | 78 |  | Do.    do.    in morning. |
| 22 | 86 | 78 | S.E. |  |
| 23 | 87 | 79 | " |  |
| 24 | 88 | 79 | " |  |
| 25 | 88 | 79 | S.E. & N.W. |  |
| 26 | 87 | 78 | " |  |
| 27 | 86 | 78 | " |  |
| 28 | 86 | 78 | " | Cloudy, and rain. |

Mean temperature of the month 78°.58; maximum 88°; minimum 74°; monthly range 14°. Greatest daily range 9°. Mean daily range 5°.03.

Dr. Perrine states, that his self-registering thermometer was suspended " on the east side of an open entry from north to south—ten yards each way from the outside of the building—and, being in the second story, the doors are kept open day and night,"—and he adds—" the hammock, which I recline in, both sleeping and waking, is attached to the northern wall.—Hence it is the fairest representation of the temperature, which can be obtained for an invalid."

In Campeche a fire is employed only for cooking or washing, and neither chimney nor fire-place exists in any house of Yucatan.

In the number of the "American Journal of the Medical Sciences," for May, 1834, Dr. Perrine has the following remarks, respecting the climate of Campeche. "Were it not for the disagreeable peculiarities of all Spanish countries, I should long since have recommended Campeche as a winter resort to our consumptive patients. The cities, inhabited by that race alone, are entirely divested of houses for accommodation to strangers. With a population of at least 20,000 inhabitants, there is not a single establishment entitled to the name of hotel, and the only two apologies for transient visiters are miserably dirty places, not fit for a sailors' boarding house in the north, one of which is kept by a French negro woman, and the other by an Italian sailor. Luckily, the fine temperature of the climate enables one to dispense with bed, and bedding, and a hammock slung up under a shed or any shelter from the dew is sufficient to pass the night. I am now (Feb. 3, 1834,) sitting in one, at 3 A. M., with the thermometer at 74°, which has not varied three degrees in the last three days and nights."

# TEMPERATURE OF SANTA CRUZ.

Tables of the temperature at Santa Cruz, during the months of December, 1836, and of January, February, March, April, and part of May, 1837, as observed by the Rev. Joseph Tuckerman, D. D. (From *Boston Medical and Surgical Journal*, July 12, 1837, p. 359.)

## DECEMBER, 1836.

| | 6½ A. M. | 9 A. M. | 12. | 3 P. M. | 6 P. M. | 9 P. M. | Daily variation. |
|---|---|---|---|---|---|---|---|
| 7 | 78 | 79 | 80 | 79 | 77 | 77 | 3 |
| 8 | 76 | 79 | 80 | 80 | 77½ | 78 | 4 |
| 9 | 75½ | 75½ | 75½ | 76 | 75 | 75 | 1 |
| 10 | 73¾ | 76½ | 79¼ | 79 | 77½ | 76½ | 5¼ |
| 11 | 74 | 78 | 78 | 76¾ | 76½ | 76½ | 4 |
| 12 | 75 | 75 | 79 | 79 | 77 | 76 | 4 |
| 13 | 72½ | 76 | 77½ | 76 | 76 | 75½ | 5 |
| 14 | 74 | 76 | 76 | 76½ | 74 | 75 | 2½ |
| 15 | 73 | 76 | 78¼ | 78½ | 76½ | 75 | 5½ |
| 16 | 73 | 78 | 80½ | 80 | 77 | 76½ | 7½ |
| 17 | 75 | 78 | 80½ | 80 | 78 | 77 | 5½ |
| 18 | 78 | 79 | 81½ | 80 | 77½ | 76½ | 3½ |
| 19 | 76 | 77½ | 79 | 79½ | 77½ | 78 | 3½ |
| 20 | 75 | 76½ | 79 | 79½ | 77 | 76½ | 4½ |
| 21 | 75 | 77 | 80 | 79½ | 77 | 76 | 5 |
| 22 | 75½ | 77 | 78½ | 78½ | 76 | 74½ | 4 |
| 23 | 72 | 76 | 78 | 76½ | 74 | 74½ | 6 |
| 24 | 73¼ | 76½ | 78 | 77¾ | 76 | 73½ | 4½ |
| 25 | 73 | 76¼ | 76¼ | 76 | 73½ | 73 | 3¼ |
| 26 | 73 | 76¼ | 77½ | 76 | 74 | 73 | 4½ |
| 27 | 73 | 74 | 74½ | 76 | 75 | 74 | 3 |
| 28 | 73 | 76 | 78 | 77 | 75½ | 74 | 5 |
| 29 | 72 | 74½ | 76 | 77½ | 76½ | 74 | 5½ |
| 30 | 70 | 73 | 75 | 76¼ | 74 | 73 | 6¼ |
| 31 | 73½ | 75 | 76¼ | 76¾ | 75 | 74 | 3¼ |

Extremes of temperature in twenty-six days, 70, and 81½.

Greatest variation on any day, 7½ degrees. The least variation on any day, 1 degree.

The mean temperature of this month, 75¾ degrees.

Frequent small showers fell during this month, but no one which continued longer than from five to ten minutes. These showers came with short premonition of their approach; and great care was required, while taking a ride or drive, not to be wet by them.

## JANUARY, 1837.

| | 6½ A. M. | 9 A. M. | 12. | 3 P. M. | 6 P. M. | 9 P. M. | Daily variation. |
|---|---|---|---|---|---|---|---|
| 1 | 71½ | 74½ | 77 | 76½ | 74 | 73 | 5½ |
| 2 | 72 | 74½ | 78 | 78 | 76 | 75 | 6 |
| 3 | 76 | 76½ | 80 | 80½ | 78 | 78 | 4½ |
| 4 | 74 | 75 | 75½ | 76½ | 76 | 76 | 2½ |
| 5 | 76½ | 77½ | 80 | 80 | 78¾ | 77½ | 3½ |
| 6 | 76 | 78½ | 80½ | 81 | 79 | 78 | 5 |
| 7 | 76 | 79 | 80 | 81 | 79 | 77 | 5 |
| 8 | 76 | 75 | 76½ | 78 | 78 | 77 | 3 |
| 9 | 74 | 77 | 80 | 78 | 78 | 75½ | 6 |
| 10 | 74 | 77 | 80½ | 79 | 77½ | 76 | 5 |
| 11 | 74 | 78½ | 80 | 78½ | 76 | 75¼ | 6 |
| 12 | 75 | 77 | 78½ | 78½ | 76¼ | 76 | 3½ |
| 13 | 74 | 77½ | 78½ | 78½ | 76 | 75 | 4½ |
| 14 | 74 | 77 | 78 | 78½ | 75 | 74½ | 4½ |
| 15 | 74 | 78 | 78½ | 78½ | 78½ | 77 | 4½ |
| 16 | 73½ | 77½ | 77½ | 77½ | 76 | 75 | 4½ |
| 17 | 73 | 77½ | 79 | 79 | 76 | 75 | 6 |
| 18 | 74 | 78 | 78 | 78 | 77 | 76½ | 4 |
| 19 | 74 | 80 | 80½ | 79½ | 79 | 78 | 6½ |
| 20 | 75 | 79 | 80 | 80 | 78 | 76 | 5 |
| 21 | 74¾ | 79 | 80 | 79 | 78 | 76 | 5½ |
| 22 | 73 | 78 | 80¼ | 80½ | 80 | 76 | 7½ |
| 23 | 73 | 76 | 77 | 80 | 78 | 76 | 7 |
| 24 | 76 | 79 | 80½ | 80 | 78 | 76 | 4½ |
| 25 | 76 | 77 | 78½ | 78 | 76½ | 76 | 2½ |
| 26 | 75½ | 77 | 80½ | 79¾ | 77 | 76 | 5 |
| 27 | 76 | 78 | 80½ | 80 | 76 | 76½ | 4½ |
| 28 | 75½ | 77 | 77½ | 77 | 76 | 75½ | 2 |
| 29 | 74½ | 77 | 80¾ | 79 | 78 | 78 | 6¼ |
| 30 | 76 | 78½ | 81¾ | 80 | 77 | 78 | 5¼ |
| 31 | 76 | 78 | 81 | 80½ | 77 | 76 | 5 |

The extremes of temperature this month were 71½, and 81¾.

The greatest variation of temperature on any day was 7½ degrees. The smallest variation on any day was 2½ degrees.

The mean temperature of the month was 76.

Frequent small showers occurred in this, as in the preceding month, but with less frequency at its close.

Dr. Tuckerman passed the months of December and January at Frederickstœd, or West End. During that time, he lived in No. 10 Strand Street, and his thermometer was suspended in the coolest part of the hall of that house. The house fronts west, and is open also to the east; and has a constant draft through its hall whenever the wind is favourable to a passage through it.

## FEBRUARY, 1837.

| | 6½ A. M. | 9 A. M. | 12. | 3 P. M. | 6 P. M. | 9 P. M. | Daily variation. |
|---|---|---|---|---|---|---|---|
| 1 | 77 | 79½ | 82 | 81½ | 76½ | 76 | 6 |
| 2 | 74½ | 78 | 81 | 79 | 76½ | 76 | 6½ |
| 3 | 75 | 78 | 81 | 79½ | 76 | 76 | 6 |
| 4 | 75½ | 77 | 77½ | 79 | 76 | 76 | 3½ |
| 5 | 74 | 77½ | 78 | 79 | 76 | 76 | 5 |
| 6 | 74½ | 78 | 81 | 80½ | 78 | 76 | 6 |
| 7 | 74 | 77 | 80 | 79 | 78 | 76 | 6 |
| 8 | 74½ | 77½ | 80 | 77½ | 77½ | 74 | 5½ |
| 9 | 74½ | 78 | 81 | 80 | 78 | 76½ | 6½ |
| 10 | 75½ | 78½ | 81½ | 81 | 78 | 76 | 6 |
| 11 | 75 | 77 | 80 | 78 | 76 | 75 | 5 |
| 12 | 74 | 78 | 81½ | 79 | 77½ | 76 | 6½ |
| 13 | 75 | 78½ | 81 | 81 | 78 | 75½ | 6 |
| 14 | 75½ | 76 | 79 | 74½ | 74 | 73 | 3½ |
| 15 | 74 | 76 | 79 | 76 | 75½ | 76 | 5 |
| 16 | 74½ | 78 | 79 | 78½ | 75 | 75 | 4½ |
| 17 | 76 | 78 | 80 | 80 | 77 | 76 | 4 |
| 18 | 75½ | 78 | 80¼ | 79 | 77 | 75 | 4¾ |
| 19 | 74 | 79 | 79 | 78¼ | 74 | 73½ | 5 |
| 20 | 74 | 77¾ | 79 | 79 | 77 | 74 | 5 |
| 21 | 74 | 73½ | 76½ | 76 | 77 | 75 | 3 |
| 22 | 73 | 75 | 79 | 79½ | 76 | 74 | 6½ |
| 23 | 73 | 79 | 80½ | 80 | 76 | 76 | 7½ |
| 24 | 73½ | 76 | 80 | 81 | 76½ | 75 | 7½ |
| 25 | 73½ | 79½ | 81½ | 78 | 76 | 75½ | 8 |
| 26 | 74 | 79 | 81½ | 82 | 76½ | 75 | 8 |
| 27 | 74 | 78 | 80 | 78½ | 76 | 75 | 6 |
| 28 | 74 | 77½ | 80 | 77½ | 76 | 74 | 6 |

On the 1st day of this month Dr. Tuckerman removed to Bassin, the eastern town of this island; and, till the 22d of the month, lived in a house there upon elevated ground. He thought the air of Bassin drier, and more grateful to the feelings, than that of West End. On the 22d he removed to the Pearl estate, a bleak and almost altogether comfortless situation. There he remained three weeks, and in that time lost more strength than he had gained in the preceding six or eight weeks.

The extremes of temperature this month were 73, and 82.

The greatest variation of temperature on any day was 8 degrees. The smallest was 3 degrees.

The mean temperature of the month was 77½ degrees.

There were two short but heavy showers in this month; one on the 8th, and the other on the 14th. Otherwise the weather was clear and very beautiful.

## TEMPERATURE OF SANTA CRUZ.

### MARCH, 1837.

| | 6½ A. M. | 9 A. M. | 12. | 3 P. M. | 6 P. M. | 9 P. M. | Daily variation. |
|---|---|---|---|---|---|---|---|
| 1 | 74 | 80 | 80½ | 80 | 77 | 75 | 6½ |
| 2 | 74 | 76¾ | 79 | 78 | 75½ | 74 | 5 |
| 3 | 72 | 77½ | 80 | 79½ | 75 | 74 | 8 |
| 4 | 73 | 78½ | 80 | 79¾ | 76 | 74 | 7 |
| 5 | 72½ | 78½ | 80 | 80 | 76 | 75 | 7½ |
| 6 | 73 | 75 | 79 | 79 | 76 | 74 | 6 |
| 7 | 71 | 75 | 77½ | 76¼ | 73½ | 72½ | 6½ |
| 8 | 70 | 74 | 77 | 76 | 73½ | 72 | 7 |
| 9 | 68½ | 74 | 78 | 77 | 75 | 72 | 9½ |
| 10 | 71 | 74 | 77 | 76 | 74 | 74 | 6 |
| 11 | 72 | 77 | 77½ | 80 | 76 | 74 | 8 |
| 12 | 72 | 75 | 77 | 77½ | 75 | 74 | 5½ |
| 13 | 71½ | 75 | 79 | 78 | 74 | 73 | 7½ |
| 14 | 71½ | 74 | 74½ | 75 | 74 | 74 | 3½ |
| 15 | 74 | 76 | 77 | 78 | 76 | 75 | 4 |
| 16 | 74 | 75 | 76 | 77 | 76 | 74½ | 3 |
| 17 | 74 | 78 | 80½ | 80 | 78 | 76 | 6½ |
| 18 | 76 | 79 | 79 | 78½ | 77 | 76 | 3 |
| 19 | 74 | 76 | 76½ | 76½ | 75 | 75 | 2½ |
| 20 | 75 | 75½ | 76 | 77 | 76 | 75 | 2 |
| 21 | 74 | 76 | 77½ | 79½ | 75 | 74 | 5½ |
| 22 | 74 | 76 | 79 | 78 | 75 | 73 | 6 |
| 23 | 70½ | 77 | 77 | 76 | 74½ | 74 | 6½ |
| 24 | 67½ | 78 | 82 | 78½ | 76 | 74 | 14½ |
| 25 | 72 | 77 | 80 | 78 | 76 | 74½ | 8 |
| 26 | 74 | 78 | 78 | 78 | 75½ | 74 | 4 |
| 27 | 73½ | 79½ | 79 | 78½ | 76½ | 76 | 5½ |
| 28 | 76 | 80 | 82 | 81½ | 77 | 77 | 6 |
| 29 | 77 | 82 | 84½ | 83½ | 80 | 79 | 7½ |
| 30 | 79 | 80 | 84 | 78 | 76½ | 75 | 9 |
| 31 | 75½ | 76 | 77 | 77 | 75 | 74 | 3 |

A cold northerly wind prevailed from about the 7th, to the 21st of this month. On the 30th there was a heavy rain, which continued to fall for three hours. Perhaps not a sixth part so much had fallen in the preceding four months.

On the 14th of this month, Dr. Tuckerman returned to the house, in Bassin, which he had left three weeks before.

The extremes of temperature this month were 67½, and 84½.

The greatest variation of temperature on any day was 14½ degrees. The smallest variation was 2 degrees.

The mean temperature of the month was 74.

### APRIL, 1837.

| | 6½ A. M. | 9 A. M. | 12. | 3 P. M. | 6 P. M. | 9 P. M. | Daily variation. |
|---|---|---|---|---|---|---|---|
| 1 | 74 | 77½ | 78 | 77 | 74 | 73 | 5 |
| 2 | 76 | 79 | 78 | 78 | 76½ | 74½ | 4½ |
| 3 | 75½ | 79½ | 81 | 79 | 76 | 75 | 6 |
| 4 | 75½ | 78½ | 80 | 80 | 77 | 76 | 4½ |
| 5 | 78 | 83 | 85 | 85 | 80 | 78 | 7 |
| 6 | 77 | 78 | 78 | 81 | 78½ | 76½ | 4½ |
| 7 | 76½ | 79 | 80 | 79 | 78 | 77 | 3½ |
| 8 | 77 | 79 | 81 | 83 | 79 | 78 | 6 |
| 9 | 79½ | 83 | 84 | 85 | 80 | 78 | 7 |
| 10 | 78 | 80 | 83 | 83 | 81 | 79 | 5 |
| 11 | 77½ | 81½ | 81 | 80 | 78 | 78 | 3½ |
| 12 | 78 | 80 | 80 | 80 | 78½ | 78½ | 2 |
| 13 | 76 | 79 | 78 | 79 | 78 | 77 | 3 |
| 14 | 77 | 82 | 82 | 82½ | 80½ | 78½ | 5½ |
| 15 | 78 | 83 | 84 | 83 | 81 | 79½ | 6 |
| 16 | 79½ | 81½ | 84 | 84 | 81 | 79 | 5 |
| 17 | 78 | 80 | 83½ | 81½ | 80 | 79 | 5½ |
| 18 | 78½ | 81½ | 83 | 82 | 80 | 79 | 5½ |
| 19 | 78 | 80 | 82 | 82 | 80 | 78 | 4 |
| 20 | 77 | 82 | 83 | 81 | 80 | 78 | 6 |
| 21 | 77 | 79½ | 80 | 79 | 79½ | 80 | 3 |
| 22 | 78½ | 81 | 80 | 80 | 79 | 78 | 3 |
| 23 | 77 | 80 | 80 | 80 | 79 | 78 | 3 |
| 24 | 78½ | 81 | 81 | 80 | 80½ | 78½ | 2½ |
| 25 | 79½ | 83½ | 83 | 83 | 80 | 77 | 6 |
| 26 | 76 | 82 | 83½ | 82 | 80 | 78 | 7½ |
| 27 | 78 | 83 | 84 | 83 | 81 | 78½ | 6 |
| 28 | 78 | 81 | 84 | 82 | 78 | 79½ | 6 |
| 29 | 77 | 79½ | 80 | 80 | 79 | 78½ | 3 |
| 30 | 76½ | 80 | 84 | 82 | 80 | 77 | 7½ |

On the 25th of this month Dr. Tuckerman left Bassin, and returned to West End. At the time of leaving Bassin, the country around it had the appearance of almost utter sterility. The canes were yellow from exhaustion of their moisture, the grass was nearly burnt up, and a number of cattle had died from want of water. At West End he found a beautiful verdure, for frequent small showers had fallen there. But the air had become unelastic, and they all withered under its influence.

The extremes of temperature this month were 73, and 85.

The greatest variation of temperature on any day was 7½. The least variation, 2.

The mean temperature of this month was 76.

## MAY, 1837.

| | 6½ A. M. | 9 A. M. | 12. | 3 P. M. | 6 P. M. | 9 P. M. | Daily variation. |
|---|---|---|---|---|---|---|---|
| 1 | 78 | 82 | 84 | 82 | 79 | 78 | 6 |
| 2 | 77 | 82 | 84 | 81½ | 79 | 77½ | 7 |
| 3 | 78 | 81 | 82 | 81½ | 80 | 77 | 5 |
| 4 | 78 | 81 | 82 | 81 | 79 | 77 | 5 |
| 5 | 76 | 84 | 85 | 83½ | 80 | 78 | 9 |
| 6 | 76 | 82 | 82 | 82 | 80 | 77 | 6 |
| 7 | 76 | 82 | 83 | 82 | 79 | 77 | 7 |

The extremes of temperature in the first week in May were 76, and 85.
The greatest variation of temperature on any day was 9, and the least variation 5 degrees.
The mean temperature of this week was 80 1-2.

# TABLE OF DIGESTIBILITY OF ALIMENTS.

TABLE of the time required for the Stomachal Digestion of different alimentary substances,—as exhibited in the case of the individual with a fistulous opening in the stomach,—arranged alphabetically from the results of experiments by Dr. Beaumont.

The most digestible substances are taken as the standard, which has been arbitrarily fixed at 1,000; and, accordingly, *aponeurosis*, the first article in the table, requiring 3 hours, whilst *pigs' feet soused, rice, &c.*, require but one, its digestibility, compared with that of these aliments, is as 333 to 1000; and so of the others.

It need scarcely be said, that all these tabular results apply, in strictness, to the individual concerned only; yet they afford useful comparative views, which, with exceptions depending upon individual peculiarities, may be regarded as approximations, applicable to mankind in general.

| ALIMENTS. | Form of preparation. | Time required for stomachal digestion. | Ratio of digestibility compared with the most digestible articles in the table.* |
|---|---|---|---|
| | | h. m. | |
| Aponeurosis, | boiled | 3 | 333 |
| Apples, mellow, | raw | 2 | 500 |
| Do sour, hard, | do | 2 50 | 352 |
| Do sweet, mellow, | do | 1 50 | 545 |
| Barley, | boiled | 2 | 500 |
| Bass, striped, fresh, | broiled | 3 | 333 |
| Beans, pod, | boiled | 2 30 | 400 |
| Do and green corn, | do | 3 45 | 266 |
| Beef, fresh, lean, rare, | roasted | 3 | 333 |
| Do do do dry, | do | 3 30 | 285 |
| Do do steak, | broiled | 3 | 333 |
| Do with salt only, | boiled | 2 45 | 363 |
| Do with mustard, &c., | do | 3 30 | 285 |
| Do | fried | 4 | 250 |
| Do old, hard salted, | boiled | 4 15 | 235 |
| Beets, | boiled | 3 45 | 266 |
| Brains, animal, | boiled | 1 45 | 571 |
| Bread, corn, | baked | 3 15 | 302 |
| Do wheat, fresh, | baked | 3 30 | 285 |

\* Pigs' feet soused, rice, and tripe soused, being the most digestible articles in the table, are estimated at 1,000.

# APPENDIX.

| ALIMENTS. | Form of preparation. | Time required for stomachal digestion. | Ratio of digestibility compared with the most digestible articles in the table. |
|---|---|---|---|
| | | *h. m.* | |
| Butter,* - - - - | melted | 3 30 | 285 |
| Cabbage, head, - - - | raw | 2 30 | 400 |
| Do with vinegar, - - | do | 2 | 500 |
| Do - - - - - | boiled | 4 30 | 222 |
| Cake, corn, - - - - | baked | 3 | 333 |
| Do sponge - - - - | do | 2 30 | 400 |
| Carrot, orange, - - - | boiled | 3 15 | 302 |
| Cartilage, - - - - | do | 4 15 | 235 |
| Catfish, fresh, - - - | fried | 3 30 | 285 |
| Cheese, old, strong, - - | raw | 3 30 | 285 |
| Chicken, full grown, - - | fricasseed | 2 45 | 363 |
| Codfish, cured dry, - - - | boiled | 2 | 500 |
| Corn (green) and beans, - | do | 3 45 | 266 |
| Custard, - - - - - | baked | 2 45 | 363 |
| Duck, domesticated, - - | roasted | 4 | 250 |
| Do wild, - - - - | do | 4 30 | 222 |
| Dumpling, apple, - - - | boiled | 3 | 333 |
| Eggs, fresh, - - - - | hard boiled | 3 30 | 285 |
| Do do - - - - | soft boiled | 3 | 333 |
| Do do - - - - | fried | 3 30 | 285 |
| Do do - - - - | roasted | 2 15 | 444 |
| Do do - - - - | raw | 2 | 500 |
| Do do - - - - | whipped | 1 30 | 666 |
| Flounder, fresh, - - - | fried | 3 30 | 285 |
| Fowls, domestic, - - - | boiled | 4 | 250 |
| Do do - - - - | roasted | 4 | 250 |
| Gelatin, - - - - | boiled | 2 30 | 400 |
| Goose, wild, - - - - | roasted | 2 30 | 400 |
| Heart, animal, - - - | fried | 4 | 250 |
| Lamb, fresh, - - - - | broiled | 2 30 | 400 |
| Liver, beef's, fresh, - - | do | 2 | 500 |
| Marrow, spinal, animal, - - | do | 2 40 | 375 |
| Meat and vegetables, - - | hashed | 2 30 | 400 |
| Milk, - - - - - | boiled | 2 | 500 |
| Do - - - - - | raw | 2 15 | 444 |
| Mutton, fresh, - - - - | roasted | 3 15 | 307 |
| Do do - - - - | broiled | 3 | 333 |
| Do do - - - - | boiled | 3 | 333 |

\* In the case of oils, and other substances of similar nature, which undergo little digestion in the stomach, the time merely indicates the period that elapsed before they were sent on into the duodenum.

# TABLE OF DIGESTIBILITY. 457

| ALIMENTS. | Form of preparation. | Time required for stomachal digestion. | Ratio of digestibility compared with the most digestible articles in the table. |
|---|---|---|---|
| | | h. m. | |
| Oysters, fresh, | raw | 2 55 | 342 |
| Do do | roasted | 3 15 | 307 |
| Do do | stewed | 3 30 | 285 |
| Parsnips, | boiled | 2 30 | 400 |
| Pig, sucking, | roasted | 2 30 | 400 |
| Pigs' feet, soused, | boiled | 1 | 1000 |
| Pork, fat and lean, | roasted | 5 15 | 190 |
| Do recently salted | boiled | 4 30 | 222 |
| Do do | fried | 4 15 | 235 |
| Do do | broiled | 3 15 | 302 |
| Do do | raw | 3 | 333 |
| Do do | stewed | 3 | 333 |
| Potatoes, Irish, | boiled | 3 30 | 285 |
| Do do | roasted | 2 30 | 400 |
| Do do | baked | 2 30 | 400 |
| Rice, | boiled | 1 | 1000 |
| Sago, | do | 1 45 | 571 |
| Salmon, salted, | do | 4 | 250 |
| Sausage, fresh, | broiled | 3 20 | 300 |
| Soup, barley, | boiled | 1 30 | 666 |
| Do bean, | do | 3 | 333 |
| Do beef, vegetables and bread, | do | 4 | 250 |
| Do chicken, | do | 3 | 333 |
| Do marrow bones, | do | 4 15 | 235 |
| Do mutton, | do | 3 30 | 285 |
| Do oyster, | do | 3 30 | 285 |
| Suet, beef, fresh, | do | 5 30 | 181 |
| Do mutton, | do | 4 30 | 222 |
| Tapioca, | do | 2 | 500 |
| Tendon, boiled, | do | 5 30 | 181 |
| Tripe, soused, | do | 1 | 1000 |
| Trout, salmon, fresh, | do | 1 30 | 666 |
| Do do | fried | 1 30 | 666 |
| Turkey, domestic, | roasted | 2 30 | 400 |
| Do do | boiled | 2 25 | 511 |
| Do wild | roasted | 2 18 | 435 |
| Turnips, flat, | boiled | 3 30 | 285 |
| Veal, fresh, | broiled | 4 | 250 |
| Do do | fried | 4 30 | 222 |
| Vegetables and meat, hashed, | warmed | 2 30 | 400 |
| Venison, steak, | broiled | 1 35 | 631 |

# INDEX.

Ablution, 369.
Acid, 200.
Acorn, 257.
Affusion, 369.
Agarics, 261.
Air abstracts moisture from the body, 39.—Admixture of sea and land, for the consumptive, 173.—An irritant to wounded or burnt surfaces, 41.—At great elevations, 15, 41.—Change of, advantages of, 124.—Changes in the, by respiration, 59.—Confined, 61.—Diminished density of the, 17.—Great density of the, 16.—Hygrometric state of the, 38.—Moist, the ready vehicle of exhalations, 42.—Of cities, unwholesome, 116.—Pressure of the, in the diving-bell, 17.—Properties of the, 15.—Temperature of the, 23.
Albumen, nutritive properties of, 193.
Alcohol, proportion of, in wines, 311.
Alcoholic liquors, abuse of, 305.
Ale, 318.
Alimentary regimen, 322.
Aliments, animal, 204.—Classification of, 191.—Comparative digestibility of, 457.—Composition of, 181.—Definition of, 179.—Modified by cookery, 273.—Varieties of, 183.—Vegetable, 246.
Allantotoxicum, 207.
Almond, 257.
Animal aliments, 204.
Animal and vegetable bodies, much alike in their elements, 188.
Animal, age of, influences the meat, 209.—Food of, influences the meat, 211.—Iufluenced by climate, 212.—Influenced by fatness or leanness, 213.—Influenced by incipient decomposition, 213.—Influenced by the mode of slaughtering, 214.—Sex of, influences the meat, 211.
Anchovy, 271.

Aniseed, 271.
Anointing, 373.
Ant, white, 235.
Aria cattiva, 67.
Arrow root, 197.
Arum, 278.
Asparagus, 259, 260.
Ass eaten by the Romans, 208.
Atmosphere, 13.—Constitution of the, 58.—Hygrometric state of the, 38.—Electrical condition of the, 53.—Influence of, on health, 13.—Moist, the ready vehicle of exhalations, 42.—Pressure of the, 15.—Pressure of the, in mines, 17.—Sudden change of pressure of the, 21.—Temperature of the, 23.
Atmospheric changes, announced by animals, 57.—Electricity, 53.—Vicissitudes, 43.—Vicissitudes, not always noxious, 58.—Vitiations, 47.
Azores, as a winter retreat, 151.

Bacon, poisonous, 207.—Roman, 212.
Baking, 276.
Baltimore, temperature of, 441.
Barley bread, 250.
Barley water, 295.
Barometer, average height of the, 21.—Range of the, 16.
Bath, animal, 359.—Cold, 360.—Dry, 359.—Electric, 359.—Foot, 359.—General, 359.—Half, 359.—Hand, 359.—Head, 359.—Hip, 359, 370.—Hot, 364.—Shower, 359.—Spout, 370.—Tepid, 365.—Vapour, 368.—Russian, described, 47.—Warm, 363.
Bathing, 358.—Duration of, 367.—General effects of, 359.—Manner of, 366.—Practices accessory to, 371.—Sea, 365.—Time of, 367.
Bay leaves, 271.
Bean, 256.—Kidney, 256.
Beds, air, 394.

## INDEX. 459

Beef, 210.
Beer, 318.
Beet, 257.
Beriberi, ignorance of the cause of, 92.
Bermudas, as a winter retreat, 151.
Bilge water of ships, does not induce disease, 82.
Birds as aliments, 218.—Classification of, 219.—Effect of age, sex, food, &c., on, 219.—Particular parts of, prized, 221.
Bitter, a great condiment, 266.
Black assize of Oxford, 60.
Black hole of Calcutta, 60.
Blutwurste, 207.
Boar, wild, 207.
Bogs, soil of, insalubrious, 97.
Boiling, 276.
Bonnyclabber, 243.
Boletus, 260.
Boots, 353.
Boxing, 385.
Braces, 354.
Bread, 249.
Bread, barley, 250.—Buckwheat, 252.—Cassava, 252.— Corn, 251. — Millet, 252.— Oaten, 252. — Potato, 251. — Rice, 251.—Rye, 250.—Wheaten, 249.
Breakfast, 324.—Powder, Hunt's, 302.
Breeches, 353.
Broccoli, 260.
Broiling, 276.
Buckwheat, 252.
Bull-baiting, object of, 216.
Burgundy, 314.
Burns, irritated by air, 41.
Butter, 243.—As a condiment, 273.
Buttermilk, 244.

Cabbage, 259, 260.
Calisthenics, 382.
Campeche, temperature of, 503.
Canaries, as a winter retreat, 150.
Capers, 270.
Capon, 219.
Carbonic acid, effects of, 60.
Carburetted hydrogen, effects of, 62.
Caraway, 271.
Carolina, South, as a winter retreat, 171.
Carriage exercise, 387.
Carrot, 257.
Casein, 195.
Cassava bread, 252.—Flour, 198.
Castagnacio, 257.
Caterpillar, 235.
Caudle, 295.
Cauliflower, 260.
Caviare, 229.
Celery, 259.
Cemeteries, rural, 79.
Centipedes, 235.

Cepe, 262.
Champagne, 313.
Champignon, 260.
Change of air, advantages of, 124.
Chantiers, d'equarrisage, 77.
Chase, the, 384.
Cheese, 195.—Poisonous, 243.
Chemise, 351.
Chestnut, 257.
Chewing, 337.
Children, in manufactories, health of, 53.
Chili, climate of, for the consumptive, 154.
Chincapin, 257.
Chocolate, 303.
Chocolat des ignorans, 303.—de Santé, 303.—à la vanille, 303.
Choke-damp, 62.
Cholera, its prevalence in certain places, 65.—Supposed to be produced by fruits, &c., 263.—Supposed to be induced by rice, 255, 263.
Cholera infantum, a great scourge of cities, 114.
Cider, 318.
Cimblins, 260.
Cincture, 352.
Cinnamon, 271.
Cities, air of, unwholesome, 116.—Improved salubrity of, 117.—Mortality of, 111.
Citron, 271.
Clam, 234.
Claret, 314.
Climate, warm, in certain diseases, 28.
Clothing, 341.—Colour of, 346.—Shape of, 350.—Substances used for, 342.— Warm, importance of, 342.
Cloves, 271.
Clupea thryssa, poisonous, 226.
Coats, 353.
Cockle, 234.
Cocoa, 303.
Cod, 232.—Salted, 271.
Cod sounds, 228.
Coffee, 298.—Substitutes for, 302.
Cold, excessive, destructive to the aged, 33.—Of Russia, 35.—Application of, when heated, not necessarily dangerous, 46.
Colour of clothing, 348.
Condiments, 266.—Aromatic, 271.—Oily, 267.
Constantia, 316.
Constitutio aeris, what, 14, 64.
Consumption, mortality from, in Baltimore, &c., 173.
Consumptive, benefited by warm climate, 301.—Exercise useful to the, 382. —Winter residence for the, 144.

Contagion, modified by the air, 43.
Contagious diseases, 65.—Our ignorance of, 93.
Coonti root, 197.
Cookery, effects of, on aliments, 273.
Cooks, their estimation of old, 274.
Coriander, 271.
Corn bread, 251.
Corn, Indian, 255.—Diseased, 255.—Supposed to induce pellagra, 93, 251.
Corporeal occupations, 405.
Corset, 354.
Cossus, as food of the ancients, 235.
Cotton clothing, 342.
Countries, improved salubrity of, 119.
Crab, 235.
Cradle, exercise of the, 390.
Cravat, 351.
Cream, 241.—Corstorphin, 243.
Cress, 259.
Cretinism, ignorance of the cause of, 92.
Crimping, 231.
Crustacea, 235.
Cucumbers, 259.
Culinary processes, 273.—Loss by, 277.
Cumana, as a winter retreat, 154.
Cumin, 271.
Curry, Indian, 254.
Cuttle fish, 234.

Dancing, 384.
Dash, 370.
Declaiming, 385.
Deer, 207.
Digestibility, comparative of different aliments, 455.
Digestive operations, 191.—Texture, 202.
Dinner, 324.
Dirt does not produce endemic diseases, 92.
Dissecting-room, air of the, 77.
Dissection, wounds from, 81.
Diving Bell, pressure of the air in the, 17.
Dog, 207.
Dormouse, 208.
Douche, 370.
Douse, 370.
Drinks, 280.—Absorption of, 281.—Cold, 284.—Digestion of, 281.—Hot, 285.
Duck, 219.—Canvassback, 219.

Earth, unctuous, eaten by the Ottomaques, 183.
Eels, 226, 232.
Eggs, 245.—Of various birds, 246.
Electricity, atmospheric, 53.
Elephantiasis, ignorance of the cause of, 92.
Elephantophagi, 189.

Emanations, animal, 63.—Mineral, &c., 64.—Vegetable, effects of, 69.
Emotions, effects of the, 477.—Regulated indulgence of the, useful, 480.
Endemics, 65.—Our ignorance of, 94.
Endemic fever, 65.
Endemico-epidemics, 65.
England, as a winter retreat, 147.
Epidemics, 65.—Our ignorance of, 94.
Epidemic influences, 65.—Our ignorance of, 93.
Epidemico-contagious diseases, 64.
Etiolation, 51.
Exercise, 376.—Active, 377.—In a carriage, 387.—On horseback, 386.—In a litter, 387.—In a palanquin, 388.—In sailing, 387.—In a sedan chair, 387.—Passive, 386.—Should be combined with amusement, 378.—Travelling, 378.—Violent, effects of, 378.—Of the infant, 389.

Factories, influence of, on health, 56, 409.
Farinaceous vegetables, 248.
Fat, nutritive properties of, 194.
Fecula, 197.
Fencing, 384.
Fennel, 231.
Fever, endemic, 65.—Yellow, where prevalent, 14
Fibrin, nutritive properties of, 193.
Fire-damp, 62.
Fish, as food, 223.—Almost every part eaten, 228.—Castration of, 230.—Constituents of, 223.—Effects of age, sex, &c., on, 229.—Fancied spermatopoietic power of, 223.—Forbidden, 224.—Not improved by keeping, 231.—Nutritive properties of, 228.—Poisonous, 226.—Salted, 269.
Fish eaters, 223.
Flagellation, 371.
Flamingo, tongue of the, 221.
Flannel, 343.—Jacket, 343, 351.
Flesh, muscular, constituents of, 208.
Florida, Cape, as a winter residence, 164.
Flounder, 232.
Food, 179.—Of animals differs, 185.—Of a country, regulated by its productions, 190.—Of man, mixed, 186.—Of man ought to vary, 187.—Natural, of man, 189.—Poisonous, 205.—Putrescent, not unwholesome, 76.
Fowls, 220.—Barn door, 205,—Fattening of, 220.
France, as a winter retreat, 144.
Friction, 371.
Frog, 222.—Bull, 223.
Frontignan, 316.

Fruits, 262.—Farinaceous, 265.—How cooked, 278.—Preserved, 265.
Frying, 276.
Fungi, 261.
Fur clothing, 346.

Garlic, 258, 271.
Garters, 353.
Gastric juice, analysis of the, 191.—Antiseptic, 191.—Dissolves alimentary matters, 191.—Not in the stomach when empty, 191.
Gelatin, nutritive properties of, 194.
Geophagists, 183.
Georgia, as a winter retreat, 171.
Germantown, mean temperature of, 495.
Gestation, 386.
Ginger, 271.
Girdle, 352.
Gluten, 200.
Goat, 207.
Goitre, where prevalent, 14.—Ignorance of the causes of, 92.
Goose, 219.
Grouse, poisonous, 220.
Gruel, 295.
Gum, 198.
Gutspinning, not unwholesome, 77.
Gymnastics, 382.

Haddock, salted, 271.
Hare, 207.
Harmattan wind, 43.
Havannah, as a winter retreat, 153.
Heat, destructive to infants, 138.—Elevated, destructive to the aged, 33.—Of stoves, inconvenience from the, 41.
Heavenly bodies, influence of the, 132.
Hedgehog, 207.
Heimweh, 36.
Hemp clothing, 342.—Preparation of, not necessarily morbific, 85.
Herrings, 232.—Salted, 271.
Hickory nut, 257.
Hock, 313.
Hog, 207.
Horse, 207.
Horseback, exercise, 386.
Horse radish, 271.
Hygiène, what, 13.
Hydropathy, 374.
Hygrometric state of the air, 38.
Hylophagi, 189.

Ickari, 229.
Ichthyophagi, 223.
Imperial, 304.
Inaction, bad effects of, 390.
Indigo, preparation of, not necessarily morbific, 85.
Indolence, bad effects of, 390.

Influenza, ignorance of the causes of, 93.
Infusions, animal and vegetable, 294.
Ink fish, 234.
Insects as food, 235.
Interments in cities, 79.
Isinglass, 228.
Italy, as a winter retreat, 144.

Kernels, as food, 257.
Kipper, poisonous, 229.
Knacker's operations, not unwholesome, 76.
Kneading, 371.
Kohlsalat, 258.
Koumiss, 245.

Lait de poule, 246.
Lakes, northern, a summer residence, 175.
Lamb, 210.
Leaping, 383.
Leberwurste, 207.
Leek, 258, 271.
Leguminous vegetables, 256.
Lemon juice, 271.
Lemon peel, 271.
Lemonade, 294.
Lettuce, 259.
Light, effects of, 51.—Intense, injures the eyes, 53.—Necessary for full development, 52.—Privation of, 53.
Limpet, 234.
Linen clothing, 342.
Liqueurs, 321.
Liquors, fermented, simple, 305.—Malt, 318. — Spirituous, 320. — Spirituous, abuse of, 305.
Literary occupations, longevous, 412.
Literary persons, regimen of, 325.
Litter, 387.
Lizard, 222.
Lobster, 235.
Locality, influence of on health, 13, 95.
Locust, 235.
Longevity and mortality not in an exact ratio, 108.—Of counties of Virginia, &c., 108.
Lunar influence, 133.
Lunel, 363.

Macaroni, 253.
Mace, 271.
Madeira, as a winter retreat, 148.
Madeira (wine), 315.—Cape, 363.—Sicily, 315.
Maladie du pays, 36.
Malaria, 67.—After draining, 86.—Conceived not to exist as a specific poison, 86.—Does not arise from animal putrefaction, 75.—Does not arise from vegetable putrefaction, 69.—Heavier

than air, 91.—Laws that govern, 90.—
Nature of, 89.—Not produced by aqueous decomposition, 82.—Not produced by sulphuretted hydrogen, 89.—On elevations, 43.—May be fenced in, 91.—
Our ignorance of, 87, 89.—Prevented from extending by woods, 91.
Malarious soil, deposition regarding a, 431.
Malmsey, 315.
Malt liquors, 318.
Mantle, 353.
Manufactories, effect of, on the health of children and others, 53, 409.
Marsh poison, 67.
Marshy districts, seats of disease, 97.—Miasm, 67.
Massage, 371.
Mastication, necessity of, 326.
Materia alimentaria, 179.
Mattee, 298.
Meals, number of, 323.
Meats, salted, 269.—Unwholesome, 207.
Melon, 265.
Mental occupations, 405.
Milk, 236.—Constituents of, 239.—Of different animals, 239.—Sometimes poisonous, 241.
Millet, 252.
Mineral springs, 373.
Mines, pressure of the air in, 17.
Mobile, as a winter retreat, 169.
Mollusca, 237.
Monomania, a sea voyage useful in, 389.
Montefiascone, 316.
Moon, influence of the, on health, 133.
Moral, its influence on the *physique*, 426.
Mortality and longevity not in an exact ratio, 108.—At different seasons, 138—Of different cities, 111.—Of various countries, 101.—Of town and country, difference between, 111.
Morbus oryzeus, 255, 263.
Moselle wines, 315.
Mucilage, 198.
Mullet, prized by the ancients, 232.
Muscat, 316.
Mushroom, 261.
Mussel, 234.
Mustard, 271.—Seed, 273.
Mutton, 210.

Nicci, 257.
Nightingale, tongue of the, 221.
Nostalgia, 36.
Nutmeg, 271.
Nuts, 257.

Oaten bread, 252.
Occupations, different effects of, 406.—literary, not prejudicial, 412.

Oil, as a condiment, 273.—Nutritive properties of, 194.
Olera, 257.
Onion, 258, 271.
Opossum, 207.
Orange peel, 271.
Orange, 265.
Osmazome, nutritive properties of, 194.
Ostrich, brains of the, 221.
Ox, 207.
Oysters, 233.

Palanquin, 386.
Palmetto, saw, 197.
Pantaloons, 353.
Parsnip, 257.
Partridge, 218.—Poisonous, 220.
Passions, effects of the, 426.
Pastry, indigestible, 253.
Peacock, brain of, 221.
Peas, 256.
Peatmosses, soil of, insalubrious, 97.
Pellagra, ignorance of the cause of, 92.—Said to be induced by Indian corn, 93, 251.—Where prevalent, 314.
Pensacola, as a winter retreat, 169.
Pepper, 271.
Periwinkle, 234.
Perry, 318.
Perspiration modified by the air, 32.
Peru exempt from consumption, 154.
Physique, influenced by the *moral*, 426.
Pickles, 270.
Pimento, 271.
Plague, on ignorance and the cause of, 92.
Plague, cold, 81.
Planetary influence, 132.
Plum, 265.
Polenta, 256, 257.
Pork, 210, 212.—Sardinian, 212.—Virginia, 212.
Port, 314.
Porter, 318.
Potato, 250.—Bread, 251.—Sweet, 254.
Pot herbs, 257.
Poulard, 219.
Prawn, 235.
Principle, nutritive, 187.
Puddings, various, 253.
Pulse, 256.
Puppies, 208.

Quadrupeds, as food, 207.

Rabbit, 207.—Welsh, 242.
Radish, 258.
Reading aloud, 385.
Regimen, alimentary, 322.—Change of, 324.
Reptiles, as aliments, 222.

# INDEX.

Respiration, effects of, on the air, 58.
Rhenish wines, 315.
Rice, 254.—Disease, 255, 263.—Supposed to induce cholera, 255, 263.—Water, 295.
Riding, in a carriage, 387.
Riding on horseback, 386.
River bottoms, often unhealthy, 97.
Roasting, 275.
Robes, 353.
Rock, 232.
Rockbutter, eaten in Thuringia, 183.
Roe of the sturgeon, &c., 228.
Running, 383.
Rye bread, 250.—Diseased, 255.—Spurred, 255.

Sack, 315.
Sage, 271.
Sago, 263.—French, 197.—Portland Island, 197.
Sailing, 389.
St. Augustine, as a winter retreat, 157.—Temperature of, 441.
Salads, 258.
Salep, 198, 263.
Salmon, cured, 229.
Salsafy, 258.
Salt, 267.—Effects of its privation, 268.
Salted meats, 269.
Salubrity, improved, of cities, 118.—Improved, of countries, 117.
Sauces, 279.
Sauerkraut, 258.
Sausages, poisonous, 207.
Scalds, irritated by air, 41.
Scheraaz, 315.
Schmierkäse, 243.
Scuppernong wine, 317.
Sea voyage, 389.—In Consumption, 154.
Seasons, change of, necessary, 49.—Effects of the, on health, 137.—Mortality at different, 138.
Sedan chair, 387.
Sedentary habits, injurious, 391.
Serum or Whey, 244, 303.
Shallot, 258, 271.
Shampooing, 371.
Sheep, 207.
Shellbark nut, 257.
Shell fish, as aliments, 232.
Sherry, 315.
Shirt, 351.
Shoes, 353.
Shrimp, 235.
Siesta, the, 403.
Silk clothing, 393.
Singing, 385.
Sleep, 392.—Duration of, 400.—Influenced by the state of the bed, &c., 399. —Objects of, 392.—Too much, bad effects of, 392.

Sleeping chamber, best condition of, 394.
Slip, 243.
Smoking, 387.
Snail, 234.
Snuffing, 335.
Soda water, 304.
Soils, comparative salubrity of, 95.
Sole, 232.
Sol-lunar influence, 132.
Sorocco, 19.
Spinach, 259, 260.
Spirituous liquors, 320.
Spout bath, 370.
Sprat, 232.—Yellow billed, poisonous, 226
Springs, mineral, 373.
Squashes, 259, 260.
Starch, 197.
Steatite, eaten in New Scotland, 183.
Stock, 351.
Stockings, 352.
Stomach, fistulous opening in the, 191.
Struthiophagi, 189.
Sturgeon, roe of, 228.
Sugar, 199, 267.
Sugar of milk, 245.
Sulphuretted hydrogen, effects of, 63.
Summer residence for the consumptive, 175.
Supper, 324.
Swathing, 355.
Sweetmeats, 265.
Swim bladder, pressure on the, 16.

Tailors, liable to fistula ani, 391.
Tampa Bay, Florida, as a winter retreat, 157.
Tarro patches, not unhealthy, 73.
Tapioca, 271.
Tea, 296, 324.—Balm, 298.—Sage, 298.—Sassafras, 298.
Teeth, affected by drinks, 285.
Temperature, atmospheric, observed at sea, 155.—Depressed, 32.—Elevated, 23 —Equability of, for the consumptive, 144.—Highest of different climates, 24.—Mean of certain winter retreats, 144.—Of the Atmosphere, 23.—Of Baltimore, 441.—Of Campeche, 449.—Of Germantown, 441.—Of the sea at its surface, 155.—Of St. Augustine, table of the, 441.—Of Santa Cruz, 451.—Of the seasons in different places of America, Europe, &c., 447.
Tent, 316.
Terrapin, 222.
Thyme, 271.
Toast, hot buttered, 273.
Toast water, 294.
Tobacco, 329.—Medical virtues of, 331.— Opposition to, 332.
Tokay, 316.
Tomatoes, 259, 260.

## 464                    INDEX.

Tous-les-mois, 198.
Trades, different effects of, 405.
Training, 327.
Transpiration, modified by the air, 32.
Travelling, effects of, 125.—On the mind, 378.
Trowsers, 353.
Truffle, 266.
Turbaries, influence of, on health, 97.
Turbot, 232.
Turnip, 258.
Turtle, 222.

Veal, 241.
Vegetables, as aliments, 246.—Farinaceous, 248.—How cooked, 277.—Leguminous, 256.
Venison, 211.
Vera Cruz, as a winter retreat, 154.
Verjuice, 270.
Vermicelli, 253.
Vicissitudes, atmospheric, 43. — Atmospheric, not always noxious, 47.—From cold to heat, 46.—From heat to cold, 48.
Vin de grave, 317.
Vina cocta, 316.
Vinegar, 270.—Acts upon fibrin, 217.
Vinegar, raspberry, 294.
Vinegar, strawberry, 293.
Viper, 222.
Vitiations, atmospheric, 58.
Voyage, exercise during a, 389.

Waistcoats, 353.
Walking exercise, 383.
Walnut, 237.
Warmth, importance of, 395.
Wassercur, 374.

Watchfulness, effects of, 392.
Water, 286.—Barley, 295.—Distillation of, 294.—Fresh and salt, admixture of, esteemed unhealthy, 171.—Iced, 284.— Lake, 289.—Large masses of, regarded healthy, 198. Marsh, 290.—Nutritive properties of, 184.—Preservation of, 292.—Purification of, 292.—Qualities of, 286.—Rain, 287.—Rice, 295.—River, 288.—Snow, 289.—Spring, 288.— Of the Thames, peculiarities of the, 182.—Toast, 294.—Well, 288.
Weather, unseasonable, fancied effects of, 175.
West Indies, as a winter retreat, 153.
Western Islands, as a winter retreat, 151.
Wheat, flour of, 248.
Whelk, 234.
Whey, 244, 303.
Whiting, 232.
Winds, effects of, 131.
Wine, 308.—Analysis of, 309.—Brisk, 313.—Madeira, 315.—Proportion of alcohol in, 358.—Of Alicant, 315.—Of the Bordelais, 314.—Burgundy, 314.— Of the Canaries, 315.—Claret, 314.— Of Cyprus, 316.—Domestic, 317.—Of the Moselle, 315.—Of Oporto, 314.— Of the Rhine, 315.—Of the Rhone, 313. —Of Rota, 315.—Of Spain and Portugal, 315.—Spanish, 315.—Sweet, 316.
Winter residence for the consumptive, 144.
Woodcock, 218.—Trail of the, 221.
Woollen clothing, 342.
Wounds, irritated by air, 41.
Wrestling, 335.
Wuerstfettsauere, 207.
Wurstgift, 207.

THE END.

# PUBLIC HEALTH IN AMERICA

*An Arno Press Collection*

Ackerknecht, Erwin H[einz]. **Malaria In the Upper Mississippi Valley: 1760-1900.** 1945

Bowditch, Henry I[ngersoll]. **Consumption In New England Or, Locality One of Its Chief Causes** and **Is Consumption Contagious, Or Communicated By One Person to Another In Any Manner?** 1862/1864. Two Vols. in One.

Buck, Albert H[enry] (Editor). **A Treatise On Hygiene and Public Health.** 1879. Two Vols.

Boston Medical Commission. **The Sanitary Condition of Boston: The Report of a Medical Commission.** 1875

Budd, William. **Typhoid Fever: Its Nature, Mode of Spreading, and Prevention.** 1931

Chapin, Charles V[alue]. **A Report On State Public Health Work,** Based On a Survey of State Boards of Health: Made Under the Direction of the Council on Health and Public Instruction of the American Medical Association. [1915]

Davis, Michael M[arks], Jr. and Andrew R[obert] Warner. **Dispensaries:** Their Management and Development. 1918

Dublin, Louis I[srael] and Alfred J. Lotka. **The Money Value of a Man.** 1930

Dunglison, Robley. **Human Health.** 1844

Emerson, Haven. **Local Health Units for the Nation.** 1945

Emerson, Haven. **A Monograph On the Epidemic of Poliomyelitis (Infantile Paralysis) In New York City In 1916.** 1917

Fish, Hamilton. **Report of the Select Committee of the Senate of the United States On the Sickness and Mortality On Board Emigrant Ships.** 1854

Frost, Wade Hampton. **The Papers of Wade Hampton Frost, M.D.:** A Contribution to Epidemiological Method. 1941

Gardner, Mary Sewall. **Public Health Nursing.** 1916

Greenwood, Major. **Epidemics and Crowd Diseases:** An Introduction to the Study of Epidemiology. 1935

Greenwood, Major. **Medical Statistics From Graunt to Farr.** 1948

Hartley, Robert M. **An Historical, Scientific and Practical Essay On Milk, As an Article of Human Sustenance:** With a Consideration of the Effects Consequent Upon the Unnatural Methods of Producing It for the Supply of Large Cities. 1842

Hill, Hibbert Winslow. **The New Public Health.** 1916

Knopf, S. Adolphus. **Tuberculosis As a Disease of the Masses & How To Combat It.** 1908

MacNutt, J[oseph] Scott. **A Manual for Health Officers.** 1915

Richards, Ellen H. [Swallow]. **Euthenics:** The Science of Controllable Environment. 1910

Richardson, Joseph G[ibbons]. **Long Life and How To Reach It.** 1886

Rumsey, Henry Wyldbore. **Essays On State Medicine.** 1856

Shryock, Richard Harrison. **National Tuberculosis Association 1904-1954:** A Study of the Voluntary Health Movement In the United States. 1957

Simon, John. **Filth-Diseases and Their Prevention.** 1876

Sternberg, George M[iller]. **Sanitary Lessons of the War and Other Papers.** 1912

Straus, Lina Gutherz. **Disease In Milk:** The Remedy Pasteurization. The Life Work of Nathan Straus. 1917

Wanklyn, J[ames] Alfred and Ernest Theophron Chapman. **Water Analysis:** A Practical Treatise on the Examination of Potable Water. 1884

Whipple, George C. **State Sanitation:** A Review of the Work of the Massachusetts State Board of Health. 1917. Two Vols. in One.

**Selections From Public Health Reports and Papers Presented at the Meetings of the American Public Health Association (1873-1883). 1977**

**Selections From Public Health Reports and Papers Presented at the Meetings of the American Public Health Association (1884-1907). 1977**

Animalcular and Cryptogamic Theories On the Origins of Fevers. 1977

The Carrier State. 1977

Clean Water and the Health of the Cities. 1977

The First American Medical Association Reports On Public Hygiene In American Cities. 1977

Selections from the Health-Education Series. 1977

Health In the Southern United States. 1977

Health In the Twentieth Century. 1977

The Health of Women and Children. 1977

Minutes and Proceedings from the First, Second, Third and Fourth National Quarantine and Sanitary Conventions. 1977. Four Vols. in Two.

Selections from the Journal of the Massachusetts Association of Boards of Health (1891-1904). 1977

Sewering the Cities. 1977

Smallpox In Colonial America. 1977

Yellow Fever Studies. 1977

| DATE DUE | | | |
|---|---|---|---|
| ~~8 1975~~ | | | |
| | | | |
| | | | |
| | | | |
| | | | |
| | | | |
| | | | |
| | | | |
| | | | |
| | | | |
| | | | |
| | | | |
| | | | |
| | | | |
| | | | |
| | | | |

DEMCO 38-297